Toward a Theory of Psychosomatic Disorders

Proceedings of the 11th European Conference on Psychosomatic Research
Heidelberg, September 14–17, 1976

Toward a Theory of Psychosomatic Disorders

Alexithymia, Pensée opératoire,
Psychosomatisches Phänomen

Editors: *W. Bräutigam and M. von Rad,* Heidelberg

39 figures and 47 tables, 1977

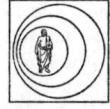

S. Karger · Basel · München · Paris · London · New York · Sydney

Reprint from 'Psychotherapy and Psychosomatics', Vol. 28, No. 1–4, 1977

Cataloging in Publication
European Conference on Psychosomatic Research, 11th, Heidelberg, 1976
Toward a theory of psychosomatic disorders : alexithymia : pensée opératoire : psychosomatisches Phänomen : proceedings of the 11th European Conference on Psychosomatic Research, Heidelberg, September 14–17, 1976.
editors, W. Bräutigam and M. von Rad. — Basel; New York: Karger, 1977.
(Psychotherapy and psychosomatics : v. 28)
1. Psychophysiologic Disorders – congresses I. Bräutigam, Walter, ed. II. Rad, M. von, ed. III. Title IV. Series
W1 PS86K v. 28
WM 90 E89 1976t
ISBN 3–8055–2747–0

Contents

Contents

Theories

Therapeutic Approaches

Varia

Retrospective View on the Conference

Address to the 11th European Conference on Psychosomatic Research

The new rules for medical licensure, which after many years of deliberation were signed into law by me as President of the Federal Republic of Germany, established medical psychology, sociology and psychosomatic medicine as legitimate subjects of medical – theoretical as well as clinical – training. Thus, a new emphasis was provided. No longer do natural science and technology alone determine the training and self-assessment of doctors.

The great developments of medical science, especially of medical techniques, must not blind us to one recognizable danger: the more emphasis we put on laboratories and apparatuses, the greater becomes the danger that the individual with his personal sufferings and problems disappears from view. Psychosomatic medicine has the great task of countering this danger. Many patients, particularly among the socially and educationally disadvantaged, can express their undue burdens, conflicts and suppressed needs only in a coded body language. Their complaints couched in psysical pains and psychosomatic symptoms, need to be listened to and understood by doctors. These doctors must ask themselves, whether their concepts, diagnostic methods and therapeutic tools are appropriate for these types of illnesses.

However, physicians, psychotherapists of psychosomatic patients, no less than other helping professions face the question, whether their efforts being expensive reach only the financially better situated rather than the great masses of those harmed physically or mentally by conflicts in their families, at their places of work or by social inequities. The fact that our national health insurance is presently covering the costs of psychotherapeutic treatments signals progress along a path we must continue. When patients and doctors learn to verbalize, understand and treat physical complaints resulting from psychosocial conflicts, then the great number of these patients will no longer need to complain vainly and repetitively in front of insensitive and expensive apparatuses.

As a young science, psychosomatic medicine needs the open exchange of experience, as practised in universities and hospitals of all countries. In Germany the development of psychosomatic medicine is very closely connected with the University of Heidelberg; here were its origins. The names of *Ludolf Krehl, Richard Siebeck* and particularly of *Viktor von Weizsäcker* stand for those of an era and doctors that were open to and even enriched psychosocial viewpoints and psychoanalytic theory and practice. Many hopes and new beginnings were destroyed by our country's political decline after 1933, and many doctors were forced to emigrate. In the meantime, psychosomatic medicine has been fully accepted in Anglo-Saxon countries. It is very gratifying that scientists from these countries and the whole world have come to Heidelberg. I welcome your 11th European Conference on Psychosomatic Research. To this conference I attach the hope that psychosomatic medicine, at universities and in medical practice, will help to alleviate the suffering of the sick in our time.

May 12, 1976

Gustav W. Heinemann

Former President of the Federal Republic of Germany 1969–1974

Introduction

Towards a Theory of Psychosomatic Disorders

W. Bräutigam and M. von Rad

Psychosomatic medicine had its origin in psychoanalysis at the beginning of this century and has only struck out on its own in the last few decades. Psychoanalysts were the first to trace causal and theoretical connections between mental conflicts or situational stresses and physical symptoms. Today it is still the subjective dimension – a person's experience of his own inner life history – as reflected in the psychoanalytical situation and in the course of psychotherapy, which is the corner stone of clinical research.

The first attempts to define psychosomatic disorders were variants of concepts stemming from neurosis theory; the physical symptom was seen as a special case of neurotic conversion and was attributed to the psyche. However, the question of whether psychosomatic medicine can 'emancipate' itself from psychoanalysis has been in existence for a long time: must it not give its research into aetiology, its concepts and theories and its methods of treatment more well-defined contours, if it is to exist as a separate entity?

One thing seems to us to be an established fact in psychosomatics as opposed to neurosis psychology: a psychosomatic medicine conscious of its own individuality sees its circumstances and its existential justification to a much lesser degree purely in the conditions of psychogenesis. This can be seen most clearly in the field of somato-psychosomatic problems. Here, the question arises of how primary physical disorders are psychologically assimilated and their subsequent course influenced by this psychological reaction. The experience of physical sickness is open to multi-factorial interpretation with regard to its origin, and invites a number of independent somatic and psychological theoretical approaches. Today we attempt to understand physical sickness in the interaction of somatic and psychic influences.

From a historical point of view, a differentiation can perhaps be made between two different developmental tendencies in psychosomatic medicine which exist in a fruitful opposition to each other and which have proved to be relevant questions in research. The one direction tends more towards specifying a disease, locating an internal or external conflict, or a trait of personality – the other seeks to determine the common denominator of various psychosomatic diseases and to comprehend and work on this aspect. This last approach, which is the more recent, was magnificently formulated in the work of *Jürgen Ruesch,* to which far too little attention has been paid. Shortly after the second world war, *Ruesch* very accurately described the affective disorder in communication and the restricted fantasy life, the object dependency and the overadapted social behaviour of the 'infantile personality' as the 'core problem' of psychosomatic patients.

Thus, it is against this background, but in a new terminological guise – pensée opératoire, alexithymia, psychosomatic phenomenon – that the 11th European Conference presents an old problem as its main theme: the specific hypothesis of whether and to what extent psychosomatic patients can be differentiated from psychoneurotic ones.

We are thoroughly convinced that the hypothesis of alexithymia is not only an interesting, hotly disputed, clinical observation. We hope, rather, that the particular point of view it represents will act as a kind of 'paradigm' to support the discussion and substantiation of the present psychosomatic theories and research approaches. It seems to us that the alexithymia hypothesis is open to the question whether the course of the disease should be viewed more from the aspect of the psychosocial situation of being ill – that is in respect of certain separation and loss reactions – or from the aspect of personality features which can be objectified in psychological tests. It also seems to beg the question of whether and to what extent the disease is determined by a predisposing factor to be sought in the organic systems, or whether a proneness to certain types of reactions should be looked for. Other elements which must be considered are linguistic hypotheses and family dynamics, which point to a connection between individual, family and social factors.

Scientific progress in our branch of medicine must always return to the central experience of observation of the patient. Advances are made in stages, in which the duality of experience and observation coalesces to create certain key concepts and hypotheses. We expect today, more than in earlier times, that hypotheses be presented in a systematic, comprehensible fashion which makes them capable of being repeated and tested critically by others. Every researcher must permit himself and others the possibility of confirming a statement or of correcting it. The ever-present question is: what forms of investigation are most appropriate to the various statements and theories; introspective or observational, accompanying treatment, or purely experimental, retrospective with regard to the patient's biography, or prospective, anticipating the future?

One aspect requiring further attention is the relationship between research and therapy, a particularly crucial point. It is true to say that from the very beginning, therapy has not been merely a testing-ground for hypotheses; the therapeutic situation has rather – particularly in psychosomatic medicine, been a constant source of observation and new theories in its own right. For this reason we thought it fitting at the 11th European Conference on Psychosomatic Research to treat the concept of alexithymia from three viewpoints: (1) observation; (2) aetiology and evolution of theory and (3) therapy.

This volume does not only contain contributions by the prominent champions of the alexithymia theory. The large number of papers devoted to clinical observation and to objectification are of particular value. Remarkable statements are also made by authors who are sceptical of the alexithymia hypothesis, and will remain so. We are very much in need of their criticism and their intimations if we are to make our observations, our theoretical approach and our research methods as good as they could be. We hope that the reprinting of part of the discussion will give the reader an impression of the frankness with which it was conducted and also give him the opportunity to check his own standpoint by means of a 'dialogue' with the authors.

In the description of the alexithimic psychosomatic patient with his emotional defence system and his concretistic way of thinking, a human being is being classified as a type. Here as so often, typological description seems not far removed from caricature, the psychosomatic patient becomes a strange species of humanity who seemingly does not exist among us. However, as therapists, we should never dissociate ourselves too completely from the patient, and should never forget when speaking of the peculiarities of our patients that we are all just as susceptible to psychosomatic illness as they are. There is scarcely anyone among us who will never encounter a situation where his psychological assimilation faculties are no longer able to cope and he reacts psychosomatically. Even if it is tempting – at least at the present stage of our knowledge – to see the psychosomatic patient as a 'type', we should still attempt to progress towards regarding the psychosomatic reaction as a situation where the psychological defence mechanism is overtaxed and where any one of us might fall back on physical reaction.

Basic Concepts of Psychosomatic Medicine

Proc. 11th Eur. Conf. Psychosom. Res., Heidelberg 1976
Psychother. Psychosom. *28:* 1–12 (1977)

The Languages of Psychosomatic Medicine

Chase Patterson Kimball[1]

The comments which I am about to make may seem self-obvious and, if so, my only explanation for them is that sometimes the self-obvious needs to be stated and restated. I think that it is timely that we consider these in our chosen field of psychosomatic medicine.

The Problem of Reality

First of all, we share with all hyphenated (the English wisely retain hyphens) disciplines the problem of bridging two language systems each with its own idiosyncratic syntaxes and conceptual orientation. Not only may their origins and histories be different, but their developments as formal conceptual approaches may be widely separated in time in terms of the evolution and sophistication of man's thinking. So there is first of all a *temporal* gap between our somatic concepts and our psychological constructs, representing fundamentally different philosophical orientations (1). The philosophical basis of somatic medicine seems to be rooted in a concrete belief in the realness of matter and of rigid laws relating to matter, a belief that characterized 19th century physics but which is largely shunned by 20th century physicists. Despite the molecular biological revolution, the practice of medicine in which most of us are schooled is a 19th century one. It is one based on the realness of matter and the laws governing it. It assiduously seems to have ignored the concurrent philosophical reflections of *Berkeley,* the Anglican Bishop, of

[1] Professor of Psychiatry and Medicine, Division of Biological Sciences and in the College, University of Chicago, Chicago, Ill.

Royce and *William James*. Only occasionally does someone like *David Wilson* in a recent paper published in Perspectives in Biology and Medicine (2) reflect that science is a grand super-structure tenuously supported on shifting sands. It adheres most often to a single cause→single effect theory of causation which is linear and two-dimensional rather than cyclical and three-dimensional.

It is more often than not addressed almost entirely to the time-limited here and now approach rather than to an evolutionary developmental one. Curiously, few of our mentors (including Freud) in the evolution of psychological medicine have given up a belief in the primacy of somatic medicine. Always, it seems, we somewhat apologetically state that final understanding of psychological processes will be forthcoming when we know more about brain neurochemistry!

The Problem of Mixed Languages

The problems of juxtaposing and linking two language systems together inevitably leads to new complexities. The first of these is that of causation, specific and primary. It seems a fundamental nature of man, whether she/he speaks in terms of science or religion to need to seek for specific and single causes of events or happenings. In a global sense, this rigid adherence may have done in 19th century religion. In psychosomatic medicine there has developed a more or less fundamental formula linking an environmental event to a psychological reaction to physiologic process (fig. 1). It seems to me that there are several difficulties with this formula.

The first is that of *vectors:* it is linear at a time when physics has given up straight lines. It would perhaps be better to draw these in a cyclical sequence (fig. 2). This would allow entry at any one of the three points rather than necessitating entry at the one most in agreement with a given individual's persuasion. It has particular appeal for those of us who would describe bio-socio-psychological or psycho-bio-social processes. We can expand this complexity a bit if we modify this formula to agree with most dynamic equations so that the curvilinear arrows are double-headed (fig. 3). Second, is the problem of *dimensionality:* our formula is two-dimensional in what has become a three-dimensional world. The processes we are describing are neither time nor place limited or fixated. They are not static but evolving even as we observe them and attempt to explain them. Not only do the language systems we are using have an evolutionary course but the phenomenon we are describing and attempting to explain in that description,

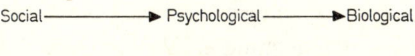

Fig. 1

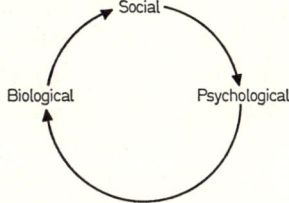

Fig. 2

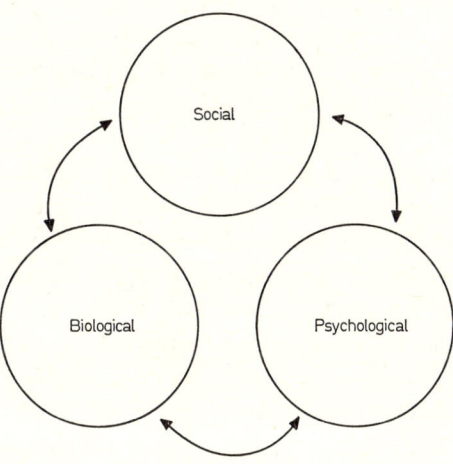

Fig. 3

specifically the illness in the patient *and* the patient, have a temporal past and future, have begun and may terminate in another place. This moves us to think in terms of three dimensions rather than two dimensions and to consider the relationship of spheres as opposed to circles (fig. 4). Third, is the problem of *correlations*. This is a more difficult area to define than the relationships of vectors and dimensions. I think this is the primary intrinsic difficulty in psychosomatic medicine. Perhaps, most simply stated it is the problem of the six blind men defining an elephant. Each examines a different part and defines the elephant in terms of that part, the trunk, the tusk, the tail, etc. (In English, there is the joke about three spinsters attempting to define a man on the basis of a sequential examination of his parts.) Actually, there are several problems here: (a) the *temporal,* i.e., change occurring in the phenomenon during the course of examination; (b) the attempt to define the whole in terms of a limited number of facets, and (c) the subjective orientations of the different examiners.

In correlations, however, there are further and perhaps more important difficulties. Most important is that if we are not examining different facets of a phenomenon at different times and attempting correlations, we are attempting to use different languages to define and explain the same phenomenon at the same time. When this is so, there should be little wonder that we can identify significantly statistical correlations between different language systems used to describe the same phenomenon. The geometric equivalent for this equation is that two things each of which is equal to a third thing are equal to each other; or more simply, things equal to a third thing are equal to each other. This might be called the problem of overlap and might look like figure 5.

In this three-dimensional or Venn diagram, we are faced with the complexity of interlocking spheres when there is diffusion at the boundaries in the phenomenological characterizations in these areas. It is these parts that lend themselves to the attempted formulations of hyphenated languages that so characterize present-day intellectual conceptualizations. These interfaces are the international market places where individuals speaking many tongues gather to exchange goods and coins for equivalences in coins and goods. X marks the spot that in financial terms may be the equivalent of the world bank where the greatest number of tongues are spoken. The analogy of the relationship between the languages of psychosomatic medicine is more one between goods and coins than between the equivalence of coins of different nationalities. In other words, a direct and specific exchange (translation) is much more complex between tongues than between coins.

The discussion of relationships becomes infinitely more complex when we begin to add to each one of our spheres the multiple different sublanguage systems that each loosely contains. In biology, we have the dynamic relativism of physics closeted with the still relatively static anatomic; in behavioral science, developmental psychology with behaviorism; in social science, cultural anthropology with economics.

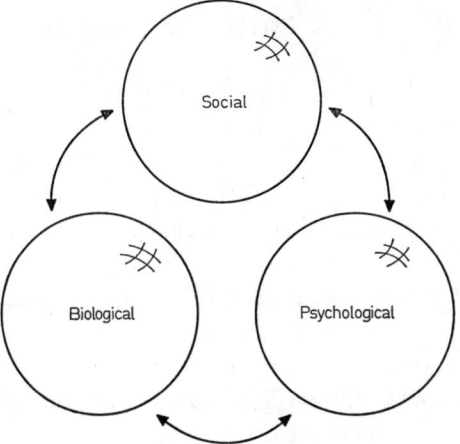

Fig. 4

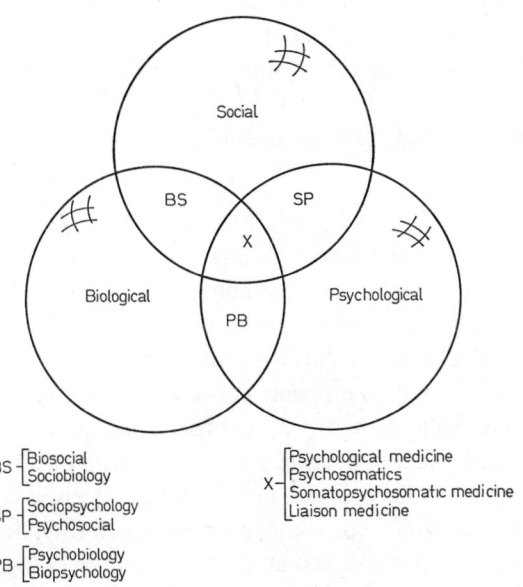

BS	Biosocial Sociobiology		X	Psychological medicine Psychosomatics Somatopsychosomatic medicine Liaison medicine
SP	Sociopsychology Psychosocial			
PB	Psychobiology Biopsychology			

Fig. 5

Evolutionary Directions for Psychosomatic Medicine

Thus far, I have belabored some of the intrinsic paradoxes and potential pitfalls of hyphenated language systems specifically as they relate to psycho-somatic medicine. We might inquire then, what are the significance of these self-obvious observations other than to cast aspersions at a noble experiment. Are there any channels or currents that beckon us out of these swirling waters?

I suggest that what we are observing in our intellectual evolution is the birth of new language systems that are questing for definition in their own right, that is, the development of its own syntax and logic apart from those from which it has evolved. If this sounds either overly optimistic or grandiose, I would merely remind you of the specific vocabulary that has evolved in our short history which is more and more the language of those of us who engage in teaching, research and patient care. We speak increasingly of the Illness Onset Situation (3) the Giving-up – Given-up State (4). Reactions to Illness, the Intensive Care Syndrome (5), a modified conversion process (6), the learning processes involved in psychological (psychosexual) development (7), of specific behavior patterns as being intrinsically a part of specific diseases (8), grief processes (9), etc. Increasingly, we need precision in defining or redefining the use of such terms as stress, symbol, specificity, denial, coping and adaptation. There remains both imprecision and contamination of meaning in the use of these and other terms in each of our language systems. Several of these are selected for illustration.

Stress

As an example of the difficulty in too rapidly translating concepts from one approach to another is that the conceptual word may have different meanings in the different context. Take for example, the idea of a social situation identified as a *stress*. This is extrapolated from what on a statistical basis most individuals within a society consider a stress because of the major readjustment that would be necessary in order to adapt to or cope with that stress and/or the secondary effects of that stress, social or psychological. But that socially conceptualized stress may not be perceived as such by the individual involved, either consciously or unconsciously. It might not be associated with secondary distress, either social or psychological.

On a secondary level, even if a stress was perceived by the individual as possibly or potentially stressful, the individual may have, based on previous experience or by natural endowment, the capacity to successfully cope with the stress to prevent distress in a psychological sense and/or strain in the physiological sense (a word recently introduced by the social stress researchers and which presumably attempts to relate to a physiological concept). On the other hand, I suppose, that a social stress might not be perceived or, if perceived, might not be acknowledged in a psychological sense. This is to say that stress is social, while distress may be reflected psychologically and/or physiologically. Even if a social stress is perceived as stressful and/or relates to psychological distress, it may not be reflected physiologically as a strain depending upon the psychological mechanisms activated by the perception and cognitive processing. We might view cognitive functioning as occurring on one or more levels including the conscious, pre-conscious, sub-conscious and unconscious.

Symbol

Moving from the social to the psychological, we exchange the complexity of the multiple social sciences and the cultural and ethnic differences that prevail among groups for the complexity of languages claiming psychological authenticity. In this context, I would divide these languages into those that belong more in biology and sociology as distinct from those of psychology which address themselves to the mind and the consideration of laws explaining those operations. Among the many terms of psychology, symbol is an important one, particularly in our consideration of stress. Whether or not a social event is perceived as stressful, whether or not it leads to psychological distress in terms of its cognitive metabolism, and whether or not it is reflected in biological strain, will depend on the significance or meaning that social event has to the perceiving organism. This will depend first upon the cognitive state of the individual; his level of arousal which depends on both biological and psychological functioning. Psychologically speaking, whether or not the event relates to a psychological distress will depend not only on its social symbolic meaning but also on its idiosyncratic personal symbolic meaning, based on that individual's previous personal experience, as reinvoked consciously or unconsciously. It is especially the relationship between the external event and the idiosyncratic symbolic meaning to the individual of that event that characterizes modern psychology and which emphasizes the uniqueness and distinctness of the individual as he has developed in and as this individuality has been secured by western civilization. The emphasis on the validity of the organism's individuality is what would characterize psychology from most other disciplines with the possible exception of genetics.

Specificity

At this point, it is timely to bring in the idea of specificity. As first introduced in psychology, the concept was related to personality and specific physiologic processes on the basis that it was frequently observed that individuals with similar personality styles, i.e., the more or less usual defensive patterns and the affects aroused by the signalling of latent conflicts by an external event. The ideal of specificity, i.e., the relationship of specific personality patterns to specific diseases has long been debunked, but it comes back to haunt us time and time again whether it be in terms of behavior pattern type A or more globally in the alexithymic personality. The nature of this relationship has intrigued many. Some have suggested that it is more in the direction of somatopsychic rather than psychosomatic while others suggest that the relationship is through a third factor common to both such as two genes frequently, but not always, inherited together. Still, a third position is that whatever event excited the psychological trauma resulting in fixation at a particular stage of development also resulted in physiologic fixation. Thus, someone with bowel dysfunction could manifest defensive patterns characteristic of anal fixation. Still others have suggested that personality patterns are not all that fixed, but may become transmuted in the course of the underlying physiologic processes that may affect brain function or are different at times of exacerbation and remission for other reasons, e.g., Engel's patients with ulcerative colitis during the constipation *vis-à-vis* the colitis phase. Hence, time and stage are also variables to be considered in our seeking of relationships between the psychological and the somatic.

The concept of specificity has also been applied to the specific conflict that the individual is bound at the time she/he develops a somatic process, suggesting that the type of process will mirror the psychosexual stage that the individual regresses to on the basis of the nature of the conflict, e.g., events that arouse latent passive defendent longings around unresolved conflicts and the defenses against these will manifest behavior reminiscent of the oral stage of development and may at the same time show physiologic processes associated with this early stage which may predilect the individual to peptic ulcer disease.

Coping and Adaptation

Psychologically speaking, we now may look at specificity related to the individual rather than to a group, i.e., a social event may be perceived as a stress, as a potential stress or not as a stress. This may depend on the threshold of perception which may be influenced by both physiological and psycho-

logical factors, influencing cognitive functions or defenses. Cognitive handling of the percept will depend also on memory on varying levels of consciousness. The extent to which recognition of a stressful event leads to coping
behavior will depend on psychological processes, i.e., the clarity that the
event is perceived, the adequacy of psychological defenses in containing
emotions and past learning. When both psychological development and learning have been optimal and/or in the presence of a supportive external milieu,
coping may be said to have occurred. This may occur with little or no
psychological distress and/or physiological strain. Coping may or may not
imply a modification in the external field evoked by the sensing individual.
Adaptation on the other hand, suggests a modified and more or less permanent response to recurring or chronic situations perceived and experienced
as stressful which successfully serves to limit both psychological stress and
physiological strain. Adaptation probably has more of a social connotation
than psychological. Both, as they are witnessed externally, are more in the
realm of the conative than the psychological.

Denial

This is perhaps the most abused of the terms suggesting the mechanisms
of repression. First, for many individuals it is misinterpreted as a conscious
mechanism and as such often equated as malingering. Second, it is often left
unclear as to what is denied, i.e., an external event, the affect related to that
event, the unconscious conflict or fantasy stimulated by the external event,
and/or the affect around the latter. In other words, a term that has had
specific definition in terms of psychology is promiscuously used and misused
in other language systems to identify some other process. In terms of this
word alone, there is sufficient justification for maintaining the purity of our
language systems.

The Present Synthesis

Few of us think of the patient sustaining a myocardial infarction or a
schizophrenic process as being any less psychosomatic than peptic ulcer
disease, hyperthyroidism, rheumatoid arthritis, neurodermatitis, asthma,
ulcerative colitis or essential hypertension. We would no more deny a
psychological or social dimension of this process in this person than we
would a physiological one. We insist of ourselves and our students an
examination and definition in each of these areas of the patient's complaint.

We speak a bit less of correlating descriptions defining a phenomenon in two dimensions or of serial linear relationships, and more in terms of suggesting that what is important is the selction of that language system which is most expedient in defining a phenomenon or situation leading to a pragmatic resolution. At the same time, another language system might give us greater intellectual satisfaction or incite our curiosity to explore another dimension of the phenomenon. To this extent, we have sometimes deliberately, but I suspect more often less so, used a general systems approach in addressing a clinical problem (10). Where we can, we would identify the concurrence or coincidence (rather than defining the co-relationship) of phenomena from the context of one language system with those of other language systems. We anticipate that over time will evolve a psychosomatic medicine where the conceptualization of health and illness will at all times be defined in terms of the psychological, social and biological. And that in this way, there would begin to emerge more specific patterns in these relatioships. In this way, the psychosomatic approach of objectively looking at the interfaces and the detection of these patterns may lead to the wholistic medicine that humanity subjectively strives for and that 19th century medicine continues to frac-tionate.

Relationship to Research and Education

I have suggested some of the intrinsic difficulties in working with multiple language systems and conceptual approaches in attending to the problems of behavior especially as they pertain to disease and illness. The pertinence of these observations to present-day research will limit our emphasis on 19th century biological approaches from which we descend and allow us to be less concrete and more relativistic in attempting to define relationships between different conceptual approaches in terms of causation, direction and dimen-sion, I suggest that we need to get away from the idea that the final common pathway of behavior is through the nervous system and the brain; that such a conceptualization has intrinsic logic only within a biological context. It does nos necessarily have such a reality within a psychological system where mind, not brain, is the universe; or in an environmental system where defined entities and their laws are derived from both of these approaches and have an identity of their own. Our researches are incomplete if we fail to view our subjects and our relationship with them from the standpoint of more than one conceptual orientation (11, 12). We need to be especially cautious in attempting to define the relationships between the observations and explanations derived from one approach with those of another. Rather, we need to tolerate the frustration of identifying and accepting the concurrence of phenomenological observations explained from different conceptual orientations without necessarily implying either direct translation or specific relatedness. Necessarily, this approach in psychosomatic medicine implies sophistication for the would-be researcher in an ever-increasing knowledge of the languages of behavior without the obligation of becoming a believer in one as opposed to another. This does not mean that as mortals we need not have our favorite. This implies a never-ending pursuance of the languages of behavior: biological, psychological and social. It implies that at least some of the individuals working in this area have extensive education and clinical experience in medicine as well as systems of thought removed from the biological sciences. This suggestion is not unlike that of *Penfield* who demanded of his neurosurgery residents that they have training in general medicine, endocrinology, neurology, general surgery and psychiatry before embarking on a life-long study of neurosurgery. As always, there are hazards in such a formula inasmuch as it can be pursued perfunctorily without individual imagination and that individuals may merely convert from one orientation to another without attempted synthesis and integration.

In closing, I suggest that the significance of the psychosomatic field is less in and of itself and more as the beacon it becomes for individuals in other disciplines emphasizing the need for multidisciplinary approaches in the observation and understanding of behavior while it pursues a continual and relentless reexamination of its attempted integration, synthesis and study of relationships between phenomena viewed from different conceptual approaches.

References

1 *Wilson, D.L.:* On the nature of consciousness and of physical reality. Perspect. Biol. Med. *19:* 568–581 (1976).
2 *Langer, S.K.:* Philosophy in a new key (Harvard University Press, Cambridge 1942)·
3 *Holmes, T.H. and Rahe, R.H.:* The social readjustment rating scale. J. psychosom. Res. *11:* 213–218 (1967).
4 *Engel, G.L.:* A life setting conducive to illness. The giving-up-given-up complex. Bull. Menninger Clin. *32:* 355–365 (1968).
5 *McKegney, F.P.:* The intensive care syndrome. The definition, treatment and prevention of a new 'disease of medical progress'. Conn. Med. *30:* 633–636 (1966).

6   *Engel, G.L.:* A reconsideration of the role of conversion in somatic disease. Compreh. Psychiat. *9:* 316–326 (1968).

7   *Dollard, J. and Miller, N.:* Personality and psychotherapy (McGraw-Hill, New York 1950).

8   *Friedman, M. and Rosenman, R.H.:* Association of specific overt behavior pattern with blood and cardiovascular findings. J. Am. med. Ass. 1286–1296 (1959).

9   *Nemiah, J. and Sifneos, P.:* Affect and fantasy in patients with psychosomatic disorders; in *Hill* Modern trends in psychosomatic medicine, vol. 2, chapt. 2, pp. 26–34 (Butterworths, Laondon 1970).

10 *Grinker, R.R.:* Toward a unified theory of human behavior. An introduction to General systems theory; 2nd ed. (Basic Books, New York 1967).

11 *Kimball, C.P.:* Techniques of interviewing. I. Interviewing and the meaning of the symptom. Ann. intern. Med. *71:* 147–153 (1969).

12 *Kimball, C.P.:* Conceptual developments in psychosomatic medicine: 1939–1969. Ann. intern. Med. *73:* 307–316 (1970).

Chase Patterson Kimball, MD, University of Chicago, Department of Psychiatry, 950 E. 59th Street, *Chicago, IL 60637* (USA)

Proc. 11th Eur. Conf. Psychosom. Res., Heidelberg 1976
Psychother. Psychosom. *28:* 13–27 (1977)

Psychological Dimensions in Psychosomatic Patients[1]

Margaret Thaler Singer
University of California, Berkeley, Calif.

During the past 50 years interest has grown in the study of the relationships between man's emotions, his environment and his health. However, during the same period, there has been an almost kaleidoscopic change of views about which psychological dimensions are central and more important to study. I will stress a few important changes in the field of psychosomatic medicine and talk about current concepts which deserve more study.

Major Changes in the Field

Five important changes in psychosomatic medicine have happened recently. The areas and the direction of the changes have been as follows.

The Scope of Psychosomatic Medicine has Broadened from Studying Psychological Factors in Chronic Illness to Studying Psychological Factors in all Illness

Early research and treatment of psychosomatic illness concentrated upon patients who suffered from certain chronic and supposedly stress-connected conditions; peptic ulcer, hypertension, asthma, rheumatoid arthritis, neurodermatitis, migraine and ulcerative colitis. And these were the most frequently studied conditions.

This early work was prompted by the increasing influence of psycho-

[1] This and other recent manuscripts by the writer have been made possible by research support from the Grant Foundation, Inc., New York, to whom appreciation is extended.

analysis on psychiatry and psychology which in turn gradually had an increasing influence on many aspects of patient care in general medicine to the extent that 'psychosomatic' illnesses were perceived by some in general medicine and many lay persons as being psychogenic. General medicine lacked effective treatments for many aspects of such chronic conditions. Over time we have learned that stress and other cultural-environmnetal influences contribute to both the onset and recurrent exacerbations of such illnesses. Psychoanalytic formulations about the effects of conflict, repression and symbolic behavior were conceptualized as the psychogenic origins of a number of physical conditions especially stress connected illnesses such as asthma, e.g., 'a cry for help', or hypertension supposedly the physical expression of repressed anger. The early psychoanalysts believed that certain illnesses were symbolic expressions of unconscious psychological conflicts and their efforts were to establish these connections. Some of these early psychoanalytic psychosomaticists (*Georg Groddeck* and *Ernst Simmel* in Germany; *F. Deutsch* in Vienna; *Smith Ely Jelliffe* in the United States, and *Angel Garma* in Argentina) uncritically attempted to explain all symptoms, even visceral ones, as direct expressions of highly specific repressed ideas or fantasies. Certain of the psychoanalytic formulations about the effect of conflict, repression and symbolic behavior appeared more plausible when applied to patients with purportedly stress-connected disease.

However, in the late 30s and early 40s, these ideas were abandoned in favor of hypotheses that linked prolonged emotional stresses with the appearances of a family of chronic illnesses which then came to be regarded as 'psychosomatic'. *Alexander's* writings were seminal in bringing a 'new look' to psychosomatic medical research (*Alexander,* 1943, 1950, *Alexander and Selesmick,* 1966). He differentiated between conversion symptoms and stress reactions. Conversions symptoms were seen as unconscious attempts to resolve psychological tensions and conflicts by the substitution of a physical disability which became a symbol for an unbearable emotional state. The resulting physical symptoms were always in the sensory or voluntary motor systems and as such were thought to be amenable to the 'talking cure' which would transmute them back into psychic expression for abreaction (*Breuer and Freud,* 1895).

However, stress reactions such as hypertension, asthma and peptic ulcers were not seen by *Alexander* and co-workers as attempts to express blocked emotions, but were regarded as responses of the vegetative involuntary physiological systems. These disorders were considered to represent physiological states triggered by constant or periodically recurring emotional conflict states. The psychosomatic illnesses were perceived to be the price paid by the body for a long and painful effort to cope with a complex conflict or problem which is never entirely resolved. The stress symptoms were seen as amenable to psychoanalytically derived treatment to reduce the interpersonal or intrapsychic conflicts, some of which were regarded as relatively specific conflicts shared by those with a certain disease, e.g., dependency conflicts were felt to be central for peptic ulcer patients.

For over a decade, following *Alexander*'s work, psychosomatic research was primarily devoted to comparing various chronically ill groups such as peptic ulcer with hypertensive patients, patients with neurodermatitis and those with asthma. Efforts were directed toward finding personality traits which would distinguish groups of hypertensive patients from those suffering from ulcers, asthma, migraine and other conditions.

As more was learned about patients with these illnesses who were studied over prolonged periods, research began to center on the course of health and illness in individual patients. Research turned from asking, 'what kinds of people have ulcers' to asking 'What were the circumstances in the patient's life prior to and at the time of the onset of his illness;' or 'What was occurring before an exacerbation of illness;' or 'What circumstances contributed to the patient's recovery?'

Research efforts shifted again to the study of different ways patients *coped* with the stresses which followed changes in their lives (*Holmes and Rahe*, 1967; *Kasl and Cobb*, 1966, 1975; *Rahe*, 1972). Relationships were sought among such changes and the occurrence, exacerbation or recovery from various illness.

Thus, the sequence of research developments in psychosomatic medicine broadened medical perspectives. This allowed attention to turn to the study of psychological variables in *all* states of health and illness. Even diseases formerly thought to be purely somatic, such as the production of growth hormones, the course of cancer, and responses of the immunological system have now been included in the field of psychosomatic research (*Ader and Cohen*, 1975; *Engel*, 1962; *Engel*, 1976; *Greene et al.*, 1970; *LeShan*, 1961; *Mirsky*, 1960; *Mason*, 1968; *Amkraut and Solomon*, 1975).

Interest has Shifted from Patient's Intrapsychic Processes to their Interpersonal Transactions

There is a growing movement within psychology and psychiatry to look beyond the individual patient and the presenting problem to view the broader context of his everyday life. Most therapies have traditionally examined the intrapsychic life of the patient with psychosomatic illness, e. g., a person with physical illness believed to have psychological components influencing his general health. Earlier treatments for such patients were based upon the so-called dynamic theories of personality. These hold that memories of past experiences and subsequent fantasies and transferences (in the psychoanalytic sense) based upon them had to be explored and insight gained by the patient about how past events and relationships influenced daily behavior. This form of treatment depend on a one-to-one relationship between patient and therapist. Since the number of patients supposedly needing psychological treatment was great, and the number of therapists few, this treatment was not accessible to many. An even more overriding problem was the growing recognition by therapists and patients alike that psychoanalytically derived methods were not widely applicable because its principal successes were essentially middle class, educated and verbal patients and not readily compatible with the poorly educated, psychologically unsophisticated and poor.

For years, a number of those prominent in psychosomatic research and theory have been urging a holistic medical approach that looks beyond sick organs and ailing bodies into patients' lives. This required knowing the patient's past and the present circumstances of his life. In other words, holistic medicine looks beyond the presenting symptoms or syndrome into individualized treatment patterns based on each patient's physical, mental and environmental states. Holistic theorists have great support from those psychologists, psychiatrists and other behavioral scientists who favor a general systems theory to explain various transactions within the body, between and among people (*Von Bertalanffy, 1966*).

Some (*Engel,* 1959, 1962, 1967, 1968a, b, 1971, 1972, 1976; *Adler et al.,* 1971; *Greene et al.,* 1970, 1973, *Schmale,* 1958; *Seligman,* 1975, and others) theorize that an emotional aura affects the patient following actual or feared psychological losses (job, lover, prestige, etc.) and is the necessary precondition before any illness can develop. A personal existential outlook beyond a mood and beyond an affect state, variously termed depression, giving up, helplessness-hopelessness, was said to evolve in a pre-sick person. After being in such states for a prolonged period, it is speculated by these writers, that the body's resistance or ability to cope changes, falters or fails.

Various disease processes emerge as the product of complex interactions to social surroundings, the psyche and the soma. How long, how intense and hopeless the patient feels about the future of the experienced stressful condition determines whether and when an illness will occur. Complex interactions which occur in a brief, but unusually strong demand on a person in a chronically stressed state need to be studied when new but short term demands on him are made (*Singer, 1974*; *Mason,* 1968; *Engel,* 1968, 1971, 1972). For example, what happens when a severely depressed man who is slowed down. inactive and in the depths of hopelessness, finds he must shovel snow after a heavy storm? Is this a likely moment for a myocardial infarction, a stroke, or other illness to occur? *Greene* and *Engel's* research suggest this possibility.

Systems theory as introduced into biology by *Von Bertalanffy* (1966) has permeated psychological theory and practice. In the past 30 years, the perspective of psychosomatic medicine has shifted: (1) from attention to the malfunctioning organ; (2) to the sick person, and (3) to the person as an open biological system interacting with other open systems around him. The attention of researchers has now turned to family studies, both the family or origin and patients' marital families. Much research is being devoted to studying how major stressfull changes within family systems and within personally significant systems (at work, social life, children's lives) in which the patients transact affect them. Since this viewpoint was adopted, it was inevitable that the ways in which patients communicate with significant others also would come under intense scrutiny.

Since the Physically Ill Person is now Perceived from a Transactional and Systems Viewpoint, his Style of Communicating with others becomes Critical to Understanding his Illnesses and Selecting Correct Treatment

Communication is vital, at the interface between the patient and significant others in his life, communication often fails or becomes garbled. Therefore, interest is growing in research on conversational styles of patients. From a systems and transactional viewpoint the words people use to express their ideas and feelings, the stylistic qualities of the ways they talk to their therapists, and the conversational style they adapt with people around them, becomes essential to an understanding of the impact they have on others which in turn affects whether or not their needs are recognized, understood and met by others. Since many therapies are 'talking therapies', therapeutic conversations, the topics of therapeutic conversations, the goals of therapeutic conversations become critical to evolving therapeutic relationships and therapeutic transactions. In most instances the therapist can only guess at the patient's probable impact on others. Part of the therapeutic goal within this transactional framework is for the patient to understand and gauge how he elicits or fails to elicit what he needs others to give him and what they need from him.

Reports of Studies Correlating Personality Traits with Specific Chronic Illnesses have Decreased, and an Increasing Amount of Literature is Appearing which Deals with Different Psychotherapeutic Methods in the Treatment of All Physically Sick Patients

Much earlier research was devoted to the study of groups of persons with specific chronic diseases (hypertension, peptic ulcer, migraine, etc.) seeking to learn if patterns of traits characterized each group in contrast to the other groups (*Dunbar,* 1946). As such research became less prominent because of modest results, there was an increasing literature on psychotherapy with a vast array of physically sick people. A number of journals have appeared devoted primarily to suggesting appropriate methods of psychotherapy for different categories of physically ill people, e.g., patients in intensive care units, the terminally ill, patients on dialysis, biofeedback, autogenic training and self help methods to help patients cope with everyday stresses and strains and thereby reduce such pressure and strains in order to decrease the likelihood of stress-induced illnesses. A number of such articles have begun to appear more frequently in other medical journals and in the popular press as well.

As the Past Quarter Century has Seen Teaching Hospitals and Clinics Increase their Staffs to Enable them to Offer More psychological and Psychiatric Services to the Physically Ill, so have the General Public Become More Aware that their Health may be Influenced by their Attitudes and Responses to Changes and Stresses in their Lives

Efforts to maintain and improve all aspects of one's own health – mental as well as physical – are being more widely advocated and accepted, not only by health care professionals, but by laymen who may even become susceptible to dietary fads, mental and quasi-religious regimens. There are so many and varied therapeutic movements they have become a national obsession which threatens to engulf the consciousness of North America. This is attested to by the widespread popularity of the so-called human potential (humanistic psychology) movement. self-help growth therapies, and the spread of the so-called consciousness-expanding movement. These therapies or philosophies for change may have leaders who call themselves gurus, trainers, group leaders, masters, guides, etc. Many of these ideologically based therapies or proposed life styles contain elements of authoritarian leadership, peer control, communal living arrangements and other means of persuasion or control. In one instance, a major symbol of leave taking of one's former life is a wake, followed by a funeral in which a box is buried, supposedly containing all the oppressive aspects of one's mother, father, spouse, siblings, etc. A recent survey (Newsweek, 6 September 1976) indicated that there were more than 8,000 varieties of nontraditional therapies in North America alone.

This brief review of five of the most important trends in psychosomatic medicine: (1) its expanding horizons: (2) the shift from intrapsychic theories to transactional and systems vantage points; (3) interest in how patients communicate; (4) concern with responses to psychotherapies, and (5) a growing popular interest in mental and physical health fads, leads us into a brief discussion of four important dimensions which appear central to the evaluation of psychosomatic patients and formulating research and therapy designs. These are: (1) the patient's cognitive style; (2) the ways patients invest themselves in transactions; (3) patients attitudes about changes which have occurred in their lives and (4) designing research which includes representative samples of the population taking into account such variables as ethnicity, age, sex, social class, etc., which match the sick and the well. Most previous psychosomatic research compared neurotic chronically physically ill people with nonneurotic physically well people. This unfortunate research situation grew out of the selective referral process in which internists, allergists and other physicians referred primarily severely neurotic asthmatics, hypertensive and peptic ulcer patients, etc., whose conditions resisted medical therapy. For some years psychologists and psychiatrists based research conclusions on these biased samples. Recently, more sophisticated sampling techniques have been used. 'Yet, the current state of our knowledge regarding the interrelationships of biological, environmental and interpersonal factors is (still) so meager that enthusiasm for such studies is dampened'. (*Feingold et al.,* 1966, p. 144).

Four current constructs attempt to assess these dimensions. *Alexthymia* (*Sifneos,* 1967, 1975; *Nemiah,* 1973, 1975) is a formulation about cognitive style. Cognitive style has been studied in different research contexts than psychosomatic studies (*Gardner et al.,* 1959). *Engagement-involvement* (*Reiser et al.,* 1955; *Singer,* 1974; *Thaler-Singer et al.,* 1957; *Weiner et al.,* 1962) is a concept of how patients' invest or fail to invest themselves in transactions. *Helplessness-hopelessness* (*Engel,* 1968, 1976; *Engel and Schmale,* 1972; *Schmale,* 1958; *Seligman,* 1975) is a formulation about attitudes toward what has transpired in patient's lives and how they view the future. *Sample bias* (*Feingold et al.,* 1966) refers to whether patients are representative or not of those who are ill with the same disease processes.

We shall now look at the current status of these four constructs in psychosomatic medicine.

Alexithymia. Alexithymia is a cluster of cognitive traits. While the term alexithymia is relatively new (*Sifneos,* 1967), and recent work by *Nemiah* (1973, 1975) has centered the attention of many resaerchers on the construct, the actual trait cluster described as alexithymia has been in the literature of psychosomatics, general personality and psychopathological research for some time. In the field of psychosomatic research, *Ruesch* (1946, 1948, 1957) labeled such patients 'infantile personalities'. He called them 'the core problem of psychosomatic medicine', and wrote: 'These patients lack satisfactory means of self-expression. . . The higher symbolic functions are underdeveloped. The vocabulary range tends to be limited; fantasy elaborations in tests such as the Rorschach and TAT are primitive, unimaginative, and stereotyped. . . They seem to pay more attention to. . . bodily sensations than to their impact. . . upon others. . . They confine the content of messages to subjects of universal interest. Reference to eating, sleeping, eliminating, sex and other body functions make up the content of most messages'. (*Ruesch,* 1957, pp. 117–118). This is not far different from Nemiah's observations that 'alexithymic' personalities display (1) an inability to describe feelings in words: (2) a marked paucity of fantasy, and (3) a failure to make significant internal psychological changes in the course of psychodynamically-oriented psychotherapy (*Nemiah,* 1975). Nor do these descriptions sound far afield from some of those of the early psychoanalytic psychosomaticists (*Deutsch,* 1927) who wrote as if they felt that if they could only assist certain patients to let the repression and denial fall away, the unleashing of pent-up feelings and fantasies would free the patients of crippling conflicts, and, therefore, of the emotionally induced components of their illness. The assumption was that this process would ultimately result in dissipation of the physical illness.

Psychologists and psychiatrists continue to find themselves working with patients who suffer from chronic physical illnesses. People other than the patient tend to believe that stressful events, social interactions and the patient's psychological states contribute to exacerbation of the disease process, while calm internal states contribute to remission of physical symptoms. However, patients tend not to see these supposed connections and therefore become the bane of both medical and psychiatric practitioners' lives because treatments cure neither the physical symptoms nor eliminate their supposed psychogenic components. Currently, such patients in poor standing with the medical and psychiatric therapists are termed alexithymic.

Because the alexithymic construct is becoming prevalent and popular, it is necessary to examine its rationale. Flaws as well as merits in the logic behind the construct should be analyzed to permit research that confirms or refutes whether alexithymia is a distinct trait cluster found only among psychosomatic patients or whether it also exists in the general population.

From the descriptions given by *Sifneos* and *Nemiah,* and from my own work and that of colleagues, it is apparent that such persons as those labeled alexithymic exist. That is not in dispute. But two questions arise: (1) Are these characteristics found outside of the psychosomatic patient group? (2) Are there other personality types found among psychosomatic patients? My impression is 'yes'.

Does the alexithymic trait cluster characterize persons other than the psychosomatically ill? For years, psychologists have been referring to many people who have traits such as those attributed to the alexithymics as persons who are 'not psychologically minded'. Many studies have found that these 'not psychologically minded' people are also not responsive to traditional insight-oriented psychotherapies. A number of test instruments (*Barron,* 1953a, b; *Edwards,* 1970) have been devised which successfully predict which patients will do best in insight-oriented therapies from the ways they describe themselves on the tests. It can also be predicted whether or not they will persist in therapy (*van Atta,* 1968). Much effort could have been saved by testing these patients before therapy was begun. Had these tests been administered, better therapeutic plans would surely have been devised.

Research *is* needed comparing psychosomatic patients with healthy people to gauge the extent to which the trait cluster called alexithymia characterizes a substantial segment of the general population. At the same time, careful matching for age, education, sex, ethnic background and social class in the sick and healthy groups must be made, because the verbal characteristics attributed to the alexithymics are known to be correlated with social class and ethnicity. Therefore, well-matched groups of the sick and healthy should be studied using standardized test batteries to measure the trait clusters.

I would predict that in such research most of the alexithymic psychosomatic patients could be properly categorized and a portion of the healthy population will share with them an inability to describe feelings in words, a marked paucity of fantasy and a failure to make significant internal psychological changes in the course of psychodynamically-oriented psychotherapy.

However, what will also be common to the two groups of sick and healthy alexithymics may be that certain constellations of age, social class and ethnicity, taken together, produce the extent of the alexithymic trait cluster.

The relevance of these findings will probably be challenged. Some will say that not all people of a given social class, ethnic background and sex are alike; they therefore will try to discover the shared neurological characteristics of alexithymic behavior. It does not seem likely that alexithymia is purely a neurological malfunctioning. But for those so inclined, the adding of psychological assessment and sociological dimensions to such research is indicated if their questions are to be answered.

Are there other personality types found among psychosomatic patients. From my discussion of alexithmia, it should be clear that I think there are. However, I think that rather than research which focuses on the search for personality traits peculiar to psychosomatic patients, the shift to more process-oriented research with psychosomatic patients should be continued. Studies of processes and transactions within the ongoing lives of patients will probably produce better treatment results. Recent studies upon how people adapt to changes in their lives reveals that great changes of a positive or negative nature are stressful and often precede physical illness (*Holmes and Rahe*, 1967; *Rahe*, 1972; *Kasl and Cobb*, 1966; *Kasl et al.*, 1975). In addition, introducing the Holmes-Rahe method of assessing changes in the patient's life, the constructs of engagement-involvement, and of helplessness-hopelessness appear to be formulations of variables related to the onset or exacerbations of physical illness.

Engagement-involvement. This construct has been introduced over the years by my colleagues and me to describe that central phenomenon in all transactions in which behavioral clues suggest that a person is locking into, or not locking into, investing or not investing in a passing interaction. It includes attention, alerting arousal, affect and evocative mental associations. In the case of hypertensives, for example, the prognosis is poor for hypertensives who are easily turned on or become heavily involved in life's passing drama than those hypertensives who do not (*Singer,* 1967). In the case of ulcer patients, those who do not sufficiently engage do not seem to recover as rapidly (*Thaler-Singer et al.,* 1957). But engagement-involvement refers to more than each of these separately. The concept of engagement-involvement is offered in an effort to capture the extent of the engagement or lack of it perceived in people at specific moments, this makes transactionally oriented ratings of their interactions with others possible. It also permits us to correlate transactional behavior with whatever physiological dimensions are being concomitantly studied in psychosomatic research or following therapy.

Helplessness-hopelessness. Engel and his colleagues (*Engel,* 1959, 1962, 1967, 1968a, b, 1971, 1972, 1976; *Adler et al.,* 1971; *Schmale,* 1958) using the terms helplessness-hopelessness and *Greene et al.* (1970, 1973) using the term depression, refer to a transactional mode which can be seen transpiring between the patient and his significant others and tells us the current outlook the patient has about the possibility of change and what the future appears to have in store for him. The patient who has responded to unpleasant circumstances in life with helplessness-hopelessness and has disengaged from his own inner drives is at a vulnerable point for becoming ill. The extent of the disengagement is speculated to produce an extreme inner apathy almost as if vital life-sustaining processes are depleted. This extreme of hopelessness seems to follow a preliminary period in which the patient felt helplesss to solve problems, and help did not come. This appears to be a precondition for the extreme condition of hopelessness. The weak links in their vital chain break. The arthritic-prone become arthritic; the cancer-prone become cancerous; and so on according to this formulation.

Sample bias. The final dimension I have time to mention is sample bias. For some years, my colleagues and I have been writing about the highly selected, biased samples of patients upon which most of the psychosomatic literature is based (*Feingold et al.,* 1966).

Certain selection processes operate at the point of referral. Internists, allergists and other physicians are more likely to refer for psychotherapy certain patients with chronic conditions who have not responded to other treatments. Therefore, psychologists and psychiatrists are more likely to have referred to them as patients the following: (a) *The difficult to work with patient* who is flat, unresponsive, who responds poorly in spite of the efforts of the physician treating him. (b) *The irritable, cantankerous, uncooperative patient* whose behavior appears to be obstructing medical treatment and progress toward health. (c) *The garrulous, dramatizing, overly talkative patient* whose tendency 'to need a great deal of time' causes them to be referred to psychologists and psychiatrists because physicians regard psychologists and psychiatrists as having 'time to listen'. (d) *The patients with multiple stresses,* crises, and difficulties in their lives who could not be helped even by Solomon.

Therefore, only certain segments of each population of sick people get into psychologists' or psychiatrists' offices, and become part of research samples.

It is not surprising that some or even many psychosomatic patients do not respond to insight-oriented psychotherapy, but could respond to paradoxical intervention techniques, behavior modification and other procedures which *Haley* (1973) ,*Watzlawick et al.* (1974), *Hoebel* (1975), *Minuchin* (1974), and others are attempting. In these psychotherapy modes, insight in irrelevant to behavioral changes. The psychotherapists work directly to effect behavioral changes and the patient does not really have to understand the sources of how past trauma have contributed to the origins of their psychosomatic illness. To what extent is this therapy successful and with which patients needs further study. It is possible that not all patients will respond.

Thus, in selecting the dimensions to study in research and then to plan effective differential treatment strategies with sick people, it appears that we need to (1) take into account clusters of personality traits; (2) the types and degrees of stress; (3) the magnitude of life changes with which a particular personality is trying to cope, (4) the extent of engagement-involvement, and (5) the degree of depression or helplessness-hopelessness present.

In psychosomatic medicine, as with all pyschotherapies, there is a need for a large number of techniques. The psychological and psychiatric professions ought not to lock themselves into narrow methods of therapy based solely upon any single theory of personality and treatment.

To conclude, the psychological dimensions touched upon here need to be considered carefully in the planning of research and therapy with all physically sick patients. Finally, those of us who are therapists and researchers should become proficient in a wide range of treatment methods which can be selectively applied to patients depending on their needs. This is a very serious task indeed.

References

Ader, R. and Cohen, N.: Behaviorally conditioned immunosuppression. Psychosom. Med. *37:* 333–340 (1975).

Adler, R.; MacRitchie, K., and Engel, G.L.: Psychologic processes and ischemic stroke (occlusive cerebrovascular disease). Psychosom. Med. *33:* 1–29 (1971).

Alexander, F.: Fundamental concepts of psychosomatic research. Psychogenesis, conversion, specificity. Psychosom. Med. *5:* 205–210 (1943).

Alexander, F.: Psychosomatic medicine (Norton, New York 1950).

Alexander, F.G. and Selesnick, S.T.: The history of psychiatry (Harper & Row, New York 1966).

Amkraut, A. and Solomon, G.F.: From the symbolic stimulus to the pathophysiologic response. Immune mechanisms. Int. J. Psychiat. Med. *5:* 541–563 (1975).

Barron, F.: Some test correlates of response to psychotherapy. J. Consult. Psychol. *17:* 235–241 (1953).

Barron, F.: An ego-strength scale which predicts response to psychotherapy. J. Consult. Psychol. *17:* 327–333 (1953).

Breuer, J. and Freud, S.: Studies on hysteria (Basic Books, New York 1957), Original, 1895).

Dunbar, F.: Emotions and bodily change; 3rd ed. (Columbia University Press, New York 1946).

Edwards, A.L.: The measurement of personality traits by scales and inventories (Holt, New York 1970).

Engel, G.L.: Psychogenic pain and the pain-prone patient. Am. J. Med. *26:* 899–918 (1959).

Engel, G.L.: Psychological development in health and disease. (Saunders, Philadelphia 1962).

Engel, G.L. and Schmale, A.H.: Psychoanalytic theory of somatic disorders. Conversion, specificity and the disease onset situation. J. Am. psychoanal. Ass. *15:* 344–365 (1967).

Engel, G.L.: A reconsideration of the role of conversion in somatic disease. Comp. Psychiat *9:* 316–326 (1968a).

Engel, G.L.: A life setting conductive to illness. The giving-up, given-up complex. Ann. intern. Med. *69:* 293–300 (1968b).

Engel, G.L.: Sudden and rapid death during psychological stress. Folklore folk wisdom? Ann. intern. Med. *74:* 771–682 (1971).

Engel, G.L. and Schmale, A.H.: Conservation-withdrawal. A primary regulatory process for organismic homeostasis. Presented at Ciba Foundation Symp. Physiology, Emotion and Psychosomatic Illness. London 1972.

Engel, G.L.: The psychosomatic approach to individual susceptibility to disease. Address given at Children's Hospital, San Francisco 1976.

Feingold, B.F.; Gorman, F.J.; Singer, M.T., and Schlesinger, K.: Psychological studies of allergic women. Psychosom. Med. *24:* 195–202 (1962).

Feingold, B.F.; Singer, M.T.; Freeman, E.H., and Deskins, A.: Psychological variables in allergic disease: A critical appraisal of methodology. J. Allergy *38:* 143–155 (1966).

Framo, A.: Symptoms from a family transactional viewpoint. Int. Psychiat. Clin. *7:* 121–175 (1970).

Greene, W.A.; Conron, G.; Schalsh, D.S., and Schreiner, B.F.: Psychologic correlates of growth hormone and adrenal secretory responses of patients undergoing cardiac catheterization. Psychosom. Med. *32:* 599–614 (1970).

Greene, W.A.; Goldstein, S., and Moss, A J.: Psychological and social variables associated with sudden death from apparent coronary heart disease. Psychosom. Med. *35:* 458–459 (1973).

Haley, J.: Uncommon therapy. The psychiatric techniques of Milton H. Erickson, MD (Ballentine Books, New York 1973).

Hardyck, C.; Singer, M.T., and Harris, R.E.: Transient changes in affect and blood pressure. Arch. gen. Psychiat 7: 15–20 (1962).

Harris, R.E. and Singer, M.T.: Interaction of personality and stress in the pathogenesis of essential hypertension. Hypertension. XVI, Neural control of arterial pressure. Am. Heart Ass. 16: 104–115 (1968).

Holmes, T.H. and Rahe, R.H.: The social readjustment rating scale. J. Psychosom. Res. 11: 213–218 (1967).

Hoebel, F.C.: Coronary artery disease and family interaction, unpubl. diss. California School of Professional Psychology. San Francisco (1975).

Kasl, S.V. and Cobb, S.: Health behavior, illness behavior, and sick role behavior. Arch. envir. Hlth 12: 246–266, 531–541 (1966).

Kasl, S.V.; Gore, S., and Cobb, S.: The experience of losing a job. Reported changes in health, symptoms and illness behavior. Psychosom. Med. 37: 106–122 (1975).

LeShan: A basic psychological orientation apparently associated with malignant disease. Psychiat. Q. 35: 314–330 (1961).

Lidz, T.: General conditions of psychosomatic medicine, in *Arieti* American handbook of psychiatry, vol. 1 (Basic Books, New York 1959).

Mason, J.W.: Organization of psychoendocrine mechanisms. Psychosom. Med. 30: 565–808 (1968).

Meissner, W.W.: Family dynamics and psychosomatic processes. Family Process 5: 142–161 (1966).

Miller, G.: The psychosomatic interface; in *Rosenbaum and Beebe* Psychiatric treatment. Crisis-clinic-consultation (McGraw-Hill, New York 1975).

Minuchin, S.: Families and family therapy (Harvard University Press, Cambridge 1974).

Mirsky, I.A.: Physiologic, psychologic, and social determinants of psychosomatic disorders. Dis. nerv. Syst. 21: 950–956 (1960).

Nemiah, J.C.: Psychology and psychosomatic illness. Reflections on theory and research methodology; in *Freyberger* Topics of psychosomatic research. Proc. 9th Eur. Conf. Psychosom. Res. (Karger, Basel 1973).

Nemiah, J.C.: Denial revisisted. Reflections on psychosomatic theory. Psychother. Psychosom. 26: 140–147 (1975).

Price, D.B.; Thaler-Singer, M., and Mason, J.W.: Preoperative emotional states and adrenal cortical activity. Studies on cardiac and pulmonary surgery patients. Archs Neurol. Psychiat. 77: 646–656 (1957).

Rahe, R.H.: Subject's recent life changes and their near-future illness susceptibility; in *Lipowski* Psychosocial aspects of physical illness. Adv. psychosom. Med. ,vol. 8, pp. 2–19 (Karger, Basel 1972).

Reiser, M.F.; Thaler-Singer, M., and Weiner, H.: The experimental manipulation of projective stimuli in the study of psychophysiological responses. Psychosom. Med. 17: 480 (1955).

Ruesch, J.; Harris, R.E.; Christiansen, C.; Loeb, M.B.; Dewees, S., and Jacobson, A.: Duodenal ulcer (University of California Press, Berkeley 1948).

Ruesch, J.; Harris, R.E.; Loeb, M.B.; Christiansen, C.; Dewees, S.; Heller, S.H., and Jacobson, A.: Chronic disease and psychological invalidism. (University of California Press, Berkeley 1951).

Ruesch, J.: Disturbed communication. The clinical assessment of normal and pathological communicative behavior (Norton, New York 1957).

Schmale, A.H.: Relationship of separation and depression to disease. A report on a hospitalized medical population. Psychosom. Med. *20:* 259–277 (1958).

Seligman, M.E.P.: Helplessness (Freeman, San Francisco, 1975).

Sifneos, P.E.: Clinical observations on some patients suffering from a variety of psychosomatic diseases. Proc. 7th Eur. Conf. Psychosom. Res. (Karger, Basel 1967).

Sifneos, P.E.: Problems of psychotherapy of patients with alexithymic characteristics and physical disease. Psychother. psychosom. *26:* 65–70 (1975).

Sifneos, P.E.: Criteria for psychotherapeutic outcome. Psychother. Psychosom. *26:* 49–58 (1975).

Singer, M.T.: Presidential address. Engagement-involvement: a central phenomenon in psychophysiological research. Psychosom. Med. *36:* 1–17 (1974).

Singer, M.T.: Enduring personality styles and responses to stress. Trans. Ass. Life Ins. Med. Direct. Am. *51:* 150–166 (1967).

Thaler-Singer, M.: Effects of stressful situations on learning. Psychiat. Res. Reports, No. 3. (American Psychiatric Association, Washington 1956).

Thaler-Singer, M.; Reiser, M.F., and Weiner, H.: An exploration of the doctor-patient relationship through projective techniques. Their use in psychosomatic illness. Psychosom. Med. *19:* 228–239 (1957).

Van Atta, R.E.: Relationship of personality characteristics to persistence in psychotherapy. J. Consult. Clin. Psychol. *32:* 731–733 (1968).

Von Bertalanffy, L.: General systems theory and psychiatry; in *Arieti* American handbook of psychiatry, vol. 3 (Basic Books, New York, 1966).

Watzlawick, P.; Weakland, J.H., and Fisch, R.: Change Principles of problem formation and problem resolution. (Norton, New York 1974).

Weiner, H.; Thaler-Singer, M.; Reiser, M.F., and Mirsky, I.A.: Etiology of duodenal ulcer. Relation of specific psychological characteristics to rate of gastric secretion (serum pepsinogen). Psychosom. Med. *19:* 1–10 (1957).

Weiner, H.; Singer, M.T., and Reiser, M.F.: Cardiovascular responses and their psychological correlates. A study in healthy young adults and patients with peptic ulcer and hypertension. Psychosom. Med. *24:* 477–498 (1962).

Margaret Singer, Ph.D., 17 El Camino Real, *Berkeley, CA 94705* (USA)

Proc. 11th Eur. Conf. Psychosom. Res., Heidelberg 1976
Psychother. Psychosom. *28:* 28–35 (1977)

Suitability for Psychotherapy

II. **Unsuitability and Psychosomatic Disease**

Harley C. Shands

Many years ago, I defined 'unsuitability for psychotherapy' in operational terms in five criteria the first of which is an *inability to describe feeling* (*Shands,* 1958). In the same period I was able to demonstrate that a group of patients with rheumatoid arthritis were highly unsuitable, while a group of anxious college students were highly suitable (*Shands,* 1976a). The inability to describe feelings in psychosomatic patients was noted previously by both *Ruesch* (1948) and *MacLean* (1949); subsequently the phenomenon has been described in Greek (*Sifneos,* 1973), French (*Marty and de M'Uzan,* 1963) and German in the three titles of this symposium.

What does this inability mean? First, let me suggest we can understand the problem in freudian language as that of an 'unconscious' status of feeling. Second, I would like to demonstrate that the relation between *meaningful behavior* and *described feeling* (between 'unconscious' and 'conscious' status) is appropriately described in piagetian language as the difference between *concrete operations* and *formal operations* (*Piaget,* 1950). Then, I want to point out that the problem is clarified by reference to skinnerian behaviorist language (*Skinner,* 1963): in this context, 'feelings' exist in some unknowable 'private' context until and unless they are externalized, as for instance through scientific investigation (cf. Cannon's 'wisdom of the body') or through verbal formulation.

It is of great importance here to note that the term 'introspection' cannot have any meaning until and unless we recognize that the visual metaphor *conceals* the essential mediation of verbal description. Undescribed feelings (as for instance in 'dumb' though skillful animals) are often involved in problem-solving; Einstein once said of his own problem-solving efforts that they did not use words at all. However, he said, when he wanted to communicate the results to anyone else, he had to convert his thinking into words. So, similarly, one can only 'know' feelings consciously by converting them into description: the bizarre limitation is that unless one can do so, he cannot know *his own feelings*. That is, to have feelings in the 'introspective' sense requires *having been able* to 'externalize' these feelings in verbal patterns.

Ortega comments upon the modern psychologist who approaches ideas not as something to *think with* but as entities to be made into *objects of thought*. Thus, ideas change their status from instrument to object. Animals unconsciously 'feel' their way through many intricate behaviors – but neither we nor they can 'know' how they feel. Some human beings, on the other hand, can and do convert their 'inner' feelings into 'objects': professionally, artists are said to 'exhibit' feeling in artifacts. Some people are able to describe their feelings to others, particularly in intimate relations, and all of us have the impression that this ability is an important aspect of the general level of social integration reached. The task of 'insight' psychotherapy is that of helping 'patients' learn themselves through knowing their own feelings – but this function is generally impossible for the 'unsuitable' patient to learn (*Shands*, 1976a) because he has not learned externalization in verbalization.

In focussing upon one's feelings, it develops that one has feelings about those same feelings: one tends to be 'ashamed' or 'proud' of 'the way I feel' as well as about 'what I do'. In Piaget's language, becoming able to reflect upon one's feelings is the addition (to 'concrete operations') of a formal operational approach. Piaget speaks of formal operations as 'operations upon operations'.

If we 'turn round upon these schemata' again, we find that using this criterion allows us to differentiate two populations. Recently, *Crown et al.* (1975) reached this same conclusion from a quite different point of view. They used an index of 'neuroticism' derived from an objective test they had devised, and compared values obtained with levels of 'rheumatoid factor' in patients with rheumatoid disease. They found an inverse correlation and suggested that the psychoneurotic population and that with rheumatoid disease are quite separate; they suggest that the problem requires epidemiological investigation. Most interestingly, in their view, rheumatoid disease patients are *not* different from the general population, thus challenging the approach that assumes that there are similar conflicts in the psychoneurotic and psychosomatic groups.

This finding is of particular interest to me because when we have in the past worked out from criteria supplied by official psychoanalytic sources the sample of the population from which suitable (or 'analyzable') patients are drawn, it turns out to be *less than 2%* – about the same proportion of the population qualified to enter graduate school. The 'suitable' group clearly constitutes an elite – as otherwise indicated by the enthusiasm with which highly educated physicians and psychologists embrace personal analysis (*Shands*, 1976b).

Demographic analysis demonstrates easily that psychoanalysis and its psychotherapeutic 'relatives' appear in that time and in those countries in which the concept of 'development' is applicable. Self-investigation is a part of 'becoming modern' (*Inkeles and Smith*, 1974). Introspective self-evaluation has the goal of developing what can be called a 'theory of the self', in a way unknown as recently as two centuries ago. In a paper recently published (*Shands*, 1976c), I have explored the earliest descriptions of a 'modern' self in a state of 'secondary' or 'signal' anxiety (*Freud*, 1936) I could find; these were written by Søren Kierkegaard and Emily Dickinson in essentially modern terms in the middle of the 19th century.

When we return to the problem of the psychosomatic patient, we find that the crucial problem is that of an inability to 'know' one's inner 'world', In terms consonant with the above, the psychosomatic patient presents significant behavior of which he is quite *unconscious. Nemiah and Sifneos* (1970) note that it is not at all unusual in interviewing psychosomatic patients to observe weeping – an overt manifestation, one would think, of 'feeling'. One such patient, asked about her feeling when she wept in discussing her husband's last illness, replied, 'I felt I should have been able to keep him at home', subtly changing the whole connotation of the word.

A highly intelligent man, still relatively young, had had asthma as a child and later had a bout of persistent diarrhea that occurred during a long automobile trip in which he was forced into an intimate close association with his parents and brother. At this time he had been shown to have two small colonic ulcers. Divorced for 3 years when seen, he had had no sexual relations with anyone for that period although he was handsome, under 40, well-educated, and solvent. He showed a remarkable capacity for observing himself from outside, but he had no idea whatever that 'feelings' have visceral ('physical') correlates. He developed pain in the chest and thought he had heart trouble, although at the same time he described himself – from outside – as healthy: 'I'm in pretty good health. I'm not overweight, I don't smoke, I don't take drugs or drink too much or anything like that. I get a reasonable amount of exercise.' Characteristically and conspicuously, there was no mention of feeling good or feeling bad.

He had consulted an internist about the chest pain. The internist had examined and reassured him, but he communicated the message reported by the patient as, 'Evidently, *I looked very depressed,* and he had me come back a number of times'. When he was asked if he could attach any inner feelings to this state, he said, 'Just very lonely... I sort of say over and over to myself that I'm really depressed, that I wish I were dead, and it's true I don't get much fun out of life – but I'm not at all suicidal. It has nothing to do with that, in fact, it's sort of an escape valve.' The examiner pointed out to him that he was smiling as he said this, and he said, smiling, 'I smile too much... It's probably a way of dealing with other people... I think I was told that *if you smile other people will like you.*'

A little further along in the interview, this patient made a precise differentiation between being voluble (or 'circumstantial') (*Shands,* 1958) and being expressive: he said, of an instance in which there was a mixup in appointments with his psychoanalyst, 'I talked elaborately about what I felt and also asked him about what had really happened, and I never got any response.' When asked about 'inner feeling', in stomach, chest, limbs, head, etc., the patient answered, 'I don't think it *upset me physically...* I just feel upset... *I must have felt* hurt and angry and also at the time I was afraid I was going crazy... I was always very good about going to my appointments, and I would just go in and talk, *constantly and sort of unstoppably,* but very superficially. It wasn't that I was holding anything back, it was just *nothing was coming out except trivia...* And I really couldn't even stop talking... I talked the way a deaf person does when he doesn't want you to say anything because he'll be reminded of his deafness.'

This patient was particularly interesting because he was a good observer of himself from the outside, while showing no capacity for the kind of *introspection* the psychoanalyst-psycho-therapist expects. The instruction, 'Say what comes to mind' was literally, even compulsively, followed by this patient – but it did not lead to any benefit or to any 'insight' into the relation between overt behavior, relations to other human beings, and visceral awareness.

The extraordinary hypothesis appears that patients of this sort can be said to have no *private life* or *private world* in the sense that suitable patients appear to be continuously and acutely aware of such an inner world. A phobic patient, on the other hand, easily reports pounding of the heart, 'all gone' feelings in the stomach, dryness of the mouth, rubberiness of the knees and blurring of vision when acutely anxious. Help is available in this respect from an unexpected source, the behaviorist *Skinner* (1963).

Skinner points out that Freud demonstrated that 'mental activity did not, at least, *require* consciousness. His proofs that thinking had occurred without introspective recognition... were *operational analyses* of mental life' (italics added). He goes on to discuss the problem of 'seeing' one's own 'mental life', commenting, 'It is a difficult question, partly because it raises the question of what 'seeing' means and partly because the events seen are private. The fact of privacy cannot, of course, be questioned. Each person is... uniquely subject to certain kinds of proprioceptive and interoceptive stimulation.' Thus, *Skinner* precisely focusses on the problem of how to 'see' or to 'know' events such as those inner emotional states 'invisible to' the outside observer. In the material quoted above the patient lacks awareness of the private, 'inner' or proprioceptive-interoceptive correlates of either *exhibited* or *imagined* meaningful interpersonal behavior (such as the inner component of the aggressive act of throwing a pillow at the therapist).

Skinner proceeds to discuss the difficulty in developing self-descriptive behavior, noting the paradox that to 'know' the private, inner world is far more difficult than to know the public, outer world. The word 'conscious' (from roots meaning 'with' and 'know') implies a *communality* of experience: when something 'becomes conscious' the implication is that knowing is shared – in the psychotherapeutic enterprise therapist and patient 'know together' through the shared interpretation of shared material. *Skinner* writes, 'Instead of concluding that man can know only his subjective experiences – that he is bound forever to his private world and that the external world is only a construct – a behavioral theory of knowledge suggests that it is the private world which, if not entirely unknowable, is at least not likely to be known well. The relations between organism and environment involved in knowing are of such a sort that the privacy of the world within the skin imposes more serious limitations on personal knowledge than on scientific accessibility.' In other words it is easier for, say, *Cannon* (1932) to 'know' a person's (or animal's) emotional state through scientific investigation than it is for that person (or animal) to 'know himself'.

In this formulation, psychosomatic patients fall into the class of those who do not know their feelings, even though it is common for others to be able to 'read' them; one young man with rheumatoid arthritis said, 'On occasion, people (will) say... "Why do you look angry?" or "Why do you look so glum?" – and I don't feel this on my face. It's kind of unconscious. When people will say that it's disturbing to me because... I'm not the type of person who likes to be read that easily.' He described himself before the arthritis as a 'merciless' football player, saying 'People twice my weight wouldn't want to come up against me because they knew I worked at it'; the implication is that he took so 'objective' a view of others that he frightened them.

To this man, his body was a kind of machine that was to be trained relentlessly; at 15, he was 'squatting', lifting over 200 pounds, his own body weight at the time. He felt 'trapped' or addicted; he knew that he 'looked like a chunk'. He 'couldn't stop', but when he developed arthritis and had to give up this compulsive weight-lifting he felt that 'there was no *me*' anymore. He said he had always been aware of 'being alone', and that he was 'very unhappy' in growing up. His only recourse was 'to be the best', and 'that's why it hurt so much when I lost it'.

The poignant realization evident in highly intelligent psychosomatic patients is that 'something is missing' – but it is quite impossible for the patient to define for himself what the trouble is. Formulating the problem in terms that the patient has no private life appears to be useful; the immediately subsequent question that emerges is, 'How then is it possible for such a person to *learn* himself from the inside out?' Is it possible to *learn feeling* as an adult? Using this approach in psychotherapy with 'suitable' patients for many years has often resulted in a very positive statement from the patient who says that he has been able to 'realize' his feelings and to 'describe' them much more successfully. The therapeutic problem is then that of whether it is possible for an (unsuitable) adult to learn what he had never known. The problem may be similar to that of 'talent' as in music: it is possible to learn how to play, but without talent, the playing remains 'mechanical' and 'unfeeling'.

From a somewhat different point of view, it is probable that many psychosomatic patients can be expected to benefit greatly from a situational context in which their difficulties with socialization are understood and attempts made by therapeutically oriented persons to supply from outside the 'other' that they have not been able to internalize. In working with the rheumatologist who referred a number of these patients, it was easy to get the impression that his success is attributable to an extraordinarily well-developed but largely unconscious set of techniques for making contact and continuing support – but never explicitly so. A powerful impression affirmed is that it may be absolutely necessary for the physician-therapist to prescribe the medications used, to take the major responsibility, and to make the relevant decisions. In other words, the physician treating the psychosomatic patient has to be a 'real doctor' at the same time that he understands, probably better intuitively than consciously, the supportive-regulative function of the physician as a 'real' human relative. But, again, this is a matter of stating the obvious.

Modern physiology uses as its central notion that of *self-regulation*. Self-regulation evolves through the internalization of 'the environment' particularly in the form of anticipated reciprocal behavior between the two parties involved. Social systems evolve through regulation of the group through the activity of each other. Ultimately with the advent of the modern period, we find again that the same principle, that of self-regulation, emerges. In pre-literate societies, *Carothers* (1959) points out that: 'Behavior is minutely governed from childhood on in a host of particular, concrete situations by meticulous rules and taboos, and not on the basis of a few broad principles which require personal decision for their application.' The 'other-regulated' human being (like the young child) has much less information-processing work to do; he has relatively few decisions to make. Much suggests that it is this situation that is somehow crucial in the psychosomatic situation. The patient suffering a loss in his human 'environment' does not know how important that loss is because he cannot feel it in a meaningful way (*Shands*, 1954). He is therefore deprived of essential information, and his whole feedback system is deranged; since he 'does not know' what he has lost, he cannot replace it. He cannot grieve – and without grieving the loss remains 'unhealed' and without compensation (*Lindemann*, 1949), so that he can be considered to remain in a chronic disintegrative state that tends to induce spreading physiological effects.

References

Cannon, W.B.: The wisdom of the body (Norton, New York 1932).
Carothers, J.C.: 'Culture, psychiatry, and the written word'. Psychiatry *22:* 307–320 (1959).
Crown, S.; Crown, J.M., and Fleming, A.: Aspects of the psychology and epidemiology of rheumatoid disease. Psychol. Med. *5:* 291–299 (1975).
Freud, S.: The problem of anxiety (Norton, New York 1936).
Inkeles, A. and Smith, D.H.: Becoming modern (Harvard Univ. Press, Cambridge 1974).
Lindemann, E.: Modifications in the course of ulcerative colitis in relationship to changes in life situations and reaction patterns. ARNMD *29:* 706–723 (1949).
MacLean, P.D.: Psychosomatic disease and the visceral brain. Psychosom. Med. *11:* 338 (1949).
Marty, P. et M'Uzan, M. de: La pensée opératoire. Revue fr. Psychoanal. *27:* 345–356 (1963).
Nemiah, J.C. and Sifneos, P.E.: Psychosomatic illness. A problem in communication. Psychother. Psychosom. *18:* 154–160 (1970).

Ortega y Gasset, J.: The dehumanization of art (Doubleday, Garden City 1956).

Piaget, J.: The psychology of intelligence (Harcourt, New York 1950).

Ruesch, J.: The infantile personality. The case problem of psychosomatic medicine. Psychosom. Med. *10:* 134 (1948).

Shands, H.C.: Problems of separation in the etiology of psychosomatic disease. Bull. Muscogee County med. Soc. *1:* 9–19 (1954).

Shands, H.C.: An approach to the measurement of suitability for psychotherapy. Psychiat. Q. *32:* 500 (1958).

Shands, H.C.: How are 'psychosomatic' patients different from 'psychoneurotic' patients? Psychother. Psychosom. *26:* 270–285 (1975).

Shands, H.C.: Suitability for psychotherapy. I. Transference and formal operations. Paper prepared for 10th Int. Congr. on Psychother., Paris 1976b.

Shands, H.C.: Malinowski's mirror. Contemp. Psychoanal. *12:* 300–334 (1976c).

Sifneos, P.E.: The prevalence of 'alexithymic' characteristics in psychosomatic patients. 9th Eur. Conf. Psychosom. Res., Vienna 1972. Psychother. Psychosom. *22:* 255–262 (1973).

Skinner, B.F.: Behaviorism at fifty. Science *140:* 951–958 (1963).

Harley C. Shands, MD, Department of Psychiatry, The Roosevelt Hospital, 428 West 59th Street, *New York, NY 10019* (USA)

Proc. 11th Eur. Conf. Psychosom. Res., Heidelberg 1976
Psychother. Psychosom. *28:* 36–46 (1977)

The Observer, the Psychosomatic Phenomenon and the Setting of the Observation

P.-B. Schneider

Policlinique Psychiatrique Universitaire (Directeur: Prof. *P.-B. Schneider*), Lausanne

Professor *Bräutigam,* the President of our conference, has been so kind as to ask me to deliver a brief introductory report to today's session, which is devoted to the observation of the psychosomatic phenomenon, and more specifically to the 'pensée opératoire' and the alexithymic phenomenon. Thus, my introduction will be almost entirely descriptive or more precisely phenomenological. Nevertheless, within the framework of this description, I shall have to allude to the theories of certain authors, since the ideological standpoint of the observer may possibly modify his attitude towards observation.

Although it seems evident that the act of observing is accomplished globally, and that it involves, at the same time, the observer, the observed phenomenon, and the setting in which the observation is made, it seems preferable to me for the sake of clarity to dissociate these three elements and to treat them separately.

The Psychosomatic Phenomenon

In its wider meaning, the psychosomatic phenomenon must be seen as the simultaneous existence of a symptom, a disturbance, or a lesion within the body and a particular structure of the psychical life, whether it be static or dynamic, conflictual or not. This structure is either at an instinctive or pulsional level, or at the level of the affects or the mental life, in the restricted sense of the term.

The 'pensée opératoire' was described in 1963 by the French psychoanalysts *Marty, de M'Uzan* and *David,* but its elaboration had already been prepared by the many works of *Marty* and *Faïn* from 1950 onwards. This 'pensée opératoire' is one of the constituents of the psychosomatic structure described in '*L'investigation psychosomatique*'. Within this structure we also find the so-called blank transfer relationship, which hinders the creation of the 'romance' that is characteristic of the neurotic or genital transfer relationship. Other characteristics of this structure are the absence of a neurotic or psychotic organisation, a break with the unconscious, the negation of one's own originality and that of others. The authors find that the 'pensée opératoire' is found above all in psychosomatic patients, but it can also be found in certain character neuroses. The activity fantasizing is greatly reduced or might even be absent. The way of thinking sticks closely to 'materially present' facts and 'the usefulness of objects'; it is engulfed in actuality. This type of thought is quite literal and uses only words, not symbols. Daydreaming is absent and dreams are either absent or operative. This absence of freedom to fantasize, the paucity of both daydreaming and dreams, lead to diminished interpersonal exchanges and a drying up and sclerosis of verbal expression.

In *Marty*'s most recent works and especially in his book *Les mouvements individuels de vie et de mort – Essai d'économie psychosomatique* of which the first volume has just been published, he returns to the subject of the 'pensée opératoire (*Marty,* 1976). We shall see a little later on the setting in which he introduces the notion of 'vie opératoire'. However, he does not describe the various forms it can take on.

Without knowing the work of the French authors, *Sifneos,* then *Nemiah* describe a mental process which is very close to the 'pensée opératoire' even if it is a little different. *Sifneos* created the term of 'alexithymia' to describe it.

On the basis of their clinical observations, these authors point out a significant disorder among psychosomatic patients that concerns their expression of affects, feelings and emotions. This phenomenon may be observed in many, but not all, psychosomatic patients. It is characterized by the patients' inability, or partial inability, to describe their feelings and affects. We may wonder if they have feelings at all, or if they are not like the colour blind in that they are blind to certain feelings or to all feelings. In this respect the subjects have a limited vocabulary. They cannot describe their affects with subtle nuances and can no longer localize their feelings in specific regions of the body. Furthermore, they show a paucity of fantasies which reflect and express the quality of their inner drives or desires. Thus we see that this last characteristic brings them closer to the patient with a 'pensée opératoire'.

Whereas the French authors have been primarily interested in fantasms and the Americans in feelings and affects, their observations are very similar and seem to relate to a phenomenon which we can now consider globally.

This phenomenon concerns that mental activity which is expressed through language. This is to be strongly underlined, since it is through language alone that it may be apprehended. Thus, a linguistic problem comes to the fore. We will come back on this point later on, and it is fortunate that reports and a round table will deal with this subject during our conference. *Marty,* in his latest book has taken a strictly evolutionist point of view. For him, the evolution of man starts with inanimate matter which is already structured and culminates in the superior mental functions, in particular in its fantasmic function. The 'vie opératoire' and the 'pensée opératoire' belong to the counter evolutionary movements, a view point which I shall not develop any further. For our friends from Boston, it is also by analysing what the patients express through their language that alexithymia appears, as the etymology of the word clearly indicates.

But I have shown previously that besides its mental or psychic aspect, expressed in this case through language, the psychosomatic phenomenon is inscribed in the body. Those who study the psychosomatic phenomenon are far from agreement and the difference of opinion extend to the 'pensée opératoire' and alexithymia. In reading *Sifneos* and *Nemiah,* we see that they describe this particular aspect of the affective life as it is expressed through the language, of those persons who have what I would call 'classic' psychosomatic illnesses. On the other hand, *Marty*'s present opinion is very different. The clinical examples given at the beginning of his book define his concept of what constitutes the psychosomatic. His patients present all the illnesses that a man can have during his lifetime. It's not by chance alone that a physician practising somatic medicine in a Paris hospital, should count, among his cases, patients with myeloid leukaemia, pulmonary embolism and meningial illness involvement and that these illnesses are often fatal. Whereas, in 1963 the Parisian school limited the 'pensée opératoire' to classic psychosomatic illnesses and even excluded asthmy, *Marty*'s conceptions have evolved and if I have understood him correctly, the 'pensée opératoire', like the 'vie opératoire', can occur in any person, but more specifically in a character neurosis and behavioural neurosis. This occurs when they show what he calls an essential deterioration, culminating in an 'essential depression'. The depression is a counter evolutionary movement which is related to the death instincts. In 1972, *Marty* states this explicitly: 'The pensée opératoire, as a result of a life-long "vie opératoire", can affect those persons whom we currently class among character and behavioural neurotics and who seem to constitute the majority of the population at present in this part of the world' (*Marty,* 1970). It seems that we are far from the psychosomatic phenomenon as I described it at the beginning of my presentation, and that, basically, we are speaking not merely of the psychological mechanisms of man, but of his bio-psychology, and in a very general way at that.

We lose sight of the specific nature of the 'pensée opératoire', as a sign of a particular structure in the individual, in a more global aspect of the way in which man works. To conclude these few remarks on the psychosomatic phenomenon, we can see that the two groups of authors who have drawn our attention to the particular mental processes of certain subjects, do basically agree on the purely phenomenological description of this process. But, because of their different conceptions as to what the psychosomatic is, they disagree as to which group of subjects actually show signs of 'pensée opératoire' or alexithymia.

The Observer

Let us rapidly review certain authors who have studied or mentioned this particular type of mental process. This review will have to be incomplete since I have not investigated all the literature on the subject. But first, I should like to point out that the 'pensée opératoire' or alexithymia have not yet been recognized in psychosomatic research and very many authors do not mention them. By implication, they infer that the fantasmic life and the expression of affects through language do not show any particularities in psychosomatic patients, and thus deny the existence of this mode of thought. However, it would be surprising if these authors had not come across the same difficulties as the Bostonians and the Parisians when they tackled the psychosomatic patient.

To give honour where it is due, I should add that from experiments carried out during in-patient group therapy of psychosomatic and neurotic patients, *Bräutigam* (1972) has concluded that, compared with neurotics, psychosomatic patients seem to have less imagination and express their feelings and imaginings less well. The verbal messages have a superficial and vacuous character and the words offer little release, if any. *Bräutigam* points out the necessity of making a psycholinguistical study of these patients, and this seems to have been done. Furthermore, *Ruesch* (1948) and *MacLean* (1949) should be mentioned among the precursors of the 'pensée opératoire'. They were the first to allude to the difficulties encoutered by the psychosomatic patient in the expression of his feelings and affects, and in verbalizing his emotions in a symbolic system close to fantasm. Their findings passed practically unnoticed at the time and are not used by *Marty* and the Parisian school, who do not seem to know of their existence.

Several French authors occasionally mention the 'pensée opératoire' in one or another of their patients. The most recent is *Bergeret* (1976) who, a few months ago, presented a report entitled '*Dépressivité et dépression dans le cadre de l'économie défensive*', at the Congress of Romance language psychoanalysts in Geneva. He remarked that the 'pensée opératoire' could be a defense mechanism against essential depression, thus including a vast category of patients situated between neurosis and psychosis. In that case, the 'pensée opératoire' would constitute an efficient protective system against this deep-seated depression in patients whose regressions may go back a very long way. It is noteworthy that *Bergeret* (1976) alludes to widespread psychodynamic mechanisms and that the group of essential depressions that he describes is very large.

Assal and Zander (1975) from Lausanne, a psychiatrist and neuropsychologist, and a neurosurgeon, respectively, have studied behavioural disturbances following cerebral contusions. They found that during the recovery period, these patients presented a condition in which 'there was no longer any room in their lives for daydreaming and reflections with all the pleasant and distressing aspects they imply'. These patients' dream lives had practically disappeared. For the authors, this recovery period is reminiscent of the personality organization of a psychopath. It can either be temporary or become definitive and take on a psychopathic structure. It seems plausible to them that this diminished fantasmic life is one of the after-effects of the cerebral contusion. Here we have the description of a mental phenomenon, closely similar to the 'pensée opératoire'.

Finally, the observations of my collaborators and myself show that the 'pensée opératoire' can undoubtedly be observed in psychosomatic patients examined in certain circumstances which I shall describe in a moment. But it also exists in other patients, for example in psychopaths or in patients who are in a particular situation like a psychiatric examination, or finally in neurotics. Such was the case of a patient undergoing analysis: the 'pensée opératoire' seemed to predominate even though he had not suffered from a psychosomatic illness either in the present or in the past. After more than a year of psychoanalysis, fantasmic thoughts with a dream life began to appear little by little and is still developing. This patient was previously incapable of describing the least feeling.

This harvest is not very rich but there must certainly be other authors who have published works on the subject. In any case, it shows that a mental process close to the psychosomatic 'pensée opératoire' has been observed by some authors outside the framework of psychosomatic illnesses (essential depressions, psychopaths).

The Setting of the Observation

There is one thing that is quite obvious: the setting of the observation can permit the appearance of the desired phenomenon or, on the contrary, inhibit and block its manifestation. For example, free association can only occur if a neutral and non-directive psychological framework is established. Therefore, it seems to me indispensible to try, if possible, to describe the setting in which the 'pensée opératoire' phenomenon was observed.

The Parisian authors use an examination method described in 'L'investigation psychosomatique'. It is derived from Deutsch's technique of associative case history, and is still used by Marty in the example he gives in his latest book. Without any prior preparation, the psychoanalyst places the patient, who has been referred to him by a doctor of physical medicine, in front of a group of collaborators; they observe him in a situation of neutrality which it seems must be felt by the patient as hostile. The psychoanalyst conducting the interview tries to maintain an atmosphere of neutrality which, according to the Parisian authors, will favour the appearance of fantasms. For nearly 20 years, we have used an examination method which is very close to Marty's; but we use it for a different purpose, that of studying the suitability for psychotherapy. In such a situation the patient rarely calls up fantasies. From our experience, it seems to us that such a setting diminishes if not suppresses the imaginative life of the patient. On the other hand, it favours the appearance of defense mechanisms and emphasizes the working of the ego, in particular its autonomous functions. Nevertheless, in our examination situation, the patients' motives are very different from those of the patients examined by the Parisian authors. Their patients are suddenly placed in a situation in which they have to express their affective and fantasmic life at a time when their attention is mainly pre-occupied by their physical ailments, so that any notion of a psychological approach to their problems is far from their minds. Nemiah and Sifneos, inasmuch as they describe their methodology in detail, studied, on the one hand, the recordings of patients who showed at least two psychosomatic illnesses. These patients had not been examined for alexithymia, since it had not yet been described. *Nemiah* stated that the interview should facilitate the appearance of free association. On the other hand, *Sifneos* used a questionnaire to diagnose alexithymia. This questionnaire was filled out by the doctors who had examined psychosomatic and neurotic patients. Moreover, *Sifneos* used his clinical experience within the framework of his customary examinations. It was from a comparison of the patients hospitalized in a psychosomatic clinic and treated by psychotherapy that *Bräutigam* (1972) deduced that there was a difference, which we have described, between the groups of neurotic and psychosomatic patients. We may wonder if the deficiency or lack of fantasmic phenomena in psychosomatic patients is not related to the defense mechanisms, above all isolation and denial, which are so often seen in psychosomatic patients. It is true that *Nemiah* criticized this notion of denial.

Bergeret (1976) does not give the methodology he used to examine his patients. From an overall reading of his abundant work, one gains the impression that his patients were undergoing psychoanalytic treatment or analytically orientated psychotherapy.

Finally, we have other information about the 'pensée opératoire' from the study of *psychological tests*. The advantage of projective tests is that they put all the patients, neurotic, normal or psychosomatic, in the same examination setting. They have to carry out a task in which they cannot know the hidden or the real goal. Even though the basic situation is more favorable than that of a psychiatric or psychoanalytic investigation, the problem of motivation has to be mentioned. This motivation can vary and depends upon whether the patient desires to follow a psychological treatment (neurotic patient) or, on the contrary, is pre-occupied by his physical ailments and is looking for a magical solution, by medication, for example.

Using different projective or questionnaire tests, *Rausch de Traubenberg* examined a group of patients who were suffering from arterial hypertension and compared them with a group of ulcer patients. The results seem to confirm a certain reduction in their fantasmic life. A work by *Bonami and Rime* alludes to the 'pensée opératoire' in speaking of an approach to the pre-coronarian personality.

In my out-patient clinic, we have examined 18 ulcer patients by means of the MMPI test, the TAT and the Rorschach test. As a preliminary, we determined the intellectual level with the aid of Raven's Progressive Matrix. In those patients with a lower or mediocre intellectual levels, we obtained very poor Rorschach and TAT responses, which indicates great difficulty in expressing fantasms. It really seems that the intellectual level plays a role in the possibility of fantasmic expression through language. In the subjects with average and good intelligence, we are struck by the weakness of production in the Rorschach and the lack of originality in the contents. This difference is even more evident in the TAT. The subjects seem to try to camouflage this insufficiency in their imaginative capacities by resorting to criticism. On the whole, the wish to stick to reality and even the fear of moving away from the concrete are dominant features. We judged that this research should be pursued, but we have not yet had the possibility of doing so.

Finally *Melon* (1975) published the results of an examination of psychosomatic patients by the Rorschach test and the Szondi test. The results confirm the existence of a weakness in the fantasmic life or its non-existence. He also mentioned that the results resemble those found in psychopaths who are incapable of maintaining a conflictual relationship. The Szondi test showed the same results. The profile is similar to that of asocial psychopaths, the chronically depressed and the 'normal' with a character neurosis. According to this author, the psychosomatic and the psychopathic structures are related.

Discussion

Having completed this partial review of the works dealing with that phenomenon of the mental life known as 'alexithymia' or the 'pensée opératoire', we can now make a number of remarks:

(I) At present, we have sufficient evidence to affirm that there is a process in mental life which is characterized by the reduction, the inhibition, and the blocking of expression through language of the imaginative life, the fantasmic life, daydreams and dreams. The expression of feelings by language is also reduced, inhibited or blocked (pensée opératoire; alexithymia).

(II) The observations of the first authors who have dealt with this mental phonomenon were made on psychosomatic patients. Later on, other investigators observed the phenomenon in patients suffering from phases of essential depression or psychopathic structures, as well as in patients under examination conditions that reduce their possibilities of expressing the world of the imagination. *Marty* then extended the notion of operative modes of life and thought *(la vie et la pensée opératoires)* to man in general. In this case, operative life *(la vie opératoire)* would be a sign of mental as well as biological deterioration, portending death.

(III) The mental phenomena, 'alexithymia' and 'pensée opératoire' reveal themselves through language. A psycholinguistic study should be carried out and it may be hoped that we will have the first results today. In a previous article I alluded to the conceptions of *Piaget* and his description of the development of intelligence. What is the relationship between the 'pensée opératoire' and the operative stage of thinking in children? This is only the first question that we cannot yet answer. A second question which concerns language is the following:

In the majority of human societies, as in ours, several linguistic systems exist. The metaphoric and symbolic language is that of poetry, of fantasy and of daydreams; another language is utilitarian, or as we should say, 'operative'. For example, among the Mongols, important persons and old men use a language containing metaphors and symbols, rich in fantasy, which enables them to communicate with the spirits, whereas another inferior language is used when selling or caring for cattle. This is the language of children and women. Similar differences in language can be found in other civilizations: the language of priests who are in contact with deities; the language of the ruling class who wield power; the language of the people. The Japanese have one language for men and one for women.

The process of symbolization is linked to the fantasmic life and to poetic productions. It can readily be observed in neurotic patients and even more so in psychotics when they are positively motivated, for example, when they desire psychotherapeutic treatment. But what about the 'ordinary' man? What do we know of his language appartenance, or of his fantasmic possibilities, in particular when he finds himself in a stressing situation such as being examined by a doctor or, worse, by a psychiatrist? It seems that this phenomenon should be studied more thoroughly since fantasizing seems to depend on the socio-cultural level.

In their theoretical approach (which I shall not go into in detail), *Sifneos* and *Nemiah* lean on the theories of *MacLean* concerning the limbic system. They advance the hypothesis that there exists an agenesis or dysgenesis of this system which hinders the communication by language of affects to the neo-cortex. Shouldn't this dysgenesis (or agenesis) of the limbic system cause much deeper modifications of linguistic expression than that which is seen in psychosomatic patients? Rather than a total lack of symbolic thinking, here we have come up against something that inhibits the use of a certain language code, and more specifically the code which opens up the way to fantasms.

By studying audio-visual recordings, we have noticed that in his relationships with others, a man rarely uses the register of fantasmic thought. When he consults a physician, he remains on the operative level of thinking. Seen from another point of view, he very rarely uses an intimate relation with the doctor, prefering relationship on the level of a repair service which blocks the imaginary life.

(IV) We have already put forward the hypothesis that the 'pensée opéra-toire' facilitates the adaptation to the purely objective reality of everyday life. From this point of view, it may be seen as a useful, autonomous function of the ego that, if it is well developed, enables very practical activities to be carried out.

(V) The setting in which the examinations are performed, especially the psychosomatic investigation described by the Parisian authors, forces the psychosomatic into a psychological world against which he has, above all, an unconscious need to defend himself. He seeks to maintain the somewhat precarious psychic balance, which he had established at the price of a psycho-somatic illness.

In the same situation, on the other hand, the neurotic senses a worsening of his psychological imbalance, which existed before the examination, and this may result in an increase of fantasmic life.

(VI) We should seek to ascertain the opinion and experience of all the psychosomaticians who do not speak of the 'vie opératoire' and the 'pensée opératoire' and who see the psychosomatic patient merely as a neurotic whose fantasmic life allows his unconscious intra-psychic conflicts, which can only be fantasized, to be approached. Psychosomatic illnesses are not rare and the number of patients even greater.

(VII) The 'pensée opératoire' has also been observed by certain authors outside the field of psychosomatic medicine: in essential depressions, as a symptom of the degradation of the mental life, in psychopaths and so on. These observations indicate that the field of research should be widened.

Conclusions

We must be grateful to the Parisian authors and to *Nemiah* and *Sifneos* who have tenaciously studied mental processes and especially the expression of feelings and the fantasmic life in so-called psychosomatic patients. A new phenomenon in mental life has appeared and, however, widespread it may be, however normal or pathological it may be in character, neurophysiological in origin, or related to a deterioration of life in general, or even a defensive phenomenon found only in certain classes of patients or in all subjects, we have a veritable mine to explore.

References

Assal, G. et *Zander, E.:* Esquisse d'une histoire naturelle des troubles comportementaux à la suite de contusions cérébrales. Méd. Hygiène *33:* 1183–1186 (1975).

Bergeret, J.: Dépressivité et dépression dans le cadre de l'économie défensive. 36e Congr. psychanalystes de langues romanes (PUF, Paris 1976).

Bräutigam, W.: Psychothérapie de groupe dans un milieu hospitalier de malades psychosomatiques et névrosés. Problèmes de formation et de recherche. Psychol. méd. *4:* 230–231 (1972).

MacLean, P.D.: Psychosomatic disease and the 'visceral brain'. Recent developments bearing on the Papez theory of Emotion. Psychosom. Med. *11:* 338–353 (1949).

MacLean, P.D.: The triune brain. Emotion and scientific bias; in *Schmitt* The neurosciences. Second study program, pp. 336–344 (Rockefeller Univ. Press, New York 1970).

Marty, P.: La dépression essentielle. Revue fr. Psychanal. *32:* 595–598 (1968).

Marty, P.: Intervention. Points de vue psychanalytiques sur l'inhibition intellectuelle. Revue fr. Psychanal. *36:* 805–816 (1972).

Marty, P.: Les mouvements individuels de vie et de mort (Payot, Paris 1976).

Melon, J.: Réflexions sur la structure psychosomatique et son approche à partir des tests de Rorschach et de Szondi. Feuillets psychiat., Liège *8:* 33–46 (1975).

Nemiah, J.C.: Psychology and psychosomatic illness. Reflections on theory and research methodology. 9th Eur. Conf. Psychosom. Res., Vienna 1972. Psychother. Psychosom. *22:* 106–111 (1973).

Nemiah, J.C.: Denial revisited. Reflections on psychosomatic theory. Psychother. Psychosom. *26:* 140–147 (1975).

Schneider, P.-B.: Remarques sur les rapports de la psychanalyse avec la médecine psychosomatique. Revue fr. Psychanal. *32:* 646–677 (1968).

Schneider, P.-B.: La pensée opératoire: essai d'une approche critique à partir des affections digestives psychosomatiques. Revue Méd. psychosom. Psychol. méd. *15:* 3–14 (1973).

Sifneos, P.E.: Is dynamic psychotherapy contraindicated for a large number of patients with psychosomatic diseases? Psychother. Psychosom. *21:* 133–136 (1972–1973).

Sifneos, P.E.: The prevalence of 'alexithymic' characteristics in psychosomatic patients. Psychother. Psychosom. *22:* 255–262 (1973).

Sifneos, P.E.: A reconsideration of psychodynamic mechanisms in psychosomatic symptom formation in view of recent clinical observations. Psychother. Psychosom. *24:* 151–155 (1974).

Prof. Dr. med. *P.B. Schneider,* Rue Caroline 11 bis, *1003 Lausanne* (Switzerland)

Observations

Proc. 11th Eur. Conf. Psychosom. Res., Heidelberg 1976
Psychother. Psychosom. *28:* 47–57 (1977)

The Phenomenon of 'Alexithymia'

Observations in Neurotic and Psychosomatic Patients

Peter E. Sifneos, Roberta Apfel-Savitz and Fred H. Frankel

Department of Psychiatry, Harvard Medical School, Beth Israel Hospital, Boston, Mass.

To see the term 'alexithymia', which first appeared in print in 1972, as a part of the 11th European Conference on Psychosomatic Research gives rise to an awesome feeling, because of the senior author's responsibility for its inception. Deriving from the Greek 'a' for lack, 'lexis' for word, and 'thymos' for emotion, it has been criticized both by classicists as being inappropriate and nonrepresentative, and by some psychosomaticists as being irrelevant. Since it has been found helpful, however, by the Heidelberg organizers to grace the title of their Conference, it appears, for better or worse, that it is destined to be here to stay (1). 'Alexithymia' has been used to describe certain psychological characteristics which were observed on patients who suffer from a variety of psychosomatic diseases as well as on some individuals who are not medically ill [2].

In this paper, we shall review briefly the observations, which were first made in a Psychiatric Clinic setting, at the Massachusetts General Hospital, a teaching hospital of Harvard Medical School, during the years 1954–1967, on patients with alexithymic defects. As others have done before, the purpose of this presentation is to set these observations in a proper frame of reference for the discussion of the 'psychosomatic phenomenon', as well as for comparison purposes with neurotic or healthy individuals (3).

Because the majority of the patients who came or were referred to the clinic were neurotics complaining of psychological conflicts, patients suffering from psychosomatic diseases, being in the minority, were easy to spot and given special attention in the evaluation of their difficulties. Thus, the clinical observations about them were made as carefully and as objectively as it could be expected.

Table I

Alexithymic	Neurotic
1 *Presenting complaints* a) Endless description of physical symptoms, at times not related to an underlying medical illness	a) less emphasis on physical complaints
Example: an ulcerative colitis patient complained more about aches and pains all over his body, muscle twitches and sour stomach, than about his bloody diarrhea.	b) elaborate description of psychological difficulties (symptoms and/or interpersonal problems)
2 *Other complaints* Tension, irritability, frustration, pain, boredom, void, restlessness, agitation, nervousness	a) anxiety described in terms of fantasies and thoughts rather than in physical sensations
	b) depression described in terms of feelings of worth-lessness, guilt, during sleepless nights, etc.
3 *Thought content* Striking absence of fantasies and elaborate description of trivial environmental details (pensée opératoire) *Marty et al.* (4)	rich fantasy life marked ability to describe feelings in eloquent terms
4 *Language* Marked difficulty in finding appropriate words to describe feelings	appropriate in describing feelings
5 *Crying* a) Rare b) At times they cry copiosly but crying seems not related to an appropriate feeling such as sadness or anger	a) appropriate to specific feeling
6 *Dreaming* Rare	often

Table I (continuation)

Alexithymic	Neurotic
7 *Affect*	
Inappropriate	appropriate
8 *Activity*	
Tendency to take action impulsively	appropriate to situation
Action seems to be a predominant way of life	
9 *Interpersonal relations*	
Usually poor with a tendency at marked dependency or preference for being alone, avoiding people	specific conflicts with people but generally good interpersonal relations
10 *Personality make-up*	
Narcissistic, withdrawn, passive-aggressive, or passive-dependent, psychopathic	flexible
11 *Posture*	
Rigid	flexible
12 *Countertransference*	
The interviewer or the therapist is usually bored by the patient whom they find frightfully 'dull'	easy communication with patient whom the interviewer or therapist finds 'interesting'
13 *Relation to social, educational, economic, or cultural background*	
None	considerable

Table I, brought up to date, highlights the differences between patients with neurotic and alexithymic defects.

It should be emphasized, first of all, that special interviewing techniques are necessary in order to verify the presence or absence of these alexithymic defects, as well as the descriptions of the stimulus-bound endless details of the 'pensée opératoire'. One must persist in questioning the patient who claims not to have any feelings, and not to assume simply that such feelings must exist, but that they are being denied. In the same way, as a medical student must learn to distinguish what certain histological tissues look like, and how tubercle bacilli or streptococci appear under the microscope, so must the interviewer search for the presence of alexithymic defects during the patient's psychiatric evaluation.

Since these defects point clearly to difficulties in the general sphere of the patient's affective life, for the sake of clarity, one must define what is meant when such words as 'affect', 'feeling', and 'emotion' are used in an attempt to eliminate the confusion which is likely to result when these terms are used indiscriminately.

'Affect' is therefore defined as 'a general personal private state of being which has both biological and psychological components'. The word 'emotion' should be reserved to describe the biological side of 'affect'. Expressed by behavioral means and mediated through the limbic system by way of the hypothalamus, it has a direct effect on both the 'endocrine' and the 'autonomic nervous system', thus it plays a key role in the exchange between the body and the outside world. Experimental work on dogs shows that lesions in the dorsomedial amygdala produce profound changes in these animals who become apathetic, indifferent, and uncooperative (5).

'Feeling', on the other hand, should be reserved to include the psychological side of 'affect' as well, and must contain the subjective fantasies and thoughts which are associated with it. It is obvious from these definitions that neocortical activity is a 'sine qua non' as far as feelings are concerned, while it is not necessary for emotions. It might be concluded, therefore, that feelings are primarily human phenomena. One should use caution, however, when words are used to describe feelings or emotions, because at times the terms which are being used do not necessarily relate to the neurophysiological changes which are actually taking place (6).

Alexithymic Characteristics and Psychosomatic Illness

On the basis of a questionnaire filled out by 15 different interviewers in 1972, 25 patients suffering from a variety of psychosomatic diseases outnumbered a similar number of control patients by better than 2–1 as far as possession of alexithymic characteristics (7). More recently, a new questionnaire was designed to be filled out by the patient in addition to the one to be filled out by the interviewer, in order to make more objective the attempt to pick out the alexithymic defects (appendix A). The scoring of this question-naire has presented innumerable difficulties, but we have finally agreed upon a 6-point scale: a score of 6 depicts total absence of alexithymic characteris-tics while zero depicts complete presence of such traits. Thus, for the 17

Table II

	Scores for normal controls			Scores for psychosomatic patients		
	evaluator A (blind)	evaluator B (blind)	evaluator C	evaluator A (blind)	evaluator B (blind)	evaluator C
Normal range						
90–102	2	5				
80–90	4	3	5			
70–80	3	2	4	2		
60–70	3	2	4	1	1	2
51–60	1		1	4	3	6
	13	12	14	7	4	8
Alexithymic range						
41–51		1		2	2	6
31–41	1			3	4	1
21–31				1	1	
11–21	1	1	1	2	2	
0–11					1	
	2	2¹	1	8	10	7

	Control patients			Psychosomatic patients		
	evaluator A	evaluator B	evaluator C	evaluator A	evaluator B	evaluator C
Normals	*13*	*12*	*14*	*7*	*4*	*8*
Alexithymic	*2*	*2¹*	*1*	*8*	*10*	*7*

¹ One illegible.

questions which were asked, a total of 102 points was the highest *normal* score possible, while zero the highest *alexithymic* score.

15 patients suffering from a variety of psychosomatic diseases which included such illnesses as ulcerative colitis, peptic ulcer, thyrotoxicosis, hypertension, asthma, neurodermatitis, and rheumatoid arthritis, completed the questionnaire and were compared with 15 individuals who were randomly selected out of 105 normal controls from a psychiatric hospital staff population, consisting mostly of physicians, social workers, nurses, and other professionals in an effort to see how many of these individuals should be considered alexithymic or not.

It is of interest that there was a prevalence of alexithymic traits in more than half of the patients in the psychosomatic group as far as the scoring by all three evaluators was concerned. In contrast, the numbers were much smaller in the control group. It should also be noted that one of the control patient's answers was illegible and this may account for the low score by two evaluators and no score by the third.

Discussion

Because certain important advances have been made in the field of psychosomatic medicine within the last few decades which throw some light on both the causation and treatment of psychosomatic disease, they should be kept in mind in reference to any discussions of the role played by the alexithymic defects. In the theoretical sphere, *Engel's* 'conservation-with-drawal' theory was well documented by observations on the helplessness-hopelessness 'giving up-given up' responses. As *Lindemann* had also predicted, such responses seem to play an important role in the higher morbidity and mortality rates occurring in bereaved individuals in contrast to non-bereaved ones (8). In the neuroendocrinological area, *Selye's* (9) 'alarm reaction' with its emphasis on corticosteroid hypersecretion, and *Miller's* (10) instrumental conditioning and behavioral shaping of autonomic responses seem to point to the importance played by the endocrine and autonomic nervous system in psychosomatic symptom formation. Finally, genetically or otherwise determined deficiencies, such as elevated pepsinogen levels, mechanical obstructions, presence or absence of mucous, increased thyroid or gastrin secretions, and so on, point to the importance of physiological changes which are taking place at the peripheral organs and contribute to the production of lesions. The interplay of all these factors, therefore, may be predisposing in the etiology of psychosomatic diseases and in the appearance of their symptoms. Another well-known fact has to do with the various psychological factors which influence the onset, complicate the course, and may also play a role in the etiology of psychosomatic disorders. Since specificity which, in contrast to a universal response, is viewed as a specific type of reaction has been shown to give rise to internal psychological conflicts, it is possible that it also acts as a predisposing factor for psychosomatic symptom formation.

The question which must be raised, however, has to do with the nature of these internalized psychological conflicts and the role which they play in psychosomatic disease (11). Up to now, such conflicts were considered to be due primarily to psychological constellations in which a variety of defense mechanisms and particularly repression and denial played a leading role. The emotions which were aroused as a result of these conflicts were thought to be expressed in physical terms and were viewed as contributing to the production of psychosomatic lesions and symptoms. The observations which helped to pinpoint the alexithymic characteristics force us to reassess the above-mentioned theory. In our opinion, it is the very existence of the alexithymic defects which is responsible for the appearance of the internalized conflicts. An alexithymic individual who is faced with a potentially dangerous situation, particularly in the interpersonal sphere which requires the awareness of feelings, and who is deficient in this area by virtue of his inability to have appropriate fantasies and language to cope with it, may find himself in a progressively frustrating situation. At first totally helpless to describe any inner feelings which do not exist, he tries to deal with the problem by going into the endless details of the 'pensée opératoire'. This totally inadequate reaction gives rise to further tension and he soon finds himself in a progressively helpless situation. On the verge of giving up, he is forced either to withdraw in order to conserve himself or to take impulsive action in a final effort to correct a seemingly hopeless state of being. While all these changes take place in the psychological sphere, physiological reactions to this stress mobilize the autonomic and endocrine systems. Thus, the ensuing hyperactivity of these systems in the absence of any defects in the peripheral organs will give rise to nothing more than an awareness of inner turmoil, tension and frustration. If, on the other hand, genetically or otherwise-determined physical defects *do* exist, then a specific lesion will soon develop in the peripheral organ which is involved, and psychosomatic symptoms will ensue.

One may try to represent the presence or absence of psychosomatic lesions and symptoms as follows:

Interpersonal stress: alexithymic patient (no thoughts of fantasies)

Psychological reactions
(1) Frustration. helplessness-hopelessness (giving up) conversation-withdrawal
(2) 'Pensée opératoire'
(3) Action

Biological reactions

(1) Hyperactivity of ANS and endocrine system
(a) If peripheral defect exists – psychosomatic lesion
(b) If no peripheral defect exists – no lesion tension frustration

At this point two additional aspects should be discussed briefly although they will be dealt with specifically during the Congress in much greater detail. Suffice it to say that the first one has to do with speculation about the causes of the alexithymic characteristics themselves. Let us pose some questions. Are they due to congenital defects? Are they the result of biochemical deficiencies? Do they result from developmental arrests, familial, social or cultural? And finally, are they due to psychological constellations with an excessive utilization of defense mechanisms such as denial or repression? The answers to these questions are not known at present, but from *Heiberg's* (12) work, there seems to be some preliminary evidence that genetic factors are of basic importance. On the other hand, *Hoppe* (13) has found 'quantitative as well as qualitative paucity of dreams, fantasies and symbolization' in ten patients following commissurotomy, possibly resulting from differences between the left and right hemispheres and interruption of communications between the two. From our own work, physiological factors such as oxygen and CO_2 consumption seem to play a significant role as far as these alexithymic defects are concerned. Furthermore, it appears that lack of hypnotizability is correlated with alexithymia. It is clear, then, that more research is indicated for the investigation of *all* and not of some of the above-mentioned etiological factors.

The second point has to do with the questions about the nature of the treatment which is indicated for alexithymic patients in general, and psychosomatic ones in particular. From the experience of several investigators, psychodynamic psychotherapy or psychoanalysis are contraindicated for the treatment of many patients with psychosomatic diseases (14, 15). For the alexithymic psychosomatic patients who fall into this category different treatment modalities should be developed in order to help them deal with their specific difficulties more effectively. Such modalities may include a supportive group psychotherapeutic experience which will be reported by one of us (16). Relaxation techniques which may be systematically taught to the patient, individual supportive psychotherapy in conjunction with psychotropic medication, and other forms of treatment should also be considered.

In the final analysis, however, the best treatment will be the one which will be based on the elimination of the etiological factors responsible for the alexithymic difficulties, and which will be able either to alter them or to eradicate them completely.

References

1 *Sifneos, P.E.:* Short-term psychotherapy and emotional crisis (Harvard University Press, Cambridge 1972).
2 *Sifneos, P.E.:* Clinical observations on some patients suffering from a variety of psychosomatic diseases; in *Antonelli* Proc. 7th Eur. Conf. Psychosom. Res., Rome 1967. Acta med. psychosom. *1967:* 1–10.
3 *Shands, H.:* Suitability for psychotherapy. II. 11th Eur. Conf. Psychosom. Res., Heidelberg 1976.
4 *Marty, P.; de M'Uzan, M. et David, C.:* L'investigation psychosomatique (Presses Universitaires, Paris 1963).
5 *Fonberg, E.:* Control of emotional behavior through the hypothalamus and amygdaloid complex; in *Porter and Knight* Physiol. emotion and psychosom. illness. Ciba Found. Symp., No. 8, pp. 131–150 (Elsevier/North-Holland, Amsterdam 1972).
6 *Sifneos, P.E.:* Problems of psychotherapy of patients with alexithymic characteristics and physical disease. Psychother. Psychosom. *26:* 65–70 (1975).
7 *Sifneos, P.E.:* The prevalence of 'alexithymic' characteristics in psychosomatic patients. Psychother. Psychosom. *22:* 255–263 (1973).
8 *Engel, E.L. and Schmale, A.H.:* Conservation-withdrawal; in *Porter and Knight* Physiol. Emotion and psychosom. Illness. Ciba Found. Symp., No. 8, pp. 57–86 (Elsevier/North-Holland, Amsterdam 1972).
9 *Selye, H.:* A syndrome produced by diverse nocuous agents. Nature, Lond. *138:* 32 (1936).
10 *Miller, N.:* Learning of visceral and glandular responses. Science *163:* 434–438.
11 *Alexander, F.:* Psychosomatic medicine, chapt. 13 (Norton, New York 1950).
12 *Heiberg, A.:* Personal commun.
13 *Hoppe, K.D.:* Liaison psychiatry and psychoanalysis; in *Pasnau* Liaison psychiatry, pp. 103–109 (Grune & Stratton, New York 1975).
14 *Karush, et al.:* The response to psychotherapy in chronic ulcerative colitis. Psychosom. Med. *31:* 201–227 (1969).
15 *Nemiah, J.C.:* The psychological management and treatment of patients with peptic ulcer. Adv. Psychosom. Med., vol. 6 (Karger, Basel 1970).
16 *Savitz, R.A.:* Personal commun.

Appendix A

Beth Israel Hospital
Psychiatry Department

Questionnaire

Please answer all questions

Name _____

Address _____

Age_____ Sex_____ SMWD Sep Religion_____ Occupation_____

Education: High School   College   Prof. School

Date _____

Part I:

1. When you are upset, do you like to take action or do you prefer to think or day-dream?
2. How would you feel if a policeman arrested you for a crime you did not commit?
    b) What thoughts do you have? Please give example.
3. How would you feel if someone insulted you? ...if someone made a false accusation about you?
    b) What thoughts do you have? Please give example.
4. How would you feel if you heard a suspicious noise while you were all alone in your house at night?
    b) What thoughts do you have? Please give example.
5. How would you feel if you had an emergency and tried to make a telephone call but the line was continually busy?
    b) What thoughts do you have? Please give example.
6. How would you feel if someone cut you off in heavy traffic?
    b) What thoughts do you have? Please give example.
7. How would you feel if someone laughed at you?
    b) What thoughts do you have? Please give example.
8. How would you feel if you saw a truck coming at you at 90 m.p.h.?
    b) What thoughts do you have? Please give example.
9. How would you feel if someone called you a coward?
    b) What thoughts do you have? Please give example.
10. How would you feel if someone called you a thief?
    b) What thoughts do you have? Please give example.
11. How would you feel if someone complimented you?
    b) What thoughts do you have? Please give example.
12. How would you feel if someone said that you are the best?
    b) What thoughts do you have? Please give example.

13. How would you feel if someone you loved died suddenly?
    b) What thoughts do you have? Please give example.
14. How would you feel if someone tried to attack you with a knife?
    b) What thoughts do you have? Please give example.
15. How would you feel if someone pulled a gun on you?
    b) What thoughts do you have? Please give example.
16. How do you feel when you are hungry?
    b) What thoughts do you have? Please give example.
17. How do you feel when you are sick?
    b) What thoughts do you have? Please give example.

Please write anything else you wish about this questionnaire.

Prof. *P.E. Sifneos*, Department of Psychiatry, Harvard Medical School, Beth Israel Hospital, 330 Brookline Avenue, *Boston, MA 02215* (USA)

Proc. 11th Eur. Conf. Psychosom. Res., Heidelberg 1976
Psychother. Psychosom. *28:* 58–67 (1977)

The Contribution of the Interview Situation to the Restriction of Fantasy Life and Emotional Experience in Psychosomatic Patients

Heinz H. Wolff[1]

The term 'pensée opératoire' coined by *Marty* and co-workers (*Marty and de Muzan,* 1963; *Marty et al.,* 1963) and the term alexithymia coined by *Sifneos* (1967, 1973) are used to describe a state of mind of certain patients which is characterised by a restriction of fantasy life and emotional functioning, by an inability to describe in words what they feel, and by a tendency monotonously to recount factual details concerning actions and events in their daily life without appropriate accompanying feelings. In a series of papers *Sifneos* (1967, 1973) and *Nemiah and Sifneos* (1970) studied these phenomena and the frequency with which they occur in psychosomatic patients. *Sifneos* (1973) concluded that they are found significantly more often in patients with psychosomatic disorders, a term here used by him to include ulcerative colitis, asthma, peptic ulcer, dermatitis and rheumatoid arthritis than in patients with psychoneurotic complaints although they were present in some of the latter as well. A normal control group was not studied and the findings were based largely on observations made during diagnostic interviews rather than in the course of on-going psychotherapy.

Nemiah (1973) has suggested that these alexithymic characteristics might be due to a neurological deficit rather than of psychological and developmental origin. It is of interest that *McDougall* (1974) whose observations in contrast were based on analytical psychotherapy of psychosomatic patients concluded that these characteristics were developmentally determined and

[1] Consultant Psychiatrist and Psychotherapist, The Bethlem Royal and Maudsley Hospital, and University College Hospital, London.

hence psychodynamically understandable and that patients with the characteristics described could be brought in touch with their feelings and fantasies if 'the investigator makes vigorous efforts to stimulate associative material concerning the patient's relationships, life experience and illness'.

My interest in this field is similarly derived from psychotherapeutic work. Although I have been concerned with both psychoneurotic patients and patients with structural or functional psychosomatic symptoms who had alexithymic characteristics the following observations are mainly concerned with the latter. In a previous paper (*Wolff*, 1973) I have drawn attention to the importance, when working with patients suffering from psychosomatic symptoms, of being sensitive to the links which exist between psychic functioning, i.e., feelings and fantasies, and somatic experience in order to help patients move out of the area of preoccupation with their body into the area of psychic experience. This is essential in order to achieve what *Winnicott* (1966) has called psychosomatic integration. In the same paper I discussed some of the problems which arise in the therapist-patient relationship when one is dealing with this mind-body split; I stressed that at times the therapist has to function symbolically and at others in reality as a holding mother (*Winnicott*, 1965) who is able to respond adequately to the patient's bodily and emotional needs in order to make up for what his original mother was unable to provide.

When confronted with alexithymic patients the therapist is dealing with a different though related split. Here the split is between thinking and action on the one hand and feeling and fantasy on the other. I will later discuss the nature of relationship between this thought-feeling split, as I will call it for the time being, and the mind-body split. But I will first deal with the task the therapist has in interviews with patients who have alexithymic characteristics and whose thinking is of the mechanistic, operative kind called 'pensée opératoire'. The central issue here is the therapist's countertransference and how this is handled in the interview situation.

I must emphasise here that in line with modern psychoanalytic concepts I regard the therapist's countertransference not just as a disturbing phenomenon which unless carefully controlled interferes with the therapeutic process, but on the contrary as a vital tool in psychotherapy. As *Heimann* (1950) has put it 'the analyst's unconscious understands that of his patient. This rapport on the deep level comes to the surface in the form of feelings which the analyst notices in response to his patient in his countertransference'.

Sandler has reviewed and discussed the practical significance of the countertransference in recent papers (*Sandler et al.*, 1973; *Sandler*, 1976) and has pointed out that what the analyst experiences is often a compromise between his own personal characteristics and responses in relationships and the role into which his patient is consciously or unconsciously trying to cast him during therapeutic sessions. The analyst's or therapist's task is first to remain sensitively aware of what he is experiencing, and then to differentiate between what is derived purely from his own personality and what is a response to the patient's needs; and then to use this understanding to make the patient aware of what is going on in him and in their interaction and how this relates to his personal development, his object relationships, and his past and present needs.

In interviews with alexithymic patients the interviewer's response is almost always one of increasing boredom as the patient goes on describing various events in repetitive detail without accompanying emotions; when asked what he felt about what may, for example, have been a tragic loss he is likely to deny that he was affected by it. Instead he may discuss why it happened, saying that it 'could not be helped'; and very likely he will yet again describe in detail the same events without sadness and distress. When the interviewer tries to get through this barrier but finds himself unable to do so he will feel increasingly useless, irritable and frustrated and sometimes his anger will build up so much that it may be difficult to contain. The manner in which the interviewer deals with this negative countertransferential response will be decisive in determining whether or not the patient will continue to maintain his alexithymic posture.

There are several possibilities to be considered depending on the interviewer's professional role. If he functions as a psychiatrist with limited psychotherapeutic expertise, conducting a diagnostic interview with a psychosomatic patient he is unlikely to scrutinise his own countertransference; he may merely conclude that the patient is out of touch with his feelings, that nothing would be gained by continuing the interview and end up labelling him alexithymic. By concentrating on the patient's physical symptoms he can avoid further contact with him at a personal and psychological level. By deciding to leave the patient's further management to a physician or surgeon and to label him as unsuitable for psychotherapy he can escape from any further interaction with him which would make him feel useless and irritated; rejecting the patient in this way absolves the psychiatrist from dealing with his negative countertransference. The patient will thus retain his alexithymic posture and any physician who continues or assumes responsibility for his medical management is likely to reinforce this posture because by the nature of *his* professional attitude he is almost bound to focus the patient's interest entirely on his physical symptoms; this will help the patient further to ignore any feelings and fantasies or life experiences which might be relevant to the understanding of his illness.

In this context it could be said that those psychiatrists who are mainly concerned with descriptive phenomenology, biological explanations and with making a formal psychiatric diagnosis, and those physicians who are concerned mainly with bodily mechanisms and physical diagnosis are both functioning in an alexithymic fashion in their respective professional roles; they collude with their patients in avoiding contact on an emotional, fantasy and experiential level and reinforce their patients' alexithymic posture.

If on the other hand the interviewer is primarily functioning either as a psychotherapist or as a psychiatrist with a psychotherapeutic approach, or as a physician with a psychosomatic, person-orientated attitude the outcome of the interview may be totally different. Let me consider the approach of an analytically orientated therapist who is working with full awareness of his countertransference. As he becomes aware of his increasing frustration and irritation with the patient he will ask himself the basic psychotherapeutic question, i.e., into what role is this patient trying to cast me? The role is likely to be that of a significant parental figure. A likely possibility is that the parent, let us assume the mother, was unable to understand and to respond to her infant's and child's emotional needs, too inhibited to respond warmly to him and show him love and affection, unresponsive to his wish to play with her and imaginatively to share his make-believe and fantasies; that the mother got impatient when the child was difficult and provocative. In short, a mother – and the same could be true of the father – who rejected the child's emotional self-expression and playfulness.

A child growing up in such an atmosphere will get no encouragement or positive reinforcement to share his feelings and fantasies with those who are closest to him. The ability to do so in relation to others will decline and he will develop a false self which relates in an emotionless manner, preoccupied only with the behavioural aspects of his daily life, attempting to be rational rather than emotional, to communicate through thought and action rather than through fantasy, imagination, play and shared feelings.

The therapist will thus become aware of the fact that his patient, functioning from his false self is relating to him as he had learned to relate to his original mother and that his, the therapist's own angry countertransferential response is due to the fact that he cannot get in touch with the patient's inner or true self, his playful, imaginative feeling side. It is exactly this that the therapist or interviewer needs now tentatively to point out or interpret to the patient. He has to avoid at all costs acting out his countertransference by getting overtly angry with the patient or rejecting him. Instead, he has to move sensitively from the present battle ground, in terms of trying to force the patient to show feelings he is not aware of or cannot communicate, into shared areas of exploring the reasons why in his early life he had learned to suppress or conceal what he felt.

It has often been a relief and surprise to me when working in diagnostic or therapeutic interviews with alexithymic patients to find that the tension and my own angry feelings dissipated after I had made a comment like 'I am beginning to wonder whether you were broughtup in a family in which your parents could not respond to you or even got angry with you when you wanted them to play with you, or to share with you what you felt; for example when you were sad, frightened or angry?' Of course, many patients find even this difficult to begin with but by shifting from the present to the past and by getting them to talk about how their parents behaved towards them as children they may gradually realise the possible connection between their present inability to share with me and others what they feel and fantasise about, and their much earlier disappointment not to have been able to do so with mother or father.

Now one can embark in the therapeutic relationship on the slow and difficult task of helping one's patient get in touch with his true self, i.e., his feelings, his fantasies and his playful and creative self. If he learns to trust the therapist to accept whatever he says without getting angry with him, even if at times it is his very inability to communicate feelings, the split between thought or action and feeling or fantasy can be healed so that his alexithymic characteristics begin to diminish.

In essence, faced with an alexithymic patient the interviewer's and therapist's task is first and foremost to avoid being cast into the role of a frustrated, angry and rejecting parent figure. Instead, he has to provide a corrective experience by being a better parent than the patient's original one. He needs to understand his problems, share his difficulty of getting in touch with feelings, and gradually help him recover the ability to feel and to communicate in words what he feels.

Interpretations alone are rarely enough to bring this about because they are so often of a cognitive rather than of an affective nature. The therapist, therefore, has to be prepared to act as a model for his patient by communicating more openly than is the rule in classical analysis how he feels, and by using the sessions for creative play in terms of shared fantasies and exploration of feelings, desires and bodily sensations. *Winnicott* (1971) has expressed this clearly in his book on *Playing and Reality* where he says 'The general principle seems to me to be valid, that psychotherapy is done in the overlap of the two play areas, that of the patient and that of the therapist. If the therapist cannot play, then he is not suitable for the work. If the patient cannot play, then something needs to be done to enable the patient to become able to play, after which psychotherapy may begin. The reason why playing is essential is that it is in playing that the patient is being creative'. Using this model of *Winnicott*'s one could define the alexithymic patient as a patient who has lost the ability to play so that it becomes the therapist's task to help him regain his playfulness.

Dreams are often helpful in this work and alexithymic patients who at the start of treatment say they cannot remember any of their dreams often begin to do so when actively encouraged by the therapist to make an effort on waking to remember what they dreamt, and as relaxed playfulness and interest in fantasy life become progressively easier during the sessions.

Sometimes other psychotherapeutic methods are useful or even essential to move out of the area of alexithymia. These may include, for example, joint marital or family interviews because in the interaction with significant others the patient may more easily be provoked into expressing what he feels. Group therapy may have similar effects because in the group atmosphere and by interacting with other patients feelings and fantasies may come to the surface which the patient had not previously been aware of. Occasionally, such techniques as Gestalt therapy, psychodrama or direct attention to bodily behaviour may be very effective. Psychosomatic patients are especially prone to reveal suppressed feelings of sadness, anger and excitement non-verbally and through bodily tension and rigid bodily postures (*Reich,* 1973). *Lowen* (1958, 1975) and *Kinston and Wolff* (1975) have described how by paying detailed attention to the patient's posture and sometimes by touching him or asking him to modify his posture and breathing pattern, feelings may be released which the patient had been unaware of or suppressed for many years.

It is essential to combine these various methods with proper psycho-dynamic understanding and ongoing analytical work. Such a flexible, combined psychotherapeutic approach often makes it possible to work psychotherapeutically with alexithymic patients who had previously been thought to be unsuitable for psychotherapy. In other words alexithymia *per se* is not a contraindication to psychotherapy although there may, of course, be other contraindications.

Lastly, I come to the problem of the relation between the thought-feeling split of the alexithymic patient and the mind-body split of the psycho-somatic patient; and the related question why alexithymic characteristics are more common in psychosomatic than in psychoneurotic patients.

The main issue here is the fact that psychological splitting processes play an essential part in human development and the normal or pathological degree of splitting that has taken place will determine the individual's psychological functioning and behaviour. A newly born infant is, of course, still functioning as an organismic whole, feelings being automatically ex-pressed in bodily reactions and there being as yet no awareness in the baby of being separate from its mother who represents the environment. This state of wholeness and fusion is lost early on with the baby's growing awareness of its separateness. Mother and father are soon experienced as either gratifying or frustrating so that feelings of love and hate directed towards the same person or object are split apart; the split off feelings and fantasies may instead find expression in physical symptoms. The normal and pathological splitting mechanisms associated with these phenomena have been described by *Klein et al.* (1952).

As the capacity for thought and verbal expression develops the educa-tional process, especially in Western culture, tends to emphasize rational thinking and behaviour at the cost of repression or denial of feelings, fanta-sies and bodily self-expression, and the loss of spontaneity. The demands of society for control and adaptation imposes further restrictions on the indi-vidual and reinforces the growing split between reason and instinctual, includ-ing erotic desires, or to use psychoanalytical terms, between ego and id. Within psychoanalysis itself developments in ego-psychology have tended to over-emphasize adaptation to reality and conformity to social expectations at the cost of spontaneous id experiences and playful creativity.

These issues and the problems they give rise to have been discussed by *Freud* (1961a, b) in *The Ego and the Id* in 1923 and in *Civilisation and its Discontents* in 1929. They have since been critically examined by *Brown* (1959) in *Life Against Death* and by *Watts* (1961) in *Psychotherapy East and West*.

Another relevant fact is that every individual to some extent maintains the wish throughout life to return to the earlier way of experiencing wholeness and fusion. Whilst this wish can at best only be partially fulfilled certain temporary experiences come at least close to its fulfilment. Thus, being in love and being united with the loved person in a mutually satisfying sexual relationship comes close to such fulfilment because it is at such moments that bodily experience, shared play, feelings and fantasies, and fusion with the other one become a temporary reality. There are, of course, other experiences like moments of spontaneous togetherness, shared joy, play, creative self-expression and spiritual or mystical experiences.

In these terms, it becomes easier to understand the significance and determinants of the thought-feeling split of the alexithymic and the mind-body split of the psychosomatic patient. Over-valuation of controlled and rational ego functions and of realistic behaviour in relation to the outside world and the corresponding impoverishment of spontaneous self-expression account for the fact that some alexithymic characteristics are found to vary-ing degrees in many individuals in our society. In the extreme and pathologi-cal case meticulous pre-occupation with controlled thinking and behaviour, i.e., 'pensée opératoire', will become the predominant mode of existence. Extreme repression of instinctual needs and spontaneous emotional expe-rience then makes the successful search for re-experiencing the original state of organismic wholeness and fusion virtually impossible. It is thus not sur-prising that ultimately a sense of inner emptiness, frustration and isolation will give rise to depression, anxiety and other psychoneurotic symptoms in some alexithymic individuals.

It is significant also that the same parents who are over-anxious to control their children's id functions and thereby lay the basis for alexithymic tendencies, also tend to be over-concerned to control the child's bodily behaviour and to pay excessive attention to the child when he complains of physical symptoms. Such children will themselves by identification become anxiously pre-occupied with bodily functions and symptoms with relative neglect of mental functioning. Their up-bringing will then leave them with a mind-body split as well as a thought-feeling split. This may be one of the reasons why some alexithymic characteristics are commonly found in asso-ciation with psychosomatic symptoms.

It follows from these considerations that in psychotherapy with such patients every effort needs to be made by the means described earlier to reduce the intensity of pathological splitting in order to help them develop a more positive attitude towards their bodily, instinctual and feeling func-tions. The alexithymic patient like all of us needs to learn or re-learn to tolerate the risks and uncertainties which a more spontaneous mode of living and self-expression inevitably involves.

How far these aims can be achieved is partly determined by the degree and kind of pathological splitting the patient presents, but also by the thera-pist's own ability to function spontaneously and as an organismically inte-grated being, at least in his professional work and hopefully also in his personal life. Both therapists and patients would, I suggest, be helped in their task if Society became less restrictive and more accepting of spontaneous self-expression, though tempered by regard for the feelings of others. Such social changes might help to prevent the development of alexithymic characteristics in some of its members.

References

Brown, N.O.: Life against death (Routledge & Kegan Paul, London 1959).

Freud, S.: Civilization and its discontents. Standard ed., vol. 21, pp. 50–145 (Hogarth, London 1961a).

Freud, S.: The ego and the id. Standard ed., vol. 19, pp. 3–66 (Hogarth, London 1961b).

Heimann, P.: On counter-transference. Int. J. Psychoanal. *31:* 81–84 (1950).

Kinston, M. and Wolff, H.H.: Bodily communication and psychotherapy. A psychosomatic approach. Int. J. Psychiat. Med. *6:* 195–201 (1975).

Klein, M.: Notes on some schizoid mechanisms; in *Riviere* Developments in psychoanalysis, pp. 292–320 (Hogarth, London 1952).

Lowen, A.: The language of the body (MacMillan, London 1958).

Lowen, A.: Bioenergetics (Coward McCann & Geoghegan, New York 1975).

Marty, P. et deMuzan, M.: La pensée opératoire. Revue fr. psychoanal. *27:* suppl., p. 1345 (1963).

Marty, P.; deMuzan, M. et David, C.: L'investigation psychosomatique (Presses Universitaires, Paris 1963).

McDougall, J.: The psychosoma and the psychoanalytic process. Int. Rev. Psychoanal. *1:* 437–459 (1974).

Nemiah, J.C.: Psychology and psychosomatic illness. Reflections on theory and research methodology. Psychother. Psychosom. *22:* 106–111 (1973).

Nemiah, J.C. and Sifneos, P.E.: Affect and fantasy in patients with psychosomatic disorders; in *Hill* Modern trends in psychosomatic medicine, vol. 2, pp. 26–34 (Butterworths, London 1970).

Reich, W.: Character analysis (Vision Press, London 1973).

Sandler, J.: Countertransference and role-responsiveness. Int. Rev. Psychoanal. *3:* 43–47 (1976).

Sandler, J.; Dare, C., and Holder, A.: The patient and the analyst. The basis of the psychoanalytic process (Allen & Unwin, London 1973).

Sifneos, P.E.: Clinical observations on some patients suffering from a variety of psychosomatic diseases. Proc. 7th Eur. Conf. psychosom. Res., Rome 1967. Acta med. psychosom.

Sifneos, P.E.: The prevalence of alexithymic characteristics in psychosomatic patients. Psychother. Psychosom. *22:* 255–262 (1973).

Watts, A.W.: Psychotherapy East and West (Mentor Books, London 1961).

Winnicott, D.W.: Counter-transference. The Maturational processes and the facilitating environment, pp. 158–165 (Hogarth, London 1965).

Winnicott, D.W.: Psycho-somatic illness in its positive and negative aspects. Int. J. Psycho-
     anal. *47:* 510–516 (1966).
Winnicott, D.W.: Playing and reality (Penguin Books, Harmondsworth 1971).
Wolff, H.H.: Psychotherapy. Its place in psychosomatic management. Psychother. Psycho-
     som. *22:* 233–249 (1973).

Heinz H. Wolff, MD, Department of Psychological Medicine, University College Hospital,
Gower Street, *London WC 1* (England)

Proc. 11th Eur. Conf. Psychosom. Res., Heidelberg 1976
Psychother. Psychosom. *28:* 68–70 (1977)

Some Remarks on the Etymological and Grammatic Aspects of the Term 'Alexithymia'

George Spyros Philippopoulos

'Alexithymia', both as a technical term and as a concept has a long-standing and deeply rooted history in psychosomatic research, thanks to *Sifneos* (1–3).

As a psychiatrist, I was really pleased to learn a new term for an old subject. This very term specifies exactly the process its meaning implies. Yet, as a Greek I was somehow puzzled from the moment I heard the new term and still wonder whether it is wise for us to keep the term as it is? Perhaps we should try and find some better and more appropriate term to substitute 'alexithymia', a word which is *not* existent in the Greek language.

I am aware that an already well-established technical term cannot be easily revoked or even changed, but I should like this time to refer briefly to some etymological and grammatic aspects of this compound so that we may be able to have a more concrete gestalt of the word 'alexithymia', as well as of the term suggested below to be a better substitute.

Sifneos, proposed the term alexithymia '... for having not a better word ...'. However, the first two elements of this compound, i.e., a-lexis in Greek means help or protection. 'Alexis' (ἄλεξις), is a derivative of the verb ἀλέξω, meaning to protect, to ward off, to act as an antidote (cf. alexins, alexipharmic, alexiteric etc.).

'Alexithymia', is a misconstructed word that has joined the myriad of similar pseudo-Greek artifacts which abound in psychiatry and allied fields (cf. Dr. Caycedo's Sophrology, Bourneville's Epiloia, Abiotrophy, etc.). These pseudo-Greek artifacts have as their only recommendation the fact that they fulfill the purpose of their construction which is to help in understanding the actual meaning of the subject, the situation or the process they specify.

Table I

---

(1) Alexithymia (Ἀλεξιθυμία)
   From the Greek: a = lack, lexis = word[1], and thymos = mood, emotion
(2) Athymoalexia (Ἀθυμοαλεξία)
   From the Greek: ἄθυμος = athymic, having no affect motivation and
                         ἀλεξία = alexia[2], lack of words, inability to talk
(3) Athymolalia (Ἀθυμολαλία)
   From the Greek: ἄθυμος and λαλιά = loquacity, talkativeness

---

1 The Greek compound alexis (ἄλεξις), means help, protection. It comes from the
   bver ἀλέξω = to ward off, to protect, to act as an antidote (cf. alexins, alexi
   pharmic, alexiteric, etc.).
2 Meaning also: word blindness.
3 From the Greek verb λαλεῖν = talking too much, prattling, being loquacious.

In view of the above and also for the purpose of obtaining at the same time an etymologically and grammatically correct term, I should like to suggest an appropriate and suitable substitute for 'alexithymia', namely the Greek word A-thymo-alexia (Ἀθυμοαλεξία) and its counter complement A-thymo-lalia (Ἀθυμολαλία).

Athymoalexia, literally means an inability to express ourselves verbally, because of athymia that is lack of affective motivation, whereas athymolalia denotes exactly the reverse, i.e., talking too much, prattling, being loquacious (table I).

If we want to be exact with reference to the right meaning and correct spelling of the word then '*athymoalexia*' is the proper substitute for alexithymia. On the other hand, '*athymolalia*' should be reserved to specify the phenomenon of excessive talking which is frequently observed in some neurotic and/or psychosomatic patients when interviewed or in the process of psychotherapy. This phenomenon is due perhaps to a conscious or unconscious wish of the patient to cover-up, deny or compensate for his depressive feelings. It is as often met in clinical practice as athymoalexia, sometimes even more so.

My intervention has no chauvinistic motivations whatsoever! Neither does it aim to narrow down the meaning of *Sifneos'* unique contribution to the field of psychosomatic research. It simply aims at drawing your attention and accentuating the difficulties of communication in our specialty due, at least in part, to the event that many technical terms of Greek origin, in fact too many, have been misused, misconstructed and/or mistranslated by foreign authors who were not and are not obligated to master the Greek language!

It may also be of some help in our attempts to attain a better understanding, promote stabilization of terminology, and finally, to 'diminish friction in communicating facts and ideas' (4, 5).

References

1 *Sifneos, P.E.:* Certain common characteristics of outpatients suffering from a variety of psychosomatic illness. 7th Eur. Conf. Psychosom. Res., Rome 1967.
2 *Sifneos, P.E.:* The prevalence of alexithymic characteristics in psychosomatic patients. 9th Eur. Conf. Psychosom. Res., Vienna 1972.
3 *Sifneos, P.E.:* The problem of psychotherapy of patients with physical disease. 10th Eur. Conf. Psychosom. Res., Edinburgh 1974.
4 *English, O. and English, C.:* A comprehensive dictionary of psychological and psychoanalytical terms (Logmans, London 1958).
5 *Philippopoulos, G.S.:* A concise English-Greek glossary of psychiatric terms; 2nd ed. (Athens 1976).

George S. Philippopoulos, MD, 92, Queen Sophias Avenue, *611 Athens* (Greece)

Discussion

Dr. Mitscherlich: I would like to say something about the language of psychosomatic patients. The first point is that they very rarely use the 'I'. The second point is that when their own problems are concerned, they use bodily metaphors and express themselves on a descriptive and concrete level. The third point is that with a patient suffering from myasthenia gravis pseudoparalytica, on being questioned about unsolved separation problems (remaining within the symbiotic relationship), after a short while he smilingly said: 'My leg has gone to sleep'. Then I told him: 'You think you have solved this problem. That is to say, you have separated one part of your body from the other'. I.e., the patient is unable to verbalize on a level of abstraction that adult people usually can.

On another occasion the same patient started to conjugate nouns. He said 'Kochtöpfe, Kochtöpfst'. This mode of expression corresponds to the sensomotoric level described by *Piaget* (approx. to the 2nd year of life) of the intellectual development.

Dr. Hoppe: Admiring the eloquence of Dr. *Wolff,* I wonder why he has to go back to the nature-nurture question. It seems to me that we should rather accept an interactional 'as well as' approach. For example, I went over the associative anamnesis of some of *Felix Deutsch*'s patients and found an astonishingly great lack of fantasies, feelings and affect. I am not sure whether we should discount in our psychological understanding the genetics and biological field which *Freud* always referred to as constitutional factors. Let us realize that both, *nature and nurture,* are involved.

Next Speaker (unidentified): I would like to mention just briefly that I admire Dr. *Wolff* very much and the whole concept. I am wondering why we cannot more widely use *Freud*'s original idea about regression of emotions and so on to regression because this concept explains practically all the problems which were discussed. Secondly, I would like to mention to you one experience which was forced on me. Many years ago I was in prison for 10 months solitary confinement. No communication at all, no books, no papers, no word at all. I was recalling past experiences – I survived physically. I had no problem in that respect. At one stage a man was thrown into my cell just for a few days as a companion. He was a man who could not express himself, he was not educated and could not externalize. This man developed high blood pressure and in front of me during the 5 days came to the stage where he nearly had a brain hemorrhage. I had to break down the iron door to get to the warders of the prison to take him away. Briefly, I learned from this experience and from many others over the past 35 years I have been doing psychotherapy and psychoanality that people who can express themselves are more protected against somatic diseases than those who cannot. But there is of course a variety and fluctuation within every patient. Our aim, as Dr. *Wolff* very wisely expressed it, is that we should be able to mobilize those people who have emotional regression and we should not give up the hope that everybody can help better somatic emotions.

Dr. Gaddini: I find Dr. *Wolff*'s contribution very interesting. There are a few points I would like to make in response. One is in agreement with him when he mentions the positive value of countertransference in psychoanalysis. Quoting *Heimann, Wolff* points out that countertransference is a valuable indicator for the therapist in the case of alexithymic patients who never attain the capacity of sharing a therapeutic relationship and of communicating with the analyst the way that neurotic patients do. Interpretations are used by these patients more at a cognitive rather than at an emotional level. *Wolff* talks of their incapacity to share, as of 'lost ability to play'. This is the other point of his presentation that I would like to discuss. I do not see it as 'a lost ability' to share but as 'a never acquired' one. Some of you may know that for a number of years I have followed longitudinally a group of children focusing on their going-to-sleep pattern at the age of one and on their capacity of creative play at the age of four. We observed that those children who at the age of one were able to protect themselves 'creatively' from the anxiety of object loss they met daily in going to sleep, where those who at the age of four were able to play 'creatively' putting on scenes, pretending that objects and persons are there who are in fact not there and who can give value and dramatic life to their scenes, to master anxiety and thus get relief. I agree with Dr. *Wolff* that the capacity to play implies the capacity to share. We are both inclined to see this capacity reduced, or absent, in psychosomatic patients. But he refers to it as a 'lost capacity', whereas on the basis of my longitudinal experience which indicates creativity as a continuum, I see it as a 'never acquired' one – a failure in the maturational process.

Dr. Shands: The psychoanalytic model suggests that people have feelings 'naturally' that are then covered up or hidden by 'repression'. A great deal of evidence, especially in relation to Dr. *Gaddini*'s remarks, suggests strongly to me that feelings are learned or developed and that this development is emphasized in a middle-class education much more than in the working-class. *Bernstein*'s distinction between a 'restricted' and an 'elaborated' code has much to do with the ability to describe feelings.

Dr. Wolff: I would like to make one comment. There is, of course, a biological counterpart to every psychological experience. Studies at the biological level of abstraction provide explanations in terms of mechanisms, studies at the psychological level are concerned with meaning and the two are complementary; biological explanations cannot replace psychological understanding and vice versa. Taking the problem of alexithymia, it would, indeed be interesting to study the neurophysiological mechanisms underlying the difficulty some patients have in expressing feelings through words but such neurophysiological or neuroanatomical knowledge does not help us to understand the psychological reasons why these patients have developed these alexithymic characteristics. The phenomenon of depression may help to illustrate this further. There is now some evidence that when someone is sad or depressed there is a diminution of catecholamines in the brain. That is the biological counterpart of feeling depressed. But there is a risk of misunderstanding the significance of these biological findings. It is now sometimes claimed that someone is depressed *because* the catecholamine level in the brain is low instead of realizing that he is depressed because, for example, his mother misunderstands him or he has suffered a bereavement, and that the low catecholamine levels are the neurobiochemical counterpart of his resultant sense of depression. The danger here, as in alexithymia, is that the biological explanation is used to ignore the patient's personal experience which can then lead us to a position of psychotherapeutic nihilism.

Concerning Dr. *Gaddini*'s comment I would like to hear more about the different ways in which children play and how this correlates with the development of psychosomatic symptoms.

Proc. 11th Eur. Conf. Psychosom. Res., Heidelberg 1976
Psychother. Psychosom. *28:* 73–82 (1977)

Recent Advances in the Content Analysis of Speech and the Application of this Measurement Approach to Psychosomatic Research

Louis A. Gottschalk

Department of Psychiatry and Human Behavior, College of Medicine, University of California at Irvine, Irvine, Calif.

Introduction

This paper will summarize the theory, reliability, validity, and applications of a method of content analysis of verbal behavior to psychosomatic research. The need for such a method became apparent to the author when he was involved in psychophysiological studies correlating the relationship of varying psychological states and psychodynamics with various physiological measures, including electroencephalographic (EEG), and galvanic skin responses (GSR) (*Gottschalk,* 1955; *Gottschalk and Hambidge,* 1955). The psychological states were being assessed in a fashion typical for clinical psychiatry, from the impressionistic content analysis of speech provided by subjects encouraged to free-associate. During this study, the author realized that though the physiological measures (EEG, GSR) could be registered with relatively high precision and could be mathematized, the magnitude of the psychological states and psychodynamic conflicts derived from the subjects' speech could be assessed only in an impressionistic manner that allowed for a relatively high likelihood of distortion and/or error from the interviewer's potentially incorrect emphatic responses and inferences during the process of assessing the subject's talk. How to minimize such error variance and how to maximize the uniformity and consistency of the inferential evaluations concerning the subject's subjective experience and the relative magnitude of these psychological states and conflicts, hence, became the aim of the author for the next 15 years. What has evolved from such a goal has been the development and testing of a method of content analysis of verbal behavior based on psychoanalytic, conditioning, and linguistic theories.

Summary of the Gottschalk-Gleser Content Analysis Method

The initial goal in the development of this method was to probe the immediate emotional reactions of subjects or patients, instead of the typical or habitual ones (traits), and to minimize reactions of guarding or covering up. Hence, the instructions to elicit speech from research subjects were purposely relatively ambiguous and nonstructured; customarily, speakers were asked to tell about personal or dramatic life experiences or simply to free-associate (*Gottschalk and Hambidge,* 1955). In many early studies, standardized instructions were used also, in order to compare individuals in a standard context so that demographic and personality variables could be explored and investigated, while holding relatively constant the influence of such variables as the instructions for eliciting speech, the nature and personality of the intervieweer, the context, and the situation. The effects of varying these noninterviewee variables were subsequently investigated, one by one, after reliable and valid content analysis scales were developed.

The development of this measurement method has involved a long series of steps (*Gottschalk and Gleser,* 1969). It has required that the psychologic dimensions to be measured (for example, anxiety, hostility-outward, hostility-inward, cognitive and intellectual impairment, achievement strivings, social alienation-personal disorganization, hope, human relations, dependency, health-sickness, and so forth) be precisely defined, that the lexical cues be carefully pinpointed by which a receiver of any verbal messages infers the occurrence of any of these psychologic states, and the linguistic, principally syntactic, cues conveying intensity (for example, the word 'very' in the proper context) be specified. Next, differential weights were assigned to these semantic and linguistic cues conveying magnitude of a subjective experience whenever appropriate. Furthermore, a systematic means was arrived at of correcting for the number of words spoken per unit time so that one individual could be compared to himself on different occasions or to others with respect to the magnitude of any particular psychologic state.

This content analysis method requires that a formal scale of weighted content categories be specified for every psychologic dimension to be measured and that research technicians be trained to score these typescripts of human speech according to any one scale at an interscorer reliability of 0.85 or above. Moreover, a set of construct-validation studies had to be carried out to recheck exactly what each content analysis scale measured, and these validation studies have included the use of four kinds of criterion measures: psychologic, physiologic, pharmacologic, and biochemical. On the basis of these construct-validation studies, changes have been made in the content categories and their assigned weights of each specific scale, in the direction of maximizing the correlations between the content analysis scores with these various independent criterion measures.

The theoretical framework from which this measurement approach has developed has been an eclectic one and has included behavioral and conditioning theory, psychoanalytic clinical theory, and linguistic theory. In addition, the formulation of these psychologic states has been deeply influenced by the position that they all have biologic roots. Both the definition of each separate psychologic state and the selection of the specific verbal content items used as cues for inferring each state have been influenced by the decision that whatever psychologic state was measured by this content analysis approach should, whenever possible, be associated with some biologic characteristic of the individual in addition to some psychologic aspect or some social situation.

The content analysis technician applying this procedure to typescripts of tape-recorded speech has not had to worry about approaching the work of content analysis following one theoretical orientation or another. Rather, the technician follows a strictly empirical approach, scoring the occurrence of any content or themes in each grammatical clause of speech according to sets of various, well-delineated language categories making up each of the separate verbal behavior scales. A manual (*Gottschalk et al.,* 1969) is available which indicates what verbal categories should be looked for and how much the occurrence of each one is to be weighted. Following initial coding of content in this way, the technician, then, follows prescribed mathematical calculations leading up to a final score for the magnitude of any one psychologic state or another.

This content analysis procedure can be and has been applied to interview material – psychotherapeutic, diagnostic, or otherwise. The content analysis scales can be applied to different kinds of language materials obtained in a variety of situations in both spoken and written form. Most of the reliability and validity studies have been done on small samples of speech, 3–5 min in duration, obtained in response to standard instructions. The typed data can be broken down into equal temporal units (for example, 2- to 5-min segments). Or the units can be based on the number of words spoken by one or both participants (or more if they are present); for example, consecutive 500-word sequences of the speakers can be coded for content. Depending on the purpose or research design of the study, these content analysis scales have also been applied to dreams, projective test data (specifically, tape recordings of Thematic Apperception Test responses), to written verbal samples, and even to literature, letters, public speeches, and any other type of language material.

Relevance of this Approach to the Problem of Psychological Measurements

One of the shortcomings of any content analysis procedure is that it discards valuable data, data which might be of considerable usefulness to the usual psychosomatic researcher in his global approach to the problem of psychological assessment. A content analysis method could never supplant the broad perspectives of a clinician nor the clinician's ability to synthesize many different points of view in listening to and reacting to a variety of forces occurring in the interview process. The value in psychosomatic research of a content analysis method lies more in its capacity to give objective assessments about the magnitude of specific psychologic states. As such, high level measurement precision is reached while global interrelationships may be lost. Such precise and accurate assessments of specific psychologic dimensions may have considerable usefulness, for example, in psychosomatic research.

There are three objective methods of measuring psychological states: self-report scales, behavioral rating scales, and the objective content analysis of spoken or written language. Self-report scales give the patient an opportunity to describe his subjective distress, and since it is the patient's subjective distress that ordinarily accounts for seeking treatment, such self-report scales would appear to be a plausible criterion of treatment effects. It is customary among some developers of self-report measures (*Parloff et al.*, 1954; *Frank et al.*, 1957; *McNair and Lorr*, 1964; *Mattsson et al.*, 1969; *Derogatis et al.*, 1974) to assay the magnitude of psychological states not only from an individual's self-report directly about affects, but also from associated somatic dysfunctions, cognitive and intellectual dysfunctions or from actual performance dysfunctions. Unfortunately, a subject may respond to self-report measures in terms of his traits as much as in terms of his state. Or it may be that the patient's self-descriptions are more in terms of the kind of person the patient believes himself to be rather than descriptions of the subjective state in which he currently finds himself. Similarly, a patient may desire to please or favorably impress an interviewer and present himself in terms of an idealized person rather in terms of his real self. Moreover, the use of self-report inventories of somatic discomfort, although useful, are not sufficient measures of affects because many patients who have significant subjective affects do not suffer appreciable somatic distress. And there are patients of hypochondriacal or hysterical disposition who tend to exaggerate or perhaps use real or imagined somatic distress without experiencing appreciable affects. Similarly, impaired performance is not found in some affectively disturbed patients who, with great psychic discomfort, mobilize their energies and continue to perform well.

Psychiatric rating scales involve assessments made by a trained observer, usually a psychiatrist or clinical psychologist. Hence, the rater customarily has had some experience in measuring psychopathological phenomena and usually has had some experience and practice in administering these rating scales. The clinician is free to assess the status of the patient from a range of behavioral and affective cues, verbal and nonverbal. His judgements are less likely to be constricted by the possible distortions inherent in the self-report approach, and the rater is generally capable of accurately establishing the pattern as well as the level of severity of the patient's symptom profile. However, though the clinical interniewer gains objectivity and detachment in comparison to the self-report approach to psychological measurements, he sacrifices familiarity with the patient. His sphere of reference is limited to the immediate interview situation. Also, clinicians are not free from systematic distortions. Definite biases or orientations regarding clinical interpretation may be introduced in the formal training and cultural background of a clinician. Also, subtle personality characteristics, usually long preceding the professional training of the rater and labelled countertransference by some clinicians, may distort the perceptions and emotional reactions of the rater vis-à-vis the patient. Also, there is evidence that different interviewers may evoke varying emotional responses from the same patients (*Gottschalk,* 1971). Finally, the agreement between independent clinical observers is often only moderate.

In summary, self-report procedures have certain shortcomings, including providing a possibility of malingering of faking and the opportunity for various response-sets, such as, social desirability, acquiescence, and deviance (*Anastasi,* 1968; *Wittenborn,* 1974). Whereas, rating scales pose measurement problems involving reliability; halo effects (such as a tendency of raters to be unduly influenced by a single favorable or unfavorable trait), error of central tendency (that is, the tendency to rate persons in the middle of a scale and to avoid extreme positions), and leniency error (the reluctance of many raters to assign unfavorable ratings) (*Anastasi,* 1968; *Wittenborn,* 1967, 1972). The content analysis of an individual's speech or writing, the third alternative approach to the evaluation of psychological states is a method that avoids many of the measurement problems of self-report and rating scales used by an external observer.

In a recent study by *Gottschalk et al.* (1976), intercorrelations were obtained between the measurement scores from 35 patients (pre- and post-drug), of a content analysis scale procedure (Gottschalk-Gleser), two behavioral rating scales (Hamilton Anxiety rating scales, 1959, and the Physician Questionnaire rating scale; *Rickels and Howard,* 1970) and a self-report method (Symptom Checklist; *Parloff et al.,* 1954). The intercorrelations included a dissection of the correlations between the subscales and item components of these different measurement methods. This investigation served as a means of translating the common meanings measured by these three different kinds of psychological tools. This study showed that these different measurement scales, labelled with the same name, e.g., 'anxiety' or 'hostility' scale, do not uniformly measure similar or overlapping variables. But often some of their subscales or separate item scales do, indeed, assay associated characteristics.

There have been a series of recent developments and applications of this content analysis method that are especially relevant to psychosomatic research. These developments and applications are described below.

New content analysis scales have been developed for adults, including a human relations, hope, and object relations scale (*Gottschalk,* 1968, 1974). This content analysis procedure has been applied to children (*Gottschalk,* 1975, 1976; *Uliana,* 1976); norms have been obtained from a sample of white and black children, ages 5–16 years, and validation studies are in progress. New applications have been reported to psychophysiological (*Bell et al.,* 1971; *Gottlieb et al.,* 1967; *Karacan,* 1966; *Gottschalk,* 1968, 1975, 1976; *Gottschalk and Gleser,* 1969; *Gottschalk et al.,* 1961, 1967; *Ivey and Bardwick,* 1968; *Silbergeld et al.,* 1971) and psychobiochemical research (*Gottschalk,* 1972; *Gottschalk and Gleser,* 1969; *Gottschalk et al.,* 1965, 1966, 1969; *Silbergeld et al.,* 1975; *Stone et al.,* 1969), neuropsychopharmacological research (*Elliott et al.,* 1974; *Gottschalk and Gleser,* 1969; *Gottschalk et al.,* 1960, 1965, 1971, 1973, 1974, 1975, 1976), psychotherapy research (*Gottschalk,* 1974; *Gottschalk and Auerbach,* 1966; *Gottschalk et al.,* 1967, 1969, 1973; *Lewis,* 1971; *Luborsky et al.,* 1975; *Perley et al.,* 1971; *Witkin et al.,* 1968), and psychokinesic research (*Freedman et al.,* 1973; *Gottschalk,* 1974; *Gottschalk and Frank,* 1967; *Gottschalk and Uliana,* 1976a, b). The likely possibility of automated computerized scoring using this content analysis methods is indicated (*Gottschalk et al.,* 1975).

In conclusion, this content analysis procedure promises to continue to contribute greatly to the measurement of psychological states in psychosomatic research.

References

Anastasi, A.: Psychological testing; 3rd ed. (Macmillan, New York 1968).

Bell, A.; Stroebel, C.F., and Prior, D.D.: Interdisciplinary study of the scrotal sac and testes correlating psychophysiological and psychological observations. Psychoanal. Q. *40:* 415–434 (1971).

Derogatis, L.R.; Lipman, R.S.; Rickel, K.; Uhlenhuth, E.H., and Covi, L.: The Hopkins Symptom Checklist (HSCL). A measure of primary symptom dimensions; in *Pichat* Psychological measurements in psychopharmocology. Mod. Probl. Pharmacopsych., vol. 7, pp. 79–110 (Karger, Basel 1974).

Elliott, H.W.; Gottschalk, L.A., and Uliana, R.L.: Relationship of plasma meperidine levels to changes in anxiety and hostility. Comp. Psychiat. *15:* 249–254 (1974).

Frank, J.D.; Gliedman, L.H.; Imber, S.D.; Nash, E.H., and Stone, A.R.: Why patients leave psychotherapy. Archs Neurol. Psychiat. *77:* 283–299 (1957).

Freedman, N.; Blass, T.; Rifkin, A., and Quitkin, F.: Body movements and the verbal encoding of aggressive affect. J. Pers. Soc. Psychol. *26:* 72 (1973).

Gleser, G.C.; Gottschalk, L.A.; Fox, R., and Lippert, W.: Immediate changes in affect with chlordiazepoxide in juvenile delinquent boys. Archs gen. Psychiat. *13:* 291–295 (1965).

Gottlieb, A.A.; Gleser, G.C., and Gottschalk, L.A.: Verbal and physiological responses to hypnotic suggestion of attitudes. Psychosom. Med. *29:* 172–183 (1967).

Gottschalk, L.A.: A hope scale applicable to verbal samples. Archs gen. Psychiat. *30:* 779–785 (1974).

Gottschalk, L.A.: An objective method of measuring psychological states associated with changes in neural function. J. biol. Psychiat. *4:* 33–49 (1972).

Gottschalk, L.A.: A psychoanalytic study of hand-mouth approximation; in Psychoanalysis and contemporary science (International Universities Press, New York 1974).

Gottschalk, L.A.: Children's speech as a source of data towards the measurement of psychological states. J. Youth Adolesc. *5:* 11–36 (1976).

Gottschalk, L.A.: Differences in the content of speech of girls and boys ages six to sixteen; in *Sankar* Studies on childhood psychiatric and psychological problems (PJD Publications, Westbury 1976).

Gottschalk, L.A.: Psychologic conflict and electroencephalographic patterns. Some notes on the problem of correlating changes in paroxysmal electroencephalographic patterns with psychologic conflicts. Archs Neurol. Psychiat. *73:* 656–662 (1955).

Gottschalk, L.A.: Some applications of the psychoanalytic concept of object relatedness. Preliminary studies of a human relations scale applicable to verbal samples. Comp. Psychiat. *9:* 608–620 (1968).

Gottschalk, L.A.: Some psychoanalytic research into the communication of meaning through language. The quality and magnitude of psychological states. Br. J. med. Psychol. *44:* 131–148 (1971).

Gottschalk, L.A.: The measurement of hostile aggression through the content analysis of speech. Some biological and interpersonal aspects; in *Garattini and Sigg* Biology of aggressive behavior (Excerpta Medica Foundation, Amsterdam 1968).

Gottschalk, L.A.; Winget, C.N.; Gleser, G.C., and Springer, K.J.: The measurement of emotional changes during a psychiatric interview. A working model toward quantifying the psychoanalytic concept of affect; in *Gottschalk and Auerbach* Methods of research in psychotherapy, pp. 3–9 (Appleton-Century-Crofts, New York 1966).

Gottschalk, L.A.; Bates, D.E.; Waskow, I.E.; Katz, M.M., and Olsson, J.: Effect of amphetamine or chlorpromazine on achievement strivings scores derived from content analysis of speech. Comp. Psychiat. *12:* 430–435 (1971).

Gottschalk, L.A.; Biener, R.; Noble, E.P.; Birch, H.; Wilbert, D.E., and Heiser, J.F.: Thioridazine plasma levels and clinical response. Comp. Psychiat. *16:* 323–337 (1975).

Gottschalk, L.A.; Cleghorn, J.M.; Gleser, G.C., and Iacono, J.M.: Studies of relationships of emotions to plasma lipids. Psychosom. Med. *27:* 102–111 (1965).

Gottschalk, L.A.; Dinovo, E.C.; Biener, R.; Birch, H.; Syben, M., and Noble, E.P.: Plasma levels of mesoridazine and its metabolites and clinical response in acute schizophrenia after a single intramuscular drug dose; in *Gottschalk and Merlis* Pharmacokinetics of Psychoactive drugs. Blood levels and clinical response (Spectrum, New York 1976).

Gottschalk, L.A.; Fox, R.A., and Bates, D.E.: A study of prediction and outcome in a mental health crisis clinic. Am. J. Psychiat. *130:* 1107–1111 (1973).

Gottschalk, L.A. and Frank, E.C.: Estimating the magnitude of anxiety from speech. Behav. Sci. *12:* 289–295 (1967).

Gottschalk, L.A. and Gleser, G.C.: The measurement of psychologic states through the content analysis of verbal behavior (Univ. of California Press, Los Angeles 1969).

Gottschalk, L.A.; Gleser, G.C.; Springer, K.J.; Kaplan, S.M.; Shanon, J., and Ross, W.D.: Effects of perphenazine on verbal behavior patterns. Archs gen. Psychiat. *2:* 632–639 (1960).

Gottschalk, L.A.; Gleser, G.C.; Wylie, H.W., and Kaplan, S.D.: Effects of imipramine on anxiety and hostility levels derived from verbal communications. Psychopharmacologia *7:* 303–310 (1965).

Gottschalk, L.A. and Hambidge, G.: Verbal behavior analysis. A systematic approach to the problem of quantifying psychologic processes. J. Proj. Tech. *19:* 387–409 (1955).

Gottschalk, L.A.; Hausmann, C., and Brown, J.S.: A computerized scoring system for use with content analysis scales. Comp. Psychiat. *16:* 77–90 (1975).

Gottschalk, L.A.; Hoigaard, J.C.; Birch, H., and Rickels, K.: The measurement of psychological states. Relationships between Gottschalk-Gleser content analysis scores and Hamilton Anxiety rating scale scores, Physician Questionnaire rating scale scores and Hopkins Symptom Checklist scores; in *Gottschalk and Merlis* Pharmacokinetics of psychoactive drugs. Blood levels and clinical response (Spectrum, New York 1976).

Gottschalk, L.A.; Kaplan, S.M.; Gleser, G.C., and Winget, C.N.: Variations in magnitudes of emotions. A method applied to anxiety and hostility during phases of the menstrual cycle. Psychosom. Med. *24:* 300–311 (1962).

Gottschalk, L.A.; Kunkel, R.L.; Wohl, T.; Saenger, E., and Winget, C.N.: Total and half body irradiation. Effect on cognitive and emotional processes. Archs gen. Psychiat. *21:* 574–580 (1969).

Gottschalk, L.A.; Mayerson, P., and Gottlieb, A.: The prediction and evaluation of outcome in an emergency brief psychotherapy clinic. J. nerv. ment. Dis. *144:* 77–96 (1967).

Gottschalk, L.A.; Noble, E.P.; Stolzoff, G.E.; Bates, D.E.; Cable, C.G.; Uliana, R.L.; Birch, H., and Fleming, E.W.: Relationships of chlordiazepoxide blood levels to psychological and biochemical responses; in *Garattini, Mussini, and Randall* Benzodiazepines (Raven, New York 1973).

Gottschalk, L.A.; Springer, K.J., and Gleser, G.C.: Experiments with a method of assessing the variations in intensity of certain psychological states occurring during two psychotherapeutic interviews; in *Gottschalk* Comparative psycholinguistic analysis of two psychotherapeutic interviews (International Universities Press, New York 1961).

Gottschalk, L.A.; Stone, W.N., and Gleser, G.C.: Peripheral versus central mechanisms acounting for anti-anxiety effect of Propranolol. Psychosom. Med. *36:* 47–56 (1974).

Gottschalk, L.A.; Stone, W.N.; Gleser, G.C., and Iacono, J.M.: Anxiety and plasma free fatty acid (FFA) levels. Life Sci. *8:* 61–68 (1969).

Gottschalk, L.A.; Stone, W.N.; Gleser, G.C., and Iacono, J.M.: Anxiety levels in dreams. Relation to changes in plasma free fatty acids. Science *153:* 654–657 (1966).

Gottschalk, L.A. and Uliana, R.L.: A study of the relationship of nonverbal to verbal behavior. Effect of lip caressing on hope and oral references as expressed in the content of speech. Comp. Psychiat. *17* 135–152 (1976a).

Gottschalk, L.A. and Uliana, R.L.: Further studies on the relationship of nonverbal to verbal behavior. Effect of lip caressing on shame, hostility, and other variables as expressed in the content of speech; in *Freedman* Communicative structures and psychic structures (Plenum, New York 1976b).

Gottschalk, L.A.; Winget, C.N., and Gleser, G.C.: Manual of Instructions for using the Gottschalk-Gleser content analysis scales. Anxiety, hostility, and social alienation-personal disorganization (Univ. of California Press, Los Angeles 1969).

Hamilton, M.: The assessment of anxiety states by rating. Br. J. med. Psychol. *32:* 50–55 (1959).

Ivey, M.E. and Bardwick, J.M.: Patterns of affective fluctuation in the menstrual cycle. Psychosom. Med. *30:* 336–348 (1968).

Karacan, I.; Goodenough, D.R.; Shapiro, A., and Starker, S.: Erection cycle during sleep in relation to dream anxiety. Archs gen. Psychiat. *15:* 183–189 (1966).

Lewis, H.B.: Shame and guilt in neurosis (International Universities Press, New York 1971).

Luborsky, L.; Docherty, J.; Todd, T.; Knapp, P.; Mirsky, A., and Gottschalk, L.: A context analysis of psychological states prior to petit mal EEG paroxysms. J. Nerv. ment. Dis. *160:* 282–298 (1975).

Mattsson, N.B.; Williams, H.V.; Rickels, K., and Uhlenhuth, E.H.: Dimensions of symptom distress in anxious neurotic outpatients. Psychopharmacol. Bull. *51:* 19–32 (1969).

McNair, D.M. and Lorr, D.: An analysis of mood in neurotics. J. abnorm. soc. Psychol. *69:* 620–627 (1964).

Parloff, M.B.; Kelman, H.C., and Frank, J.D.: Comfort, effectiveness, and self-awareness as criteria of improvement in psychotherapy. Am. J. Psychiat. *3:* 343–351 (1954).

Perley, J.; Winget, C., and Placci, C.: Hope and discomfort as factors influencing treatment continuance. Comp. Psychiat. *12:* 557–563 (1971).

Rickels, K. and Howard, K.: The physician questionnaire. A useful tool in psychiatric drug research. Psychopharmacologia *17:* 338–344 (1970).

Silbergeld, S.; Brast, N., and Noble, E.P.: The menstrual cycle. A double-blind study of mood, behavior, and biochemical variables with Enovid and a placebo. Psychosom. Med. *33:* 411–428 (1971).

Silbergeld, S.; Manderscheid, R.W.; O'Neill, P.H.; Lamprect, F., and Lorentz, K.Y.: Changes in serum dopamine-beta-hydroxylase activity during group therapy. Psychosom. Med. *37:* 352–359 (1975).

Stone, W.N.; Gleser, G.C.; Gottschalk, L.A., and Iacono, J.M.: Stimulus, affect and plasma free fatty acids. Psychosom. Med. *31:* 331–341 (1969).

Uliana, R.L.: Measurements of black children's affective states and the effect of interviewer's race on affective states as measured through language behavior; unpubl. diss. (1976).

Witkin, H.A.; Lewis, H.B., and Weil, E.: Affective reactions and patient-therapist interactions among more differentiated and less differentiated patients early in therapy. J. Nerv. ment. Dis. *146:* 193–208 (1968).

Wittenborn, J.R.: Do rating scales objectify clinical impression? Comp. Psychiat. *8:* 386–392 (1967).

Wittenborn, J.R.: Reliability, validity, and objectivity of symptom-rating scales. J. nerv. ment. Dis. *154:* 79–87 (1972).

Wittenborn, J.R.: Self-report inventories as criteria for anxiety-allaying medications (unpubl. manuscript, 1974).

Louis A. Gottschalk, MD, Department of Psychiatry and Human Behavior, College of Medicine, University of California, *Irvine, CA 92664* (USA)

Proc. 11th Eur. Conf. Psychosom. Res., Heidelberg 1976
Psychother. Psychosom. *28:* 83–97 (1977)

Differences of Verbal Behaviour in Psychosomatic and Psychoneurotic Patients

M. von Rad, L. Lalucat and F. Lolas

Psychosomatische Universitätsklinik Heidelberg

This investigation was prompted by the observation – which up to now has only been explained in a clinical-casuistic way and has been the subject of many theories – of a certain pattern of symptoms, which can be seen as a typical, but not obligatory, characteristic of psychosomatic patients and which has been given varying titles: 'infantile personality' (*Ruesch,* 1948); 'pensée opératoire' (*Marty et al.,* 1963); alexithymia (*Sifneos,* 1973); psychosomatic phenomenon (*Stephanos,* 1973). It states that, in contrast to 'neurotic' patients, 'psychosomatic' patients show (1) a conspicuous lack of fantasy, (2) a typical 'concretistic' technical manner of thinking, (3) a pronounced incapability to express feelings or even to experience them, and (4) a certain type of 'object relationships' ('projective reduplication').

These observations are at present in part hotly discussed and the reason for this lies, in my opinion, in often premature attempts to place the phenomenon aetiologically – as to whether it is genetically determined (*Heiberg,* 1977), localisable in the brain (*Nemiah,* 1973), related to social status (*Brede,* 1972), explicable psychodynamically (*Marty and de M'Uzan,* 1963; *Stephanos,* 1973), or whether it is, in fact, only a product of the examination situation, of the doctor-patient relationship. What is lacking are empirical investigations which deliver reliable data on the phenomenon by means of a controlled comparison.

The almost complete absence of empirical findings on this subject – the work of *Overbeck* (1975 *and Zepf* (1976) are exceptions – naturally also reflects the almost insoluble methodological dilemma which always presents itself when hypotheses which have been won psychoanalytically are subjected to an empirical examination – and it is a dilemma which our investigation too can naturally not escape from. However, by the same token we believe we are equally justified in presenting empirical findings without a detailed aetiological arrangement or interpretation initially, so that their provisional nature itself can make its contribution towards outlining the phenomenon, while the theoretical classification is intentionally left open. This seems quite legitimate to us, *inter alia,* because the results given here only reflect a certain section of a broader investigation which has been published in part elsewhere (*Vogt et al.,* 1977; *von Rad and Viertmann,* 1976; *Viertmann,* 1976), which is not completely terminated, and will be presented later.

Using the initial suppositions mentioned above as a basis we set up a series of particular hypotheses regarding the verbal behavior of psychosomatic patients which are discussed in detail below.

We set up two comparative groups (in the sequence of their arrival in our out-patient department) each with 40 patients, with (a) wholly dominant psychic complaints ('neurotics'), and (b) somatic complaints with an organ-

Table I. Social data

	I Psychoneurotic patients	II Psychosomatic patients
Parents		
Unskilled	4	8
Independent	13	10
Employed staff	19	16
Professional people	3	4
'Social climber'	9	4
Patients		
Unskilled	1	5
Independent	6	–
Employed staff	16	23
Students	9	5
Professional people	2	2
'Social climber'	15	8
Secondary school	9	19
'O'-level	9	8
'A'-level	15	6
Mode of referral		
Spontaneous	20	8
Physician/other persons	20	32

destructive process ('psychosomatics'), who were parallelised according to (1) intelligence (measured by the Raven test), (2) age, (3) sex, and (4) approximately, social status.

Group I, neurotics, contains only classical neuroses without any important physical complaints; group II, psychosomatic patients, almost only representatives of the 'holy seven'. A condition here was that the organ-destructive psychosomatic symptom had been manifest within the last 2 years. All the patients came to our out-patient department, i.e. they were not bedridden. (For detailed information about the patient collective, in particular with regard to social status, see *von Rad and Viertmann*.)

Table II. Survey of the parallelized samples

	I Psychoneurotics patients n = 40		II Psychosomatic patients n = 40	
Diagnostic categories	narcissistic	6	peptic ulcer	14
	depressive	7	ulcerative colitis	11
	depressive-narcissistic	5	neurodermitis	5
	obsessional	4	asthma	3
	obsessional-depressive	2	psoriasis	2
	hysterical	3	others	5
	hysterical-depressive	11		
	hysterical-obsessive	2		
Age		28.1		28.9
Sex				
Male		14		16
Female		26		24
Intelligence				
Within normal range		29		29
Above normal range		11		11
Socio-economic class (without housewifes), n = 11)				
Lower class		4		8
Middle class		30		27
Mode of referral				
Spontaneous		20		8
Physician/other persons		20		32

We carried out the investigations at various levels: (1) by tests (Rorschach, Giessen and the card 3 BM of the TAT); (2) by an unfinished ('open-end') story, and (3) by an initial psychoanalytical interview.

The story we made up for the purpose of this investigation was read to the patient slowly by the tester twice and in such a way that the sex of the main character in the story agreed with that of the patient. It was stated that it was important for the story to have end. It ran as follows:

'The long walk had made him/her very tired; the rucksack weighed down on his back and his footsteps were heavy. In the morning, when they started out on their family excursion, the sun had been shining and they had all been in good spirits. Now it was late. A dark cloud came up over the horizon and he noticed that he found it a bit sinister. Looking at the cloud, mother said: "How quickly it gets dark here in the mountains – we mustn't lose any time." Only a short time later it was completely dark; a cold wistling wind blew thick fragments of mist across the path. Suddenly he was startled to find that he was alone. Before him there was a fork in the path, around him only the dark night and the howling of the wind.'

We based the draft of the story on the following considerations: (1) It should describe a concrete incident in such a way as to offer an incentive for affective participation by way of identification with the main character, while not leaving the sphere of concrete tangibility. (2) Although the setting is one of realistic action, the background of the story was purposefully left vague and undefined so that it could serve as a screen for projection. (3) The story was intended to indicate a family situation in which, however, only the mother-child relationship is explicit. The patient is thus free to continue the story using two or more persons. (4) The dramatic climax of the story is the loss of an object – in view of the fact that such loss experiences are very frequently described by many authors with regard to the precipitation of the psychosomatic process in many patients.

In making this choice of the instruments of investigation we were led by the following considerations: we wished to investigate at various levels (test alone, test in twos, doctor-patient dyad) and to investigate offshoots of 'fantasy' or 'feelings' under different (optical, acoustic, bipersonal) and less or more 'abstract' conditions or stimulants (concrete picture, more abstract story), in as far as they are reproduced in speech. TAT, story and initial interview were tape-recorded, transcribed and evaluated. The sequence of investigations was always as follows: after the first short contact in the out-patient department the patient was, as usual, asked to come in for the first test (Giessen test) and then given an appointment for another test, in which first of all the Rorschach, then the TAT and finally the 'story' was recorded. Then, at his third appointment, the patient came to a first psychoanalytical interview, the first half hour of which was also taped. The interviews were carried out in such a way that each interviewer met about the same number of patients from each group. It was agreed in a preliminary discussion that each of the six interviewers should run the conversation in his own style but should pay attention to two points: (1) he should conduct the interview concentrating on complaints, i.e. he should get as exact a picture of the complaints as possible, and (2) should ask about the patient's inner experience as the occasion arose: ('How do you feel when you are "depressive"?'; 'What was it like when...?'; 'What went on inside you when...?').

The evaluations were done by an assistant who was not familiar with the hypotheses; the only exception was that the determination of the 'affect-laden' words was done by two of the authors independently and in duplicate. As a unit for investigation we took the first 1,000 words of the *patient* in the interview in order to have the same unit for all of them. (This corresponds roughly to 10 min of an interview.) The total word count from the TAT and the 'story' was taken into account and standardised.

Hypotheses and Results

More Formal Aspects

Word Quantity in TAT and 'Story'
We assumed that the TAT and the 'story' present a different stimulus for the patient's fantasy which would be reflected in the word quantity produced. In accordance with the initial hypotheses it was to be expected that psychosomatic patients would use less words than neurotics as a consequence of their limited access to their fantasy life. In the TAT, patients from group I produced on average 165 words as compared to 132 words in group II (this shows a clear trend, but is *not* significant). In the 'story', group I patients produced on average 211, group II patients 134 words. This is a significant (almost a highly significant) difference ($p < 0.05$). We interpret this difference between TAT and 'story' as follows: the optical stimulus of the TAT picture is more concrete, more graphic, constantly present and can always be referred to, and in this way it responds better to the concretistic thought of psychosomatic patients. In comparison, continuing a story makes higher demands on abstraction capabilities, on the capacity to free oneself from an

object and abandon oneself to fantasy. It can also be assumed that, in terms of development, sight, being a modality which is closer to touch, develops earlier and requires less 'psychic structure' than hearing.

Frequency of the Words 'I' and 'One' in the Interview

As early as 1958, *Shands* demonstrated the above characteristics of psychosomatic patients in a detailed and differentiated manner (with verbatim records); and they were rediscovered later by the French school under the designation pensée opératoire and by the Boston group as alexithymia. His work gives a pointer which we have followed up on a purely formal plane here; namely, that psychosomatic patients are not in a position to use the word 'I' in a meaningful emotional context. In contrast, very different authors (*Brede*, 1972; *Mitscherlich*, 1967; *Overbeck*, 1975) have pointed out time and again that the psychosomatic patient is overadapted and makes an effort to attain outer inconspicuousness. We assumed that both hypotheses should be reflected in a complementary way at word level: that psycho-somatic patients would use the word 'I' less and the word 'one' more than neurotic patients. (The German word 'man' is not completely transferable into English; it means something like 'one', e.g. '*one* should go to school to get a high school diploma' instead of 'I should go to school...'). Group I patients use the word 'I' significantly more frequently ($p < 0.05$) than patients in group II (mean value 67 as compared to 60 times). On the other hand, group I patients used 'one' more rarely than group II patients (on average 3.4 as compared to 5 times); this is a trend in the direction expected, but is not significant.

Frequency of the Auxiliary Verbs (to Have and to Be), of verbs and of Adjectives

We assumed that the closer affinity to concrete things and to action would also be reflected in a less differentiated and simpler word usage. We therefore presumed that psychosomatic patients would use more ('simple') auxiliary verbs than neurotic patients. This was confirmed: group I patients used 61 auxiliary verbs on average, group II patients 76. This difference is highly significant ($p < 0.01$). On the other hand, there is no significant difference in the use of main verbs (87 as compared to 83). This was to be expected and our assumption that the number of adjectives and adverbs, which tend to make out the colour of the language, would differ to the dis-favour of the psychosomatic patients, was also confirmed. In the interview there are on average 36.6 adjectives as compared to 29.5 ($p < 0.01$), in the

TAT 6.7 as compared to 5.4 (*not* significant) and in the 'story' 7.8 as compared to 5.0 (p<0.05).

Frequency of Grammatically Incomplete Sentences

Prompted by *Bernstein*'s (1972) investigations on the 'restricted code', which some authors relate to the verbal behaviour of psychosomatic patients (*Bräutigam,* 1974), we assumed that psychosomatic patients would use incomplete and grammatically incorrect sentences considerably more frequently than neurotic patients. We defined incomplete and incorrect sentences by (1) lack of a subject, verb or important part of the sentence, (2) incorrect constructions of a grammatic or formal nature. This assumption was confirmed: group I patients used on average 36, group II patients on average 45 incomplete sentences. The difference is highly significant (p<0.01). (Naturally agreement in a single, merely formal, parameter is far from being proof of the assumption that psychosomatic patients use a restricted code in *Bernstein*'s sense.)

Table III. Psychoneurotic and psychosomatic patients: quantitative differences in verbal samples (structural aspects)

Patients speech sample (absolute numbers)	I Psychoneurotic patients			II Psychosomatic patients			t	p
	n	mean	SD	n	mean	SD		
Quantity								
Words (TAT)	39	165.97	109.76	35	132.35	117.68	1.27	
Words (story)	38	211.73	144.99	33	134.14	99.85	2.62	<0.05
Frequency								
I[1]	39	67.17	12.86	40	60.84	13.83	2.09	<0.05
One (man)[1]	39	3.46	4.54	40	5.05	4.71	1.52	
Auxiliary verbs[1]	39	61.58	16.72	40	76.05	13.11	4.25	<0.01
Adjectives/adverbs[1]	39	36.56	13.13	40	29.51	8.47	2.82	<0.01
Adjectives/adverbs (TAT)	39	6.28	5.23	35	5.53	3.89	1.05	
Adjectives/adverbs (story)	38	7.76	7.30	33	4.96	3.81	1.93	<0.05
Incomplete sentences[1]	39	36.23	12.75	40	44.97	14.09	2.87	<0.01

[1] Patient's first 1,000 words during the interview.

Dyadic Aspects

Frequency of Speech Sequences of Over 70 Words in the Interview

Prompted by investigations by *Overbeck* (1975), who succeeded in determining some typical differences in the verbal behaviour of neurotic and psychosomatic patients in the course of four psychotherapy treatments, we set up the hypothesis that psychosomatic patients with their pronounced dependence on concrete orientation and on help from the therapist would have more difficulty in producing long word sequences by themselves without interruption. As a unit of measure we chose continuous speech sequences by the patient of more than 70 words, in which the interviewer did not intervene and in which there were no long pauses. This magnitude, which was taken at random, corresponds to a longish unit of speech, of the kind which is liable to occur in a psychoanalytic interview; it is also the lowest limit of a word sample to which the Gottschalk-Gleser method can be applied. In the interview, group I patients used such speech sequences of over 70 words on average 4.4, group II patients 3.5 times. This difference is significant ($p < 0.05$).

Frequency of Interviewer Intervention in the Interview

On the basis of the same assumption (see above), we expected that the therapist would intervene more frequently in interviews with psychosomatic patients. They do this on average 18.7 times with group I patients and 25.1 times with group II patients – the difference is significant ($p < 0.05$) and agrees with *Overbeck*'s (1975) results. We defined as an intervention an expression by the therapist which contains at least one word (or more) – but not semiverbal expressions such as 'hm'. A variance analysis of the six individual interviewers relating to the frequency of the intervention shows that there is no difference between the interviewers in this respect, although they do differ significantly with relation to the amount of words they use. It is an open question as to whether one can relate the agreement in the interventions more to the patients and the difference in the word count more to the individual character of the interviewer. (All the interviewers are psychoanalysts or are undergoing psychoanalytical training. As members of a clinic and participants in a regular out-patient conference it can perhaps be assumed of them that they will have a certain underlying conformity in their way of conducting an initial interview.)

Frequency of 'Affect-Laden' Words in the Interview, the TAT and the 'Story'

One of the basic premises given above states that psychosomatic patients have, in contrast to neurotic patients, difficulties in expressing their feelings.

The investigation of such a complex phenomenon gives rise to many methodo-logical problems, beginning with the choice of the parameter which should be used to investigate it, which cannot be discussed individually here. Basically it is always a question of whether one should examine more 'content analyti-cally' in the classical sense at the purely verbal level or more 'pragmatically', i.e. with more relation to the context. As a trial of this kind using the Gott-schalk-Gleser procedure (with the same patients) will be presented elsewhere, we shall limit ourselves here purely to the verbal level.

We started from the hypothesis that the difficulties which psychosomatic patients have in expressing their feelings must be reflected in some way in their use of words. So we limited ourselves to the verbal level and supposed that psychosomatic patients would use less 'affect-laden' words than neurotic patients. We define as 'affect-laden' only those nouns, adjectives or verbs in which an unambiguous *manifest tone* of feeling is evident. What is decisive is that the tone of feeling explicit in the word is comprehensible without long interpretations being used; it must be direct and colloquial and have an expression of affect, of whatever kind, as a 'primary denotation'. In accor-dance with the differentiation made by *Sifneos* (1975) these would be words which express 'feelings': (e.g. fear, insecurity, hoping, suffering, sinister, happy, etc.). In a few cases of doubt we kept to the meaning given in the Wehrle-Eggers dictionary in which emotional terms are set down lexically. It is clear to us that this in no way gives a quantifying expression of the 'total affective content' of the speech samples, nor can it be taken as an indication of it, as affect can be expressed in many ways without using any affective words in the above sense. The hypothesis was merely that when psycho-somatic patients show this kind of difficulty in expressing affects one would expect to find it reflected at the simple word level *as well*.

Group I patients used 18.6, group II patients 12.9 'affect-laden' words in the interview; the difference is highly significant ($p < 0.01$). In the TAT, group I patients had 4.8 and group II patients 3.2 affect-laden words on average – this difference is not significant. In contrast to this in the 'story', group I patients had an average of 2.7 as compared to group II patients with 1.2 – this difference is significant ($p < 0.05$). If, in addition, one compares the variability of the affect-laden words used, i.e. the number of different affect-laden words in the interview, patients from group I have an average of 10.9 words, group II patients an average of 7.9 words – this difference too is highly significant ($p < 0.01$). In contrast, no difference can be found in the interviewers, on average they used 3.2 affect-laden words with group I patients and 3.3 affect-laden words with group II patients.

Table IV. Psychoneurotic and psychosomatic patients: quantitative differences in verbal samples (dyadic aspects)

Patients speech sample (absolute numbers)	I Psychoneurotic patients			II Psychosomatic patients			t	p
	n	mean	SD	n	mean	SD		
Word sequences (more than 70)[1]	39	4.44	1.96	40	3.51	1.97	2.12	<0.05
Affect-laden words[1]	39	18.67	10.29	40	12.94	7.13	2.89	<0.01
Affect-laden words (TAT)	39	4.87	4.15	35	3.28	4.35	1.62	
Affect-laden words (story)	38	2.79	3.55	33	1.25	1.90	2.39	<0.05
Affect-laden words (variability)[1]	39	10.90	4.92	40	7.92	3.94	2.96	<0.01
Interviewers speech sample (absolute numbers)								
Interventions[1]	39	18.70	10.90	40	25.10	15.50	2.09	<0.05
Affect-laden words[1]	39	3.20	3.55	40	3.30	3.78	0.13	

[1] Patients' first 1,000 words during the interview.

Here again it is interesting to note that it is only in the TAT that the differences are not significant although they follow the tendency expected. Again this could be attributed to the greater 'concreteness' and actual presence of the stimulus discussed above. In how far the high level of significance of the affect-laden words in the interview, which practically equals that of the variability of the affect-laden words, can give an indication that it is not so much the patient's vocabulary which varies, must remain an open question. In contrast we had expected that the differences between the two groups in the variability of the affect-laden words would be still greater. Another interesting point is the result that the interviewers do not use more affect-laden words with psychosomatic patients, although they intervene significantly more often in the light of the 'emptiness of the relationship'.

Discussion

We are of the opinion that the results which we here present are of too general and unspecific a nature for it to be meaningful to attach them to a certain theoretical – perhaps a metapsychological – classification. Neverthe-less, it should be kept in mind that all our findings at least do not contradict the concept of the French school (to which this investigation is indebted for its hypotheses) and, in particular, do not contradict the observations of *McDougall* (1974). However, nothing can be derived or even be considered probable on the basis of our results, be it a question of whether the psycho-somatic phenomenon should be looked as an (inherent or acquired) defi-ciency, whether massive global defence mechanisms (denial) play a decisive role, or whether the psychosomatic symptom should be seen rather as an adaptive measure produced by the ego. One may think that this is a pity, but it is not necessarily so, especially when it is realised that in the often very rigid and schematic form in which they exist at present, none of the theories indicated here have up to now been able to claim that they can explain the specifics of formation of the psychosomatic symptoms adequately. It was always the exceptions, the 'typical ulcer patient' *without* an ulcer, the asthma of Marcel Proust, and not least the experience that we ourselves can fall victim of a psychosomatic disease under certain conditions, which has made us mistrustful of one-dimensional theories, that cannot deny their proximity to the personality typologies of bygone years. Certainly very many different, and, in individual cases, varying conditions must be fulfilled – perhaps a narcissistic deficit based on the failure of the early mother-child dyad, perhaps a specific conflict, but unspecific stresses as well, vulnerability in certain areas of personality ('psychosomatic sector') possibly as a result of a partially unsuccessful desomatisation, and finally no doubt also a proneness which is present at birth (somatic predisposition) which serves as a base to give the factors mentioned above their pathogenicity. The effect of social variables, such as those of social status, with their socially specific interaction patterns, have not yet even been alluded too. In my opinion all these open questions, most of which have hardly been researched, at the present time hinder an overall theory of the development of the psychosomatic symptom that is not largely coloured by speculation.

For this reason we shall only discuss a few apparent methodological problems of the investigation here. A particular problem is the choice of speech behaviour as the object of investigation, as this is naturally dependent on social and cultural status to a high degree. Our patient collective is indeed parallelised exactly with regard to intelligence, but with regard to professions there are slight, and with regard to schooling a number of differences to the disfavour of the psychosomatic group. It is noticeable that this difference is far less marked with the patients' parents, whose verbal ability is decisive for the patients' early childhood socialisation (table I). Thus, there is a certain social discrepancy between the professional status of the parents and that of the psychosomatic patients. This difference, which – viewed in the overall context is only slight – does certainly have some significance in respect of verbal behaviour, despite the parallelised intelligence, but the total weight of it is difficult to assess. We believe, however, that this alone cannot explain the differences in the findings, which are, in part, very distinctive.

Another uncertain factor, the significance of which is hard to determine, is the way in which patients found their way to us – namely the fact that far more psychoneurotic (20) than psychosomatic (8) patients visited our clinic spontaneously. This could express a difference in motivation, which could also have influenced the course of the investigation, although none of the patients were bedridden and they all visited our out-patient department with the desire for psychotherapeutic advice or treatment. In this connection we should at least also make mention of the problem of dependence on the disease, which we have not gone into in detail here and which is also difficult to assess, but perhaps does not play such a significant role at speech level – see *Zepf*'s (1976) findings.

Our investigation also lacks a comparison with a normal population, so that no statements can be made about the direction of a possible 'pathological deviation'. Setting apart the impossibility, in principle, of putting together a 'normal group' and then investigating it by psychoanalytical interview, we would tend here to assume that the differences found between the group of neurotics and the group of psychosomatic patients (which, when taken together, are surprisingly marked) are at least as surprising as the differences which would be found between a normal population and psychosomatic patients (*Zepf*, 1976).

It should be pointed out in particular in this connection that our patient collective is an unselected cross-section of our out-patient department inasmuch as the few patients excluded from the investigation were left out simply for reasons of parallelisation or because they did not fulfil the initial criteria of the investigation. For this reason we consciously omitted a further analysis of the nosological similarities of the patients, who were certainly heterogeneous (ulcer patients in the sense of *Overbeck*'s (1975) typology would have been an example) in order to obtain a more global picture at first.

In view of the marked differences between the two groups of patients, which even we ourselves found surprising, one finding seems to us to be of particular significance. This is the absence throughout of significant results with the TAT card 3 BM. Naturally we must ask in how far the relatively monotonous card with the 'depressive' sunken figure allows relatively less play for the creative fantasy, merely in view of its outer monotony. Here, however, the closer interpretation seems to us to be that it is rather the concrete tangible presence and availability of the optical stimulus which allows the psychosomatic patient to express himself purely quantitatively in the same way as neurotic patients (rather as if he were describing a picture). This interpretation, if it is correct, would not only agree with the hypotheses concerning 'concretistic thought', it would also indirectly explain the differences which arise more clearly in the story, where these conditions of concrete availability do not exist to that degree. Perhaps the findings of significantly increased intervention frequency by the interviewer with psychosomatic patients, which also agree with *Overbeck*'s (1975) findings, can be looked on as an indirect corroboration of *Marty and de M'Uzan*'s (1963) assumption that the analyst should make an 'energetic contribution' in conversation with the psychosomatic patient.

In conclusion, it remains to be said that in the content-analytical examination of different variables using speech samples obtained in different ways, the psychosomatic phenomenon comes to the fore surprisingly clearly (both at word level and in the dyadic variables). In conformity with the specific hypotheses set-up, psychosomatic patients, in contrast to neurotic patients, are found to have (1) a lower word production in the TAT and particularly in the 'story'; (2) more auxiliary verbs, less adjectives and more grammatically incomplete sentences; (3) less use of 'I' and more use of 'one'; (4) they use fewer long speech sequences in the interview, and (5) cause the therapist to intervene more frequently, and finally (6) they use less affect-laden words, in the TAT, particularly in the 'story' and in the interview as well.

We are of the opinion that these findings support the existence of the 'psychosomatic phenomenon' and make the explanation unlikely that it is *only* a product of the interview situation or a countertransference phenomenon. It is, however, urgently necessary to test and differentiate these findings by investigations which take the context more into account. (The findings given here will be presented elsewhere using the Gottschalk-Gleser method and the same verbal sample, *von Rad et al.,* in press).

Acknowledgement

We are very much obliged to our colleagues *H. Becker, K. Brecht, G. Bürckstümmer, M. Drücke, L. Ernst, A. Hildebrandt, H. Lüdeke, K. Mayer and B. Viertmann* for their assistance and for their help in conducting the tests and the interviews.

References

Bernstein, B.: Sozialisation und Sprachverhalten (Schwann, Düsseldorf 1972).

Bräutigam, W.: Pathogenetische Theorien und Wege der Behandlung in der Psychosomatik. Nervenarzt *45:* 354–363 (1974).

Brede, K.: Sozioanalyse psychosomatischer Störungen (Athenäum, Frankfurt 1972).

Cremerius, J.: Psychosomatic disorders: class specific and/or structure-specific neuroses? Psychother. Psychosom. (in press, 1977).

Gottschalk, L.A. and Gleser, G.C.: The measurement of psychological states through the content analysis of verbal behavior (University of California Press, Berkeley 1969).

Heiberg, A.: Alexithymia – an inherited trait? Psychother. Psychosom. (in press, 1977).

Hoppe, H.: Die Trennung der Gehirnhälften. Psyche *29:* 919–940 (1975).

MacLean, P.D.: Psychosomatic disease and the 'visceral brain'. Psychosom. Med. *11:* 338–353 (1949).

Marty, P. et M'Uzan, M. de: La 'pensée opératoire'. Revue fr. Psychoanal. *27:* suppl., pp. 1345–1356 (1963).

Marty, P.; M'Uzan, M. de et David, C.: L'investigation psychosomatique. Presses univ. de France, 1963).

McDougall, J.: The psychosoma and the psychoanalytic process. Int. Rev. Psycho-Anal. *1:* 437–459 (1974).

Mitscherlich, A.: Krankheit als Konflikt. II (Suhrkamp, Frankfurt 1967).

Nemiah, J.C.: Psychology and psychosomatic illness: reflections on theory and research methodology. Psychother. Psychosom. *22:* 106–111 (1973).

Nemiah, J. and Sifneos, P.: Affect and fantasy in patients with psychosomatic disorders; in *Hill* Modern trends in psychosomatic medicine (Butterworths, London 1970a).

Nemiah, J.C. and Sifneos, P.: Psychosomatic illness: a problem in communication. Recent research in psychosomatics. Psychother. Psychosom. *18:* 154–160 (1970b).

Overbeck, G.: Objektivierende und relativierende Beiträge zur 'Pensée opératoire' der französischen Psychosomatik. Habilitationsschrift, Giessen (1975).

Overbeck, G. und Brähler, E.: Eine Beobachtung zum Sprechverhalten von Patienten mit psychosomatischen Störungen. Vorläufiger Bericht. Dynam. Psychiat. *7:* 100–108 (1974).

Rad, M. von; Drücke, M.; Knauss, W.; Lolas, F.: Alexithymia: a comparative study of verbal behavior in psychosomatic and psychoneurotic patients; in *Gottschalk* The content analysis of verbal behavior: further studies, New York Spectrum Publications (in press).

Rad, M. von und Viertmann, B.: Psychosomatische und psychoneurotische Patienten im Vergleich. III. Selbst- und Idealbild im Giessen-Test. Unpublished manuscript (1976).

Ruesch, J.: The infantile personality. Psychosom. Med. *10:* 134–144 (1948).

Shands, H.: An approach to the measurement of suitability for psychotherapy. Psychiat. Q. *32:* 501–522 (1958).

Sifneos, P.: The prevalence of 'alexithymic' characteristics in psychosomatic patients. Psychother. Psychosom. *22:* 255–262 (1973).

Sifneos, P.: Problems of psychotherapy of patients with alexithymic characteristics and physical disease. Psychother. Psychosom. *26:* 65–70 (1975).

Stephanos, S.: Analytisch-psychosomatische Therapie. Jb. Psychoanal., suppl. 1 (1973).

Viertmann, B.: Eine empirische Untersuchung zum 'psychosomatischen Phänomen' mit Hilfe des Giessen-Tests; Diss. Heidelberg (1976).

Vogt, R.; Bürckstümmer, G.; Ernst, L.; Meyer, K., and Rad, M. von: Differences of fantasy life in psychosomatic and psychoneurotic patients. Psychother. Psychosom. (in press, 1977).

Wehrle-Eggers: Deutscher Wortschatz 1 und 2 (Fischer, Frankfurt 1968).

Wolff, H.H.: The contribution of the interview situation to the apparent restriction of fantasy life and emotional experience in psychosomatic patients. Psychother. Psychosom. (in press, 1977).

Zepf, S.: Die Sozialisation des psychosomatischen Kranken (Campus, Frankfurt 1976).

Dr. *M. von Rad,* Psychosomatische Universitätsklinik, Thibautstrasse 2, *D-6900 Heidelberg* (FRG)

Proc. 11th Eur. Conf. Psychosom. Res., Heidelberg 1976
Psychother. Psychosom. *28:* 98–105 (1977)

Differences in Phantasy Life of Psychosomatic and Psychoneurotic Patients

R. Vogt, G. Bürckstümmer, L. Ernst, K. Meyer, and M. von Rad

Psychosomatische Universitätsklinik Heidelberg

Our study started from the hypothesis that had emerged from clinical experience that psychosomatic patients have a great difficulty to express their feelings, to experience psychic conflict, to have ideas in psychotherapy and that they tend to a mode of thinking which is rather poor, mechanistic, lacks emotional nuances and is dependent on the concrete situation. This was called 'pensée opératoire' by *Marty and de M'Uzan* (1963), 'alexithymia' by *Sifneos and Nemiah* (1970) and described in German psychosomatic research as 'the psychosomatic phenomenon'.

A more detailed psychological analysis of these observations seems to reveal a close relationship between the way of perceiving, imagining, feeling and thinking connected with this phenomenon and what we designate as phantasy.

If we try and disentangle the concept of phantasy from the relatively vague colloquial and clinical usage and give it a more precise definition, we had best turn to psychoanalysis which among all pyschological and psycho-pathological disciplines has by far provided most of the contributions for understanding and clarification of phantasy.

According to *Freud,* phantasy has as main metapsychological characteristics the following: from the topological aspect three different kinds of fantasies must be distinguished:

(a) The conscious daydream fantasies, which are of a wish fulfilling nature and highly structured in terms of the prevailing secondary process.

(b) Presconscious fantasies which cannot become conscious at once but under specific conditions only and which too are mainly subject to the secondary process.

(c) The unconscious fantasies (in the systematic sense) which belong to the system of the unconscious and are subject to the primary process, where – in the view of *Sandler and Nagera* (1966) – they lose their wish-fulfilling functions and, getting an increased instinctual charge, rather acquire the character of unfulfilled needs. Whenever structured fantasies appear in the unconscious, their elaborate organisation does not stem from the id, but from the ego. These sort of fantasies have preserved their differentiated form on their way from consciousness via the preconscious to the unconscious. According to *Freud,* imaginative activity is primarily an ego activity the instinctual motivation of which proceeds from the id and some inhibiting influences it has to cope with come from the super-ego.

The most essential psychic functions of phantasy are:

(1) An easier discharge of drive tension through its wish fulfilling function (*Freud,* 1900).

(2) The postponement of an immediate drive-determined reaction, as phantasy intermediates between need and action thus rendering possible trial action, id is a rehearsal of an anticipated situation at the representation and thinking level.

Imaginative activity thus becomes an eminent factor for adaptation to reality (*Beres,* 1960) as it makes the individual more independent from the concrete situation liable to provoke immediate motor action. In a similar way the imaginative faculties in the child develop parallel to his capacity to get gradually detached from the real presence of the need satisfying object and to gain autonomy. This process can only fully develop in the child when there are no serious disturbances in his relationship with his mother.

When major traumata occur in the mother-child dyad, this maturational process which implies the gradual detachment from the mother by way of introjecting her into the super-ego and the ego ideal can be so inhibited that an extreme dependence on the real presence of the mother or her substitutes remains throughout.

Yet, it is this enormous dependence on the concrete presence of the love object that is consistently described as a specific characteristic of psychosomatic patients. There is in fact a close psycho-genetic link between early disruptions of the object-relation as repeatedly stated for psychosomatic patients by various psychosomatic theories and the inhibition of phantasy development.

This psychoanalytical concept which I could but outline and which is necessarily incomplete was operationalized within the framework of the Rorschach test to a Rorschach phantasy syndrome and examined on the two experimental groups described by Dr. *von Rad.*

One group consists of 40 psychoneurotics without organic troubles, the other of 40 psychosomatics suffering from organic lesions. Both groups were parallelized with the non-verbal intelligence test – the Advanced Progressive Matrices by Raven – as to the subjects general intelligence and correspond too in terms of age, sex and social class.

Taking into account the level of intelligence when matching experimental groups has been found to be necessary as in our experience the level of intelligence in the average and subaverage domain has an impact on the distinctness of the phantasy syndrome.

These two groups were investigated into the Raven and Rorschach by *Gottfried Bürckstümmer, Karin Meyer* and *Lucia Ernst*. The number of subjects tested by each examiner was the same in both groups in order to keep constant the tester's influence we have to reckon with in the Rorschach for both groups. I then scored the protocols according to the scoring system by *Klopfer* without knowing to which group the subject belonged. This procedure was meant to avoid any falsification of scoring by our existing hypotheses which – in view of the questionable objectivity of Rorschach scoring generally constitutes one of its major risks.

The Rorschach phantasy syndrome is an operationalization of the viewpoints I just explained and was set up with the observations made by *Rorschach* (1921), *Bohm* (1957), *Klopfer* (1954, 1956, 1967), *von Zeppelin* (1969), and finally based in our personal clinical experience.

It includes the following 5 scoring categories: human movement, the proportion of form determined color responses to less form-determined color responses, the number of original responses, the total number of responses, and the variability of content.

Rorschach phantasy syndrome

M	>	3.0	M = motion (human movement)
FC: (CF + C)	>	0.5	FC = FormColor; CF = ColorForm
			C = Color
0%	>	25	0% = percentage of original responses
R	>	20	R = number of all responses
Con%	>	25	Con% = variability of content

Rorschach experience type

Sum M : Sum C

Restricted experience type

M : Sum C = 0:0 or 0:1 or 1:0 or 1:1

Dilated experience type

M : Sum C = 5:5 or more

For statistical reasons we were compelled to define index values for the fully developed phantasy. The above Rorschach phantasy syndrome displays the minimum conditions for clearly recognizable imaginative activity.

The number of M responses should be greater than 3.0, the proportion of FC:(CF + C) should be either 0.5 or more. The percentage of original responses – that means very rare responses – should be more than 25. The total number of responses given for the 10 Rorschach cards should be greater than 20. The variability of content is good if more than 25% of the content categories refer neither to man nor to animal and if these responses can be assigned to three different content categories at least.

We now have to check whether there is agreement between the psycho-analytical concept of phantasy that was briefly outlined and its operationalization to the Rorschach scores just explained.

Human movement as a concept is the most complex category of the whole Rorschach test. Rorschach himself interpreted human movement as a hint to the special emphasis laid on internal representations, values and fantasies. This interpretation was largely confirmed partly by clinical, parly by ex-perimental findings and has been further differntiated by *Klopfer* on the basis of psychoanalytical ego psychology to indicate a successful integration of id impulses into the ego resulting in the ability to postpone drive dis-charge, to engage in trial action at the representation level, and to come into contact with the emotional albeit conflict-laden sides of internal impulses. Thus, the main requirement of our theoretical definition of phantasy is fulfilled.

As to the proportion FC:(CF + C), it must be generally stressed that Rorschach considered color to be an equivalent of emotions in so far as it indicates a psychic readiness to react to environmental stimuli. The way a person treats colour in his Rorschach interpretations is supposed to be the same he treats his feelings towards the environment. The relative impact of form in color interpretations provides some clues as to the structure of and the degree of control over these feelings. From determined color responses,

FC therefore represent emotions that are controlled and adapted to the environmental conditions. They indicate the persons readiness to get involved with other people and to sympathetically understand them. The more the form component recedes and color comes to the force as in the case of CF and C, the more uncontrolled and affect-laden is the subject's behavior, the more he is dominated by a self-centered and impulsive tendency to immediately discharge psychic tensions through motor action. The proportion FC: (CF + C) thus translates the relationship between adapted and impulsive emotional life. The meaning of this proportion first points in a direction similar to that of human movement, i.e., that of polarity : postponement of drive discharge-immediate impulsive drive satisfaction, but this proportion does take into account the person's relations to the outer world thus covering another essential aspect of our theoretical definition; phantasy is constantly activated and supplied to its material by the outer world.

In fact, the elements of phantasy have been direct perceptions in the past. The number of original responses which should exceed 25% of all responses means that well-functioning imaginative activity should not only allow for collective and common concepts but for individual, i.e., rare ones as well. The total number of responses includes the quantitative factor of a certain amount of representations derived from the relatively unstructured stimulus material of the Rorschach cards. The variability of content marks a certain degree of concept abundance which a distinct imaginative faculty should be able to draw upon.

Finally, we have to discuss the experience type. It consists of the proportion of the number of responses containing human movement M to the weighted sum of color responses, sum C. As previously described, human movement answers imply a mode of experiencing mainly dependent on representations, internal values and fantasies. To designate such an attitude Rorschach adopted the term introversion from Jung. Color, on the contrary, marks the person's interest for and attitude towards the outer world and represents in Rorschach's view extraversion. The experience type includes the polar tension between the concerns for the inner and the outer world. On the whole the experience type serves as an indicator for the range of experiences available to the individual.

The Rorschach phantasy syndrome and the experience type were used to check the five hypotheses that follow:

Hypothesis 1. The distinct phantasy syndrome is significantly more frequent with psychoneurotics than with psychosomatics. For statistical reasons our sample being too small we could not base our comparison on all

five categories of the phantasy syndrome at once but had to confine ourselves to three scores at a time. According to our theoretical definition, human
movement and the proportion FC:(CF + C) being of special importance,
the reduced phantasy syndrome always contained both basic variables M
and the proportion FC:(CF + C) supplemented either by the number of
original responses or the total number of responses or the content variability.
Hypothesis 1 could be confirmed at the 5% level by inference statistical
method and at the 0.1% level by descriptive methods. The statistical method
applied is the configuration-frequency-analysis by Lienert and Krauth. This
recent statistical nonparametrical procedure, published in June 1973, is
particularly well adapted to Rorschach studies insofar as it makes possible a
precise quantitative comparison of complex syndromes without degrading
the test by the atomistic distorting approach which is accountable for the
restricted validity of so many Rorschach studies.

Hypothesis 2. With depressive and anancastic psychoneurotics, the
phantasy syndrome is significantly less distinct than with hysterical or
narcissistic forms of neuroses. Confirmation of this assumption was obtained
at the 0.1% level. Again, the statistical method used is the configuration-
frequency-analysis.This hypothesis reflects the clinical experience that the
existence of marked depressive traits may eventually alter the Rorschach
record of such neurotic persons in a way that the test reveals but the depressive traits the remainder of the personality hardly appearing any more
in the test protocol. This seems to point to certain limitations of the Rorschach technique. The clinician knows very well how to distinguish between
alexithymus and depressive traits during the interview, most probably the
Rorschach does not delineate them.

Hypothesis 3. The restricted experience type is significantly more frequent in psychosomatic than in psychoneurotics. The confirmation was
obtained at the 0.1% level. As compared to psychoneurotics, psychosomatics
would consequently have significantly restricted experience modalities in the
sphere of experiencing the self, imagination, phantasy and contact with other
people.

Hypothesis 4. The dilated experience type is found more frequently in
psychoneurotics than in psychosomatics. This assumption could be confirmed at the 5% level. Psychologically speaking, this means an abundant emotional ability to experience the self and the outer world. Psychoneurotics display these faculties to a significantly greater extent than psychosomatics.

Hypothesis 5. The simultaneous occurrence of human movement and
color in the same Rorschach interpretation is far more frequent with psycho-

neurotics than with psychosomatics. We could in fact discover such a trend which, however, is not yet statistically significant.

As the last step of the investigation, a heuristic hierarchial configuration-frequency-analysis with the Rorschach phantasy syndrome was carried out for the two groups. It yielded 22 different highly significant trait combinations for the psychoneurotics yet only 4 of them for the psychosomatics. As these results turn out to be a new modification of the hypotheses we started from, a fully valid interpretation presupposes further clarification by another investigation. Nevertheless, and despite all necessary reserves, we may well venture to assume that psychoneurotics show far more different types of fantasies than psychosomatic patients.

Finally, if we try and critically resume this study we must stress a number of points that might restrict the importance of the findings. These are the following:

(1) Unwarranted objectivity of Rorschach scoring constitutes a delicate problem the most distorting repercussions of which could be counterbalanced by scoring the protocols without knowing the respective group of the subject. However, a certain amount of uncertainty still remains and this factor need further clarification.

(2) The sample of psychosomatic patients is not yet representative of all psychosomatic troubles recognized as such. It contained an unproportionate number of patient suffering from ulcer and colitis (24 of 40) hence the generalizations we made here when speaking of a general psychosomatic syndrome need further experimental verification.

(3) In experimental investigations like the study we reported on, it is decisive to ascertain the highest possible degree of correspondence between clinical observation, the theoretical basis and specification it is given when connected to a theory of personality and finally their retranslation into an operational definition which comes up to experimental conditions.

Finally, as concerns our investigation we are not quite sure whether those clinical observations described in terms of pensée opératoire', alexithymia and psychosomatic phenomenon are sufficiently represented by the psychoanalytical concept of phantasy. Furthermore, it seems that the psychoanalytical definition of phantasy is more complex in some of its aspects than the Rorschach phantasy syndrome and vice versa.

In spite of these limitations that call for a cautious evaluation of the results reported here, this Rorschach study may be regarded as an experimental confirmation of the fact that in psychosomatic patients alexithymeous traits such as a relative lack of imaginative activity and hence a restricted ability to experience emotions and express them both in the encounter with the self and with other people are significantly more marked than in psychoneurotic patients.

References

Beres, D.: Perception, imagination and reality. Int. J. Psychoanal. *41:* 327–334 (1960).

Bohm, E.: Lehrbuch der Rorschach-Psychodiagnostik (Huber, Bern 1957, aufl. 1972).

Freud, S.: Die Traumdeutung, Vol. 2/3 GW (1900).

Klopfer et al.: Developments in the Rorschach technique, vol. 1 (World Book Company, New 1ork 1954).

Klopfer et al.: Developments in the Rorschach technique, vol. 2, (World Book Company, New York 1956).

Marty, P. et M'Uzan, M. de: La pensée opératoire. Revue fr. Psychoanal. *27:* 345–356 (1963).

Rorschach, H.: Psychodiagnostik (Bircher, Bern 1921).

Sandler, J. and Nagera, H.: Einige Aspekte der Metapsychologie der Phantasie. Psyche *20:* 188–221 (1966).

Sifneos, P.E.: The prevalence of 'alexithymic' characteristics in psychosomatic patients. Psychother. Psychosom. *22:* 255–262 (1973).

Sifneos, P.E.: A reconsideration of psychodynamic mechanisms in psychosomatic symptom formation in view of recent clinical observations. Psychother. Psychosom. *24:* 151–155 (1974).

Zeppelin, I. von: Die Rorschachtestvariablen B-Antworten und b-Antworten als Merkmale des Phantasierens und Agierens in neurotischen Abwehrprozessen. Bull. psychol. Inst. Univ. Zürich *2:* 109–119 (1969).

Dr. *Rolf Vogt,* Psychosomatische Klinik, Abteilung Medizinische Psychologie, Mönchhofstrasse 15a, *D-6900 Heidelberg 1* (FRG)

Proc. 11th Eur. Conf. Psychosom. Res., Heidelberg 1976
Psychother. Psychosom. *28:* 106–117 (1977)

How to Operationalize Alexithymic Phenomena – Some Findings from Speech Analysis and the Giessen Test (GT)

G. Overbeck

I believe it has become a matter of generally recognized clinical knowledge that in initial interviews and in psychotherapeutic treatment among patients with psychosomatic disorders there are a number of patients whose distinguishing characteristics are appropriately rendered with the term 'alexithymia' or 'pensée opératoire'. While very many subtle observations and casuistic descriptions have been offered, relatively little is known about the objectification of these characteristics in patients with psychosomatic disorders. For this reason I should like to bring forth the results, briefly summarized, of a series of my own research (a complete review is contained in *Overbeck, 1975*). which seem to objectively confirm the existence of the alexithymia or pensée opératoire. In the first part of this paper I shall present the results within a comparative framework, that is, I shall discuss the differences which seem to exist between alexithymic patients and neurotic patients. The results of the second part should serve as a contribution to the question as to whether all patients who suffer a certain psychosomatic illness show signs of the alexithymia, or whether this only holds true for certain subgroups of patients.

Part I

First we selected two patients, who, according to impressions gained in the initial interviews very clearly presented signs of what is generally understood as the alexithymia or pensée opératoire: a poor ability to fantasize, concrete thinking, and empty interpersonal relationships. We recorded the conversations with these patients in their individual therapy sessions on tape, and investigated them as part of a larger psycholinguistic research program. With the help of the Giessen Speech Analyser, a formal speech criterium was automatically investigated, namely the speech-pause-behavior of patient and therapist. For an exact explanation of the research methodology and complete results see *Overbeck et al.* (1974), *Junker et al.* (1974), *Overbeck and Brähler* (1974), and *Brähler et al.* (1974). We were interested in finding out in what way the subjective experiences of therapy form a certain objectively measureable speech-pause-behavior between patients and therapists. Alongside this attempt to substantiate casuistic observations with objective data (an additional attempt towards objectification was carried out with the same patients with the help of a session therapy report – see *Overbeck and Brähler,* 1975, 1976), we began to isolate the special features of these two therapies, which we named A1 and A2, by comparing them with two other therapies, B1

Table I. The Giessen Speech Analyser ascertains the mean duration, the absolute frequency, and the percentage of the entire therapy hour of 12 categories

1 Pauses beginning after the therapist has finished speaking and ending when the patient starts speaking (TOP)

2 Pauses beginning after the patient has finished speaking and ending when the therapist starts speaking (POT)

3 Pauses beginning after the therapist has finished speaking and anding when the therapist starts speaking (TOT)

4 Pauses beginning after the patient has finished speaking and ending when the patient starts speaking (POP)

5 Speech of the patient which begins after a pause and ends with a pause (OPO)

6 Speech of the patient which begins after a pause and ends with speech of the therapist (OPT)

7 Speech of the patient which begins after speech of the therapist and ends with a pause (TPO)

8 Speech of the patient which begins after speech of the therapist and ends with speech of the therapist (TPT)

9 Speech of the therapist which begins after speech of the patient and ends with speech of the patient (PTP)

10 Speech of the therapist which begins after speech of the patient and ends with a pause (PTO)

11 Speech of the therapist which begins after a pause and ends with speech of the patient (OTP)

12 Speech of the therapist which begins after a pause and ends with a pause (OTO)

and B2. This second group of therapies presented, as it were, the other extreme, that is, they offered a wealth of fantasy, liveliness, and dynamic interactions. In this way we obtained the following important results for therapies A1 and A2, the therapies with the alexithymic patients.

Silence Categories

(1) The amount of silence during the entire hour of therapy is on the average considerably higher throughout all therapy sessions and often amounts to between 40 and 50% of the total time (as opposed to 28–35% in the other two therapies). Similarly, the percentages of all silence categories (TOP, TOT, POP, POT) (table I) in therapies A1 and A2 were considerably above those of therapies B1 and B2 (fig. 1).

(2) The percentage of the reaction times during the entire hour of therapy with these patients amounts to nearly two to three times that of those patients in the other therapy groups (on the average 8.2–12% as opposed to 3.6–4.9%). This means that the pauses in which the patient says something after the therapist has spoken are much longer with these patients (fig. 2).

(3) The percentage of the therapist's initiative time during the entire hour of therapy is nearly twice as high (10–11.1% as opposed to 5.1–6.8%). This means that the therapist begins to speak again after a long pause which was preceded by his own speech much more often (fig. 3).

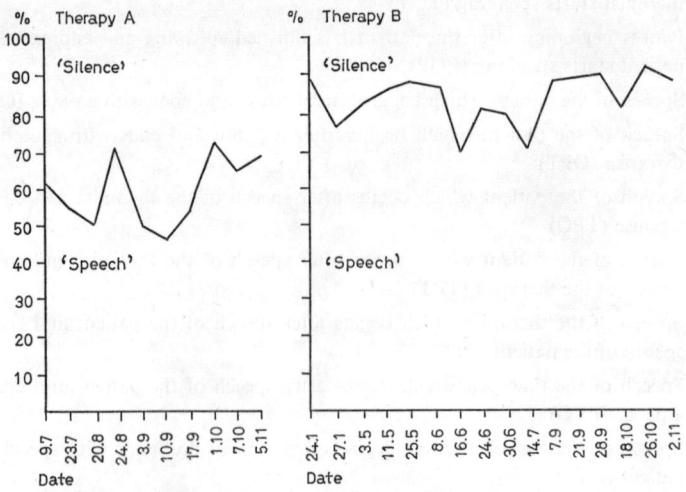

Fig. 1. Proportion of speech: silence per hour.

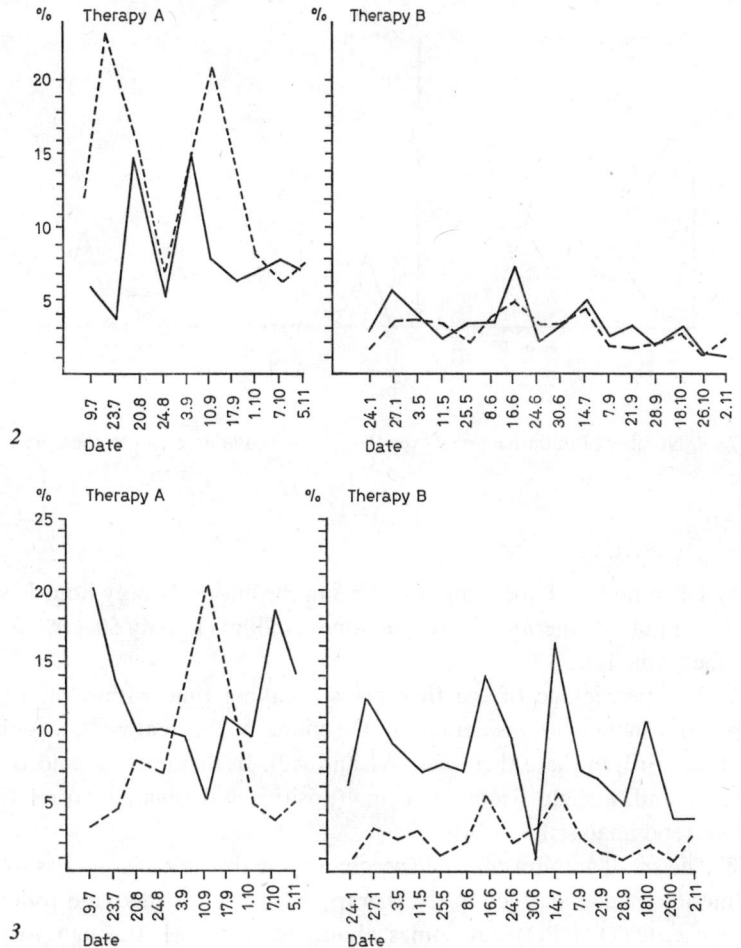

Fig. 2. Percentage of patients' (—) and therapists' (---) reaction time in total duration of conversation.

Fig. 3. Percentage of patients' (—) and therapists' (---) initiative time in total duration of conversation.

(4) The number of very long pauses (longer than 10 sec), whether after the patient's own speech or after the therapist's (initiative and reaction times) is significantly higher among these patients (fig. 4).

(5) Long pauses (longer than 10 sec) in these therapeutic sessions are ultimately broken by the therapist.

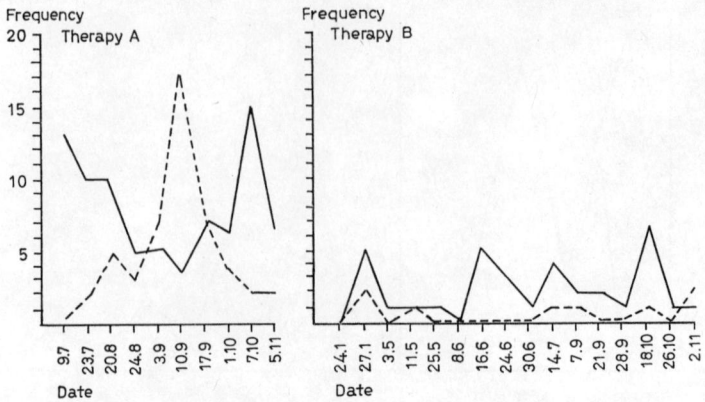

Fig. 4. Number of initiative times over 10 sec. —— = Patient; --- = therapist.

Speech Categories

(6) The amount of speaking time during the entire therapy hour is very much lower in these therapies and sometimes amounts to only 50–60% of the total time (table II).

(7) The percentage of the therapist's speaking time within the entire therapy hour increases considerably in the course of the treatment, especially in the first third, in these therapies (A1 and A2). In therapies B1 and B2 on the other hand, a slight decrease occurs (positive and negative correlations with the trend analysis).

(8) The small amount of total speech in these therapies is due less to too little 'monologueing' (speech in the therapy which is preceded and followed by a pause, OTO, OPO) but comes about, for example, through varying

Table II. Mean percentages of speech and silence

Therapy	Therapists' speech time	Patients' speech time	'Silence'	'Speech'
A 1	20.2	27.6	52.1	47.9
A 2	23.8	27.0	49.1	50.9
B 1	23.8	40.8	35.6	64.6
B 2	27.7	44.3	27.9	72.1

Table III. Influence of various speech categories on total speech time (in %)

Therapy	OPO a. OTO	Sum of cat. 6–11	Speech
A 1	36.4	11.4	47.8
A 2	35.3	15.7	51.0
B 1	43.6	21.0	64.6
B 2	41.2	30.8	72.0

scores in the 'interruption speech' (TPT, PTP) which here only amounts up to 1.4% (as opposed to 4.6%). If one also adds up and includes the remaining 'dialogue variables' (6–11), that is, all of the contributions of one partner to the conversation which are immediately followed by a contribution of the other, then the special nature of the conversation in these therapies becomes even clearer. While the 'dialogue variables' only amount to between 11.4 and 15.7% of the speech in these therapies, in the other therapies they come to almost twice as much (20.0–30.8%; table III).

The most striking aspect of the overall results of this study is the considerable proportion of silence in the therapy sessions with alexithymic patients. Even if silence in individual therapy sessions was understandable psychoanalytically, that is, in the sense of instinctual satisfaction and from the viewpoint of ego psychology (*Overbeck et al.,* 1974), these meaningful silences occurred far less often than the empty silences. Both therapist and patient experienced this as a noticeable lack of ideas, there was simply nothing to say, everything was 'normal'. Outside the therapy sessions the patients, for the most part, had *experienced* nothing, rather they had *done* this or that. After they had reported about their activities (painting, remodeling, family celebrations, club events, etc.), they also found it very difficult to experience, that is, to fantasize, have feelings, or reflect during the therapy session. The relatedness between therapist and patient increasingly faced the danger of being broken off; boredom and emptiness expanded. The therapist's speech-silence-behavior becomes understandable in view of the patient's helplessness. He helps after longer pauses which follow the patient's speech if the patient is unable to continue himself (therapist's high reaction time), begins to speak again after pauses which follow his own speech (therapist's high initiative time), and intervenes supportively in the long pauses (therapist breaks off the long pauses). This active behavior on the part of the therapist corresponds entirely to the patient's expectations of common actions.

That the therapist talks more and more in the early phase of these therapies also points to a change in the therapist towards greater speech activity. This is utilized in part by the therapist for the purpose of demonstration (c.f. 'Sprach-Con-Ego' by *El-Safti,* 1973), that is, he tries to enrich and raise the patient's barren reports to the level of experience by offering him many colorful ideas (*Freyberger,* 1976). In doing so he notices that in sessions in which he spoke a lot, the patients spoke a lot as well, when he was silent, the patients did the same. In other words, the patients followed passively, almost mechanically, the therapist's speech behavior (this affected the data objectively in such a way that the patients as well as the therapist both showed high variability in all speech and silence categories; at the same time almost all the therapist's scores correlated very highly with those of the patients (*Brähler et al.,* 1974). This subjectively experienced atmosphere of controlled, stiff, and almost automatic conversation behavior is further reinforced by the 'block speech' which forms the majority of the dialogue (you say something, then I say something, and just as much as you said). A lively conversation, on the other hand, with immediate replies, reinforcements and pressing ideas hardly comes about. This last phenomenon finds expression in the small proportion of 'dialogue' speech variables in these therapies.

Altogether one can probably find a certain objective confirmation in the results of the speech-pause-behavior of that which therapists experience in conversations with alexithymic patients. It would be premature to draw further conclusions, however, until results of investigations with larger numbers of cases become available, and other methodological problems such as differences in therapists, sex, social class, and illness are taken into consideration. This means that although one of our two alexithymic patients had essential hypertension and the other suffered a functional gastrointestinal disorder, it cannot be said that the alexithymic phenomenon stands in direct relation to the presence of the psychosomatic disorders, at least not from the results of these investigations alone, which at best provide evidence in this direction.

Part II

We are so much the more inclined to these cautious interpretations since we have more clearly seen that nor nearly all patients with psychosomatic disorders show signs of the alexithymia or pensée opératoire. I come now to the second part of my paper, namely to the question whether alexithymic patients constitute only one subgroup of patients with a psychosomatic disorder. We investigated this question further in about 90 chronic ulcer patients. On the one hand, we had observed alexithymic patients among this group; on the other hand, we had observed a diversity of other personality structures as well (*Overbeck and Biebl*, 1975; *Overbeck*, 1975; *Eckensberger et al.*, 1976). We therefore looked for a method with which the alexithymia or pensée opératoire could be objectified with larger collectives of patients. Since the Giessen test describes how a patient sees his psychic structure, his basic mood and his social relationships, this test seemed to provide hope of giving information about the question of the alexithymic phenomenon. We were eager to see whether statistical analysis on the basis of the GT would indicate the existence of such a thing as an alexithymic subgroup.

First, with the help of statistical analysis (factor analysis according to the R technique), we determined the dimensions of self-perception which play a main role among ulcer patients in the Giessen test. These are: dependency conflicts, depressive withdrawal, social failure, overadjustment, and problems in interpersonal relationships. These 5 factors never appear simultaneously and are of varying significance for the individual patient. When patients with

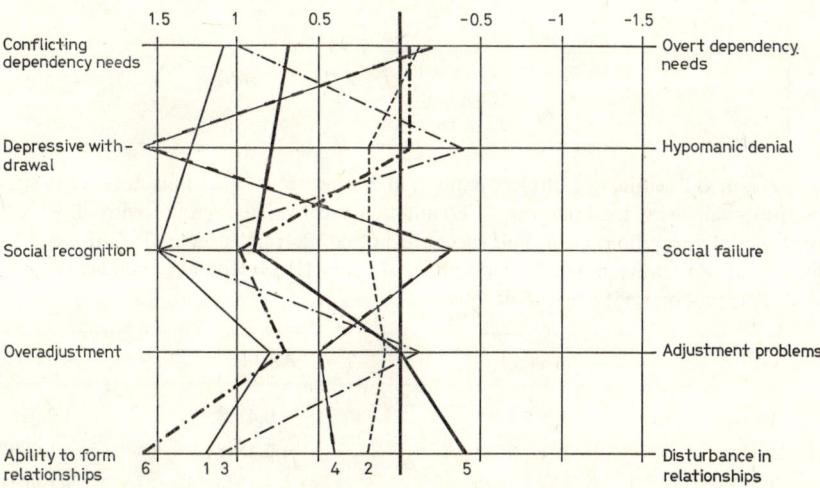

Fig. 5. GT profiles of 6 subgroups of chronic ulcer patients (selected items). Group 1: neurotic-pseudonormal (—); group 2: sociopathic (---); group 3: oral-passive (–·–); group 4: neurotic depressive (---); group 5: active-overcompensating (—); group 6: alexithymic (–·–).

similar scores are compared with regard to these 5 factors (Q-Factor-Analysis; placement according to highest loading), 6 groups of patients emerge which differ significantly from one another and which, in a few dimensions, are entirely opposing (fig. 5). In order to differentiate the self-perceptions reported among the 6 subgroups more exactly, we employed another method, the gradual discriminance analysis (–BMD 07 M). With the help of those items in the Giessen test which differentiated especially well among the 6 subgroups (18 of the 40), the ulcer patients are arranged on the basis of their self-statements in a 3-dimensional space so that their placement in one of the diagnostic subgroups with a higher rate of correct assignment becomes possible. We have labeled the 3 axes of this 3-dimensional space according to

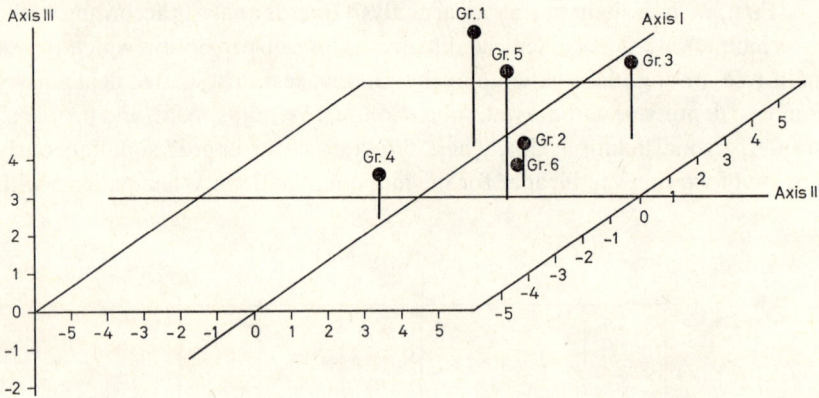

Fig. 6. GT self-images of ulcer patients in 3-dimensional discriminant space (6 subgroups by similarity, total number = 79) and numerical value of group centroid. Axis I: psychosocial integration: posit. Pol: successful; negat. Pol: failed. Axis II: Drive regulation: posit. Pol: low; negat. Pol: pronounced. Axis III: Internalised conflict-solving: posit. Pol: pronounced; negat. Pol: low.

Group	Axis I	Axis II	Axis III
1	+2.3585	−0.4178	+2.9267
2	+0.4230	+2.4598	+1.0982
3	+2.5970	+3.5526	+1.9881
4	−1.1497	−0.1959	+1.2280
5	−0.1638	+2.5662	+3.4297
6	+2.4249	+0.7241	−0.3112

combinations of certain Giessen-Test-Items as follows: Axis I – Psychosocial Integration; Axis II – Drive Regulation; Axis III – Internalized Conflict Solving (fig. 6).

On the basis of these 3 discriminant axes and the scores in the 5 factors of self-perception mentioned above, as well as additional information (*Eckensberger et al.,* 1976) on anamnesis, social class, the patient's view of his illness, and his physical ailments, we believe we have been able to identify the alexithymic ulcer patients in group 6.

Group 6 (Alexithymic Ulcer Patients)

The extraordinary thing about this group is the 'nothing' which attracts our attention in the initial interviews. The interview reports of these patients are empty, brief, and sterile. Since these patients do not experience conflicting dependency needs (Axis III) and do not openly act out (Axis II), one can assume that they do not intensely experience either their needs or their conflicts. Similarly, the patients give an uncharacteristic, diffuse picture of their bodily ailments in the BSB (a questionnaire about bodily ailments), which could point to a weak perception or an insensitivity in these patients towards their own bodies, or perhaps reflects an attitude which denies the existence of their illness, something one often finds with such patients. Patients from a relatively bad social status feel very integrated (Axis I), well adjusted (Scale 4), and especially capable of forming relationships (Scale 5). The ability to form relationships, especially emphasized by these patients, together with signs of dependency (Scale 1), draws attention to their strong needs for fusion. The patients become ill typically with small changes in family life (e.g. the son leaving home, the daughter getting married, etc.) but experience no depressive feelings (Scale 2), deny differences between themselves and family members (Scale 5) and have an unequivocal theory on bodily illness.

That these ulcer patients are indeed alexithymic patients is further confirmed by the contrast to the 5 remaining groups which we have designated sociopathic, active-overcompensating, oral-passive character neurotic, neurotic depressive, and neurotic-pseudonormal. Descriptions of these groups is beyond the scope of this paper. However, it is nevertheless important to refer once more to the diversity of subgroups among the ulcer patients. Since only *one* group showed signs of the alexithymia, but all of the ulcer patients were viewed as psychosomatic cases, I have hesitated to use the German term 'psychosomatic phenomenon', which is generally used as a synonym for the alexithymia or pensée opératoire. According to these results we can say that we have found patients with characteristics of the alexithymia or pensée opératoire among the ulcer patients we examined, but cannot designate this as a 'psychosomatic phenomenon' with its claim to a general validity for all psychosomatic disorders, since this only proved true for approximately 15% (through psychological testing) to 20% (clinical judgement) of the patients. How the alexithymia stands in relation to the development of psychosomatic illness is, in my view, still an open question (*Sifneos,* 1975). Whether the kind of illness plays a role, i.e. whether certain illnesses such as colitis exhibit especially strong manifestations of the alexithymia, or whether the severity or the duration of the psychosomatic illness decisively influences the degree of the alexithymia, are questions which still need to be clarified. Furthermore, it must also be asked to what extent (*Overbeck,* 1976) other factors such as the patients' general psychosocial development, their language development, and their belonging to a certain social class play a causative part in the formation of alexithymic characteristics.

References

Brähler, E.; Overbeck, G.; Braun, D., und Junker, H.: Was kann die automatische Analyse des Sprech-Pausen-Verhaltens (On-Off-Pattern) von Arzt und Patient für die Beurteilung von Psychotherapien leisten? Z. Psychosom. med. Psychoanal. *20:* 148–163 (1974).

Eckensberger, D.; Overbeck, G., and Biebl, W.: Subgroups of ulcer patients according to clinico-sociological, psychological test and psychotherapeutic characteristics. J. psychosom. Res. *20:* 489–499 (1976).

Eckensberger, D.; Overbeck, G. und Wolf, E.: Über ein objektivierendes Verfahren zur diagnostischen Untergruppenbildung von chronisch Ulkuskranken. Z. Psychosom. med. Psychoanal. (in press).

El-Safti, M.S.: Zum Problem der Sprache in der Psychoanalyse. Dyn. Psychiat. *6:* 87–97 (1973).

Freyberger, H.: Der Kranke ohne Organbefund. Mus. Med. *3:* 18 (1976).

Junker, H.; Overbeck, G. und Brähler, E.: Vergleich und Interpretation des formalen Sprachverhaltens (On-Off-Pattern) zweier Psychotherapien. Z. Psychother. med. Psychol. *24:* 163–175 (1974).

Overbeck, G.: Objektivierende und relativierende Beiträge zur pensée opératoire der französischen Psychosomatik. Hab.Schr., Giessen (1975).

Overbeck, G.: Das psychosomatische Symptom – psychische Defizienzerscheinung oder generative Ich-Leistung? Psyche *31:* 333–354 (1977).

Overbeck, G. und Biebl, W.: Psychosomatische Modellvorstellungen zur Pathogenese der Ulkuskrankheit. Psyche *29:* 542 (1975).

Overbeck, G. und Brähler, E.: Eine Beobachtung zum Sprechverhalten von Patienten mit psychosomatischen Störungen. Vorläufiger Bericht. Dyn. Psychiat. *7:* 100–108 (1974).

Overbeck, G. und Brähler, E.: Der Therapiesitzungsbericht (TSB) als Instrument der Psychotherapiekontrolle. Z. Psychother. med. Psychol. *25:* 187–197 (1975).
Overbeck, G. and Brähler, E.: Therapist's and patient's speech-pause behavior and the psychotherapy session. Dyn. Psychiat. *9:* 275–286 (1976).
Overbeck, G.; Brähler, E.; Braun, P. und Junker, H.: Über die Anwendung eines Sprachanalyseverfahrens (On-Off-Pattern) in einer laufenden Psychotherapie. Psyche *28:* 815–832 (1974).
Sifneos, P.: Problems of psychotherapy of patients with alexithymic characteristics and physical disease. Psychother. Psychosom. *26:* 65 (1975).

Prof. Dr. med. *G. Overbeck,* Universitätskliniken, Funktionsbereich Psychosomatik, Theodor-Stern-Kai 7 (Haus 13B), *D-6000 Frankfurt/Main* 70 (FRG)

Discussion

Dr. König: I have one short question I would like to put to Dr. *von Rad*. Among your psychoneurotic patients you have several obsessionals. I would expect that obsessionals react in a somewhat similar way to psychosomatic patients. Would you agree with this or did you not have enough obsessionals to make a comparison?

Dr. von Rad: This is a question that we have also been dealing with and Dr. *Vogt* is at present making a similar study based on the 'Rorschach'. I would say today that patients with obsessional neurosis differ very much on the basic word level. For example they say: 'I'm frightened, this terrible knife is frightening me.' These are a series of 'affect-laden words' and one also may hardly notic anything of the affect during the examination process. If a different level of examination is chosen – for example a method which relates more to the context as with the Gottschalk-Gleser method – the difference could then be less. I certainly feel that then there would also still be an evident difference.

Dr. Huebschmann: Here are two questions for Dr. *von Rad*. I would like to ask him if he can give us an interpretation of the significant difference of the speech behavior between neurotic and psychosomatic patients. I would suggest to introduce the term of alienation, of self-alienation (Selbstentfremdung) for psychosomatic patients. Secondly, I want to ask Dr. *von Rad* if he can report on changes of this speech behavior, of this self-alienation in the course of psychotherapy. I have found that recovery of psychosomatic patients is often announced by a change of speech – for instance, they begin to say 'I' instead of 'one'.

Dr. von Rad: As to the first question, I am of the opinion that we have to collect data from the most different observation conditions for a lengthy period of time before any funded reports can be made. Nevertheless, when we talk about this now, we have to remember that we are speculating. The problem of alexithymia can certainly be explained under the term of 'self-alienation'. It is at any rate buried so deeply in the body that it seems to have lost the contact to speech. We, however, do not know what the reason for this is, whether this is only applicable to psychosomatic patients or also to the underprivileged, etc. Regarding the second question, I have the same experience in therapy with psychosomatic patients as you. If one works with them regularly and, which is important, over a long period also giving them sufficient time to learn – even to learn to speak – they then slowly start identifications amongst other patients, also start cooperating with the therapists and finally a good many of them at least are able to reach their feelings which they then express. Generally this starts by simply repeating words without feeling much, but they gradually reach a stage when they can express their feelings using words and this is especially made much easier when they are in group therapy together with others who help them do so.

Dr. Wolff: I have only one brief comment to make. This concerns Dr. *von Rad*'s observations on the patient's use of the word 'I' or 'one' in analytical psychotherapy. One of the rules of gestalt therapy is useful here; if a patient says 'one' he is told to repeat the sentence, substituting the word 'I' for 'one'. This can also be done in analytical therapy and this is an example of how different forms of psychotherapy can be integrated with each other to help the patients get in touch with their own feelings.

Unidentified Speaker: You have talked about the fact that patients use words but without affect. I have observed patients who cannot understand the meaning of words and suddenly grab the body with psychosomatic symptoms. One patient with colitis ulcerosa when talking to me came to the point of pain. Pain as a child, and at the same moment the word 'pace' came into his speech with which the patient got up and went out fetching a diary, so he must percept something of the meaning but he reacts suddenly with the body. This is the other side of affect and fantasy and I mean that this patient is one of this group who has alexithymia. But he understands something more, it is not nothing that he understands.

Dr. Mitscherlich: I want to know something about how in a group your patients speak about other persons because I realize they are able to say words just as how we express our feelings of taste, our capability to realize that that means a corporal meaning and not symbolic.

Dr. von Rad: In this respect I would like to refer you to Dr. *Sellschopp*'s paper and especially agree with the colleague who brought up the expressive content of body movement. In earlier papers Dr. *Sellschopp* and I have talked about the special importance of such 'scenic arrangements'. With psychosomatic patients especially, we feel it extremely necessary to grab hold of these 'scenic arrangements' in group meetings and to make sense of their meaning. As an example, to say 'what is your hand doing at this very moment and what is it telling you?' or, 'you are opening the window – has this anything to do with the depressed silence?' It is our opinion that the concrete objective contribution of such scenic arrangements can build a bridge which helps one come into contact with unknown fantasies.

Dr. Gottschalk: I hesitate to make any comment because I think I seem to be among the more sceptical people about the relationship of the alexithymic syndrom's being specific to psychosomatic disorders. I recognize the syndrome exists, but the more I consider the issue, like Dr. *Overbeck* and a few others, I do not know that it has anything specifically to do with so-called psychosomatic disorders or somatic-psychic disorders. But what I do find extremely interesting is the heuristic value, the stimulation for research, in this hypothesis. It seems to me, however, to be quite premature at this point to seriously concern ourselves with genetic or environmental factors with psychosomatic disorders from the viewpoint of alexithymia. But that is just one personal opinion. It is just as interesting to me to see people, for instance, with psychoneurotic disorders who have many emotions and who do not know much about their psychodynamics, but they express them very openly. In fact, such people are overreactors, and some do not have any somatic disorders and some do. In the latter case, the connection between psychological and somatic phenomena are not realized and, as Dr. *von Rad* was indicating, their right hand does not know what their left hand is doing.

There is no question about phenomena of that sort so anyway I find this conference extremely interesting, provoking and stimulating us all to do more research on these matters.

Chairman: Dr. Aitken: Ladies and gentlemen, just before we close, I would like to make a comment or two. I was very struck at my reaction when Dr. *Mitscherlich* spoke in the earlier part of the session in German when I had no knowledge of the language and consequently did not understand the words she was saying, but I felt that I understood their meaning from the way in which she expressed herself. This seems to be a very appropriate response to note in relation to the topic that we have under discussion.

I do not think it matters whether we are talking about repression in *Freud*'s terms, or 'pensée opératoire', or alexithymia or even if we like to call it athymolexia, I think we are describing something which people have a feeling exists. However, this does create a challenge as Dr. *Gottschalk* said very clearly, because if we are going to describe something that exists, we must be sure that we have methods to do so which are reliable, i.e., which will produce consistent results, and which are valid, i.e., which will describe what it is though is being described. Such observations must be done in a sample of people that very clearly represent something meaningful and not just in a sample of people that happen to knock on the doors of doctors for a variety of reasons that might be very different from what are imagined to be so.

This is not in any way to belittle the contribution of *Peter Sifneos* and *John Nemiah* who have stimulated a worldwide interest in a new phenomenon in recent years, perhaps at a time when psychosomatic medicine was a bit devoid of a heuristic hypothesis to test; perhaps also at a time when many psychiatrists have become a bit disillusioned about the behavioral and pharmacological growth of the 60s, and indeed perhaps even more disillusioned about the psychoanalytic growth of the 50s. Now we are in the 70s, many of us have a feeling that there is something definite there to be described in order to understand better what our patients indeed have wrong with them, in the hope that we can develop more effective therapeutic methods that will relieve them of distress. That conclusion should hearten us all to make further observations.

Now I want to close this session by thanking our speakers for their contribution to the session.

Proc. 11th Eur. Conf. Psychosom. Res., Heidelberg 1976
Psychother. Psychosom. *28:* 121–126 (1977)

Neurosis and Psychosomatic Disorders: Aspects of Differentiation

Frode Larsen and Truls-Eirik Mogstad

In comparing psychosomatic disorders to neurosis, *our* bias has – over quite some time – been going in the direction of *differences* rather than similarities. This may be important since it influences the approach to such conditions. On the other hand, such a point of view may fail to shed any new light on the real problems, since suitable differentiating definitions of the conditions mentioned, will logically imply the difference between them from the beginning, so that one would have an easy job working out the self-affirmative study.

To counteract this bias, we have tried to control clinical evaluation through reassessment in supervision, so that what we are going to present to you, will at least be our present views upon some differences between neurosis and psychosomatic disorders.

Furthermore: since the practical handling of these conditions in a psychosomatic consultation service set-up, are by far the most important issue to us, this retrospective study on differentiation between two groups of frequently referred patients may have its value anyhow. The biographic parameters are partly hard, partly semi-soft and partly wholly soft data, some of them surely disputable psychosocial constructs. And the material does not systematically offer information on variables like 'alexithymia' 'pensees operatoires', pattern of muscular functioning or results of psychological personality tests. We should also inform you that our rating rather goes along lines of *forced choice:* meaning that mixed conditions of neurotic and psychosomatic disturbances are rated as mainly neurotic or mainly psychosomatic, whereby is omitted very important aspects of every day work.

As to *definition:* by *psychosomatic disorders* we shall mean mainly *vegetative* disturbances – with or without structural organic complications, that through thorough medical examination and clinical psychosomatic evaluation, are assumed to rest upon a tendency of the organism to develop such troubles from various *psychosocial precipitating causes*. By *neurotic* we shall mean *psychoneurotic* – diagnosis resting on the presumed identification of premorbid neurotic personality traits, actual intrapsychic conflicts, physical symptom formation affecting locomotor and sensory functions of the organism, symbolism of symptoms, primary and secondary gains, to enumerate a few. Now, according to Freudian definition anxiety neurosis hardly complies with true psychoneurosis, also since autonomous disturbances in this condition are so obvious. A fairly high number of anxiety neuroses in our material may tend to reduce the differences between our group of psychosomatic disturbances as compared to the one of neuroses as a whole. Depressions and neurasthenic states are omitted from the material. We do not consider these nosologic categories as psychoneurosis at all.

The study then, is a comparative biographic study in retrospect, comprising 244 patients referred to the Psychosomatic Department of the National Hospital of Norway, Oslo. The 3 groups compared comprise all the patients aged 20–45 years, referred during the years of 1973, 1974 and 1975, respectively carrying the diagnoses of psychosomatic disorders, anxiety neurosis and conversion neurosis: all diagnoses were based on 1–3 extensive interviews by experienced psychiatrists with re-evaluation through supervision.

In consequence of the clinical experience that patients suffering vegetative ailments and disorders in many respects seem different from neurotics, we formed the hypothesis that a biographic study of clinical material would demonstrate significant differences between such patient groups. The statistics offered are all worked out by means of χ^2-scores.

Variables and Results

The material consists of 121 cases labelled 'psychosomatic' and 123 labelled 'neurotic', a fairly even number. There are more women than men in the neurotic group (table I). Age limits are chosen to rule out adolescent and climacteric reactions.

Origin of referrals in our present situation shows an obvious dominance from neurology and gastroenterology. The referrals' rationals given by the somatic doctors are: (1) psychogenesis?. (2) obvious nervousness, (3) patients own wish, (4) others, meaning less extensive consultations. The results show that psychosomatic patients are generally considered calmer and mentally

Table I. 244 cases between 20 and 45 years of age

Diagnosis	Males	Females	Total
Psychosomatic disturbances	51	70	121
Anxiety neurosis	21	31	123
Conversion neurosis	21	50	
Total	93	151	244

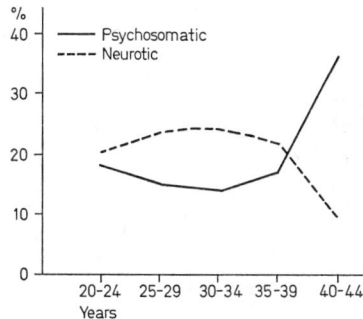

Fig. 1. Age distribution.

sound. Neurotics are generally spotted as 'functional' by the somatic staff, meaning something like hysteric. As already touched upon by several speakers of this Conference, the psychosomatic patients quite firmly stick to the somatic version of their illness, illustrated by the figure of only 2% of them coming to the psychiatric interview according to their own decision.

Concerning life biographic data, age distribution within the 20–45 years of age scale is shown in figure 1. Neurosis, on the whole, occurring comparatively early – psychosomatic disturbances comparatively later in life. On the whole, Level of education shows no obvious difference between the groups. A tendency towards upward mobility on social group ranking is rather strong at the hand of those with psychosomatic disturbances (p<0.025). As to marital status (fig. 2), the impression would be that neurotics stay unmarried and divorce more often than do the psychosomatic patients. When correlated to sex, almost the entire difference is counted for by the women.

Concerning premorbid sexual functioning (fig. 3) it would seem that psychosomatic patients more frequently exhibit orgastic functioning than do

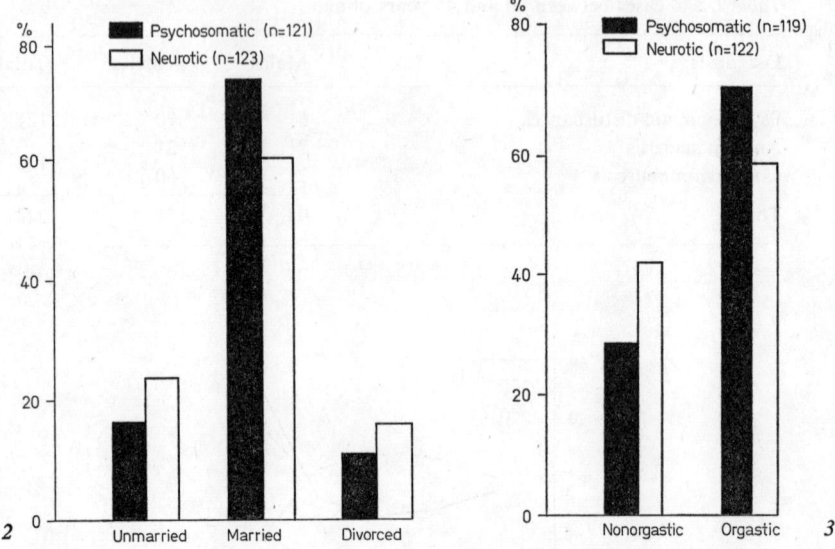

Fig. 2. Marital status.
Fig. 3. Premorbid sexual function.

neurotics (p<0.05). Additional information would show non-orgastic functioning to be more frequent in women. But then, would men lie more often about it?

Our early biographic data concern firstly parents social position in the patients childhood. This parameter possibly demonstrates a slight overall preponderance of psychosomatic disturbances in patients coming from lower social classes as compared with neurotics (the results are, however, not statistically significant at the 0.1 level).

Sibling position would also indicate a hardly significant, although interesting point, in demonstrating a slight tendency that the oldest children more often have neurosis, contrary to the youngest children which more often have psychosomatic disturbances.

Family dynamics in childhhod do not, in our technique, differentiate neurotics from psychosomatically sick persons (fig. 4). The presence of family dynamic pathology may be obvious in both cases.

Further family features like broken homes before the age of 15, alcohol abuse, orphan homes and stepparents do not demonstrate any differentiating patterns in the two groups compared, but the numbers are small.

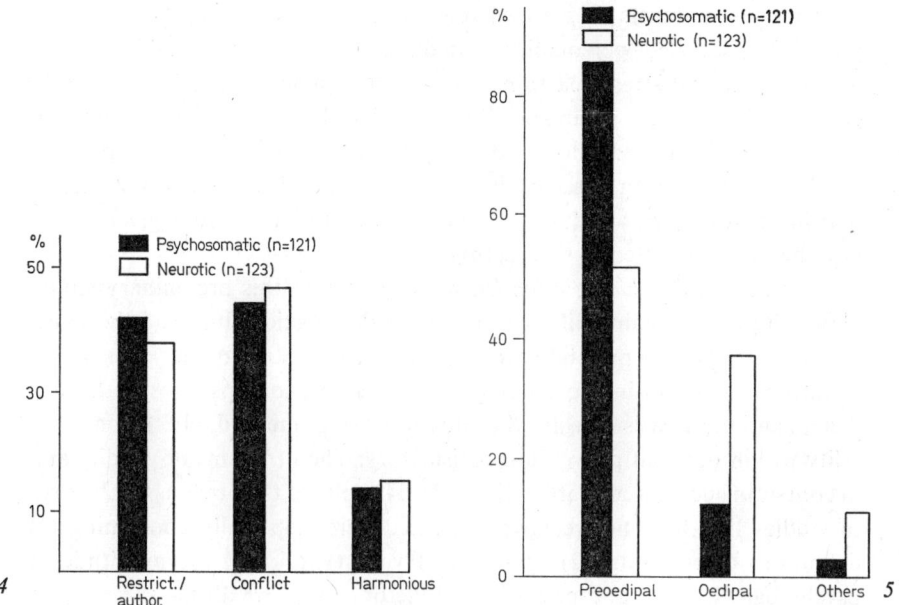

Fig. 4. Family dynamics in childhood.
Fig. 5. Personality function.

As to environmental factors, urban upbringing, contrary to rural, does not differentiate. Migration of the family before the patients age of 15 suggests a rather higher rate of outer change in neurotics as compared to the psychosomatic group (35 and 21%, respectively).

Lastly our soft data constructs. The first one is personality functioning, scored along lines of psychoanalytic theory, and in this connection generously divided into preoedipal and oedipal modes of overall style of coping (fig. 5). Figure 5 shows the relative distribution of these two types of personality functioning – with a striking preponderance of preoedipal coping characteristics in the people with psychosomatic disturbances, and as strikingly oedipal (or phallic) personality functioning in neurotics. Statistical elaboration reveals a $p < 0.01$ using a χ^2-score.

Finally there is stress. Primarily a large group of different types of stress ending up, as we did, with only two of them, namely exogenous and endogenous groups of stress sources. Endogenous intends to suggest that the patient's style of personality functioning in itself brings about the situation that he perceives or reacts to with what we call stress. It could perhaps more properly be labelled 'personality related'. Exogenous stress would mean, so to speak, natural stress reactions, due to the oncoming burdens of life in general, like physical traumata, illness, loss, isolation, etc. Exogenous and personality related stress do not differentiate between the groups of patients compared. In addition, it seems that typical exogenous stress plays the minor part in the total stress picture (11 figures illustrating the results given above have had to be omitted in this report).

By way of *concluding remarks,* we suggest that this preliminary study, although perhaps mainly illustrating a local diagnostic culture, all the same, goes in favour of the possibility to differentiate neurotic from psychosomatic disturbances, according to biographic data on various psychosocial parameters and on a basis of clinical evaluation. As to method, checks on reliability within our unit prove quite satisfactory. The problems of validity are, of course, in such a study rather disturbing. In spite of the obvious weaknesses in studies like the one we have presented here, especially concerning (1) definitions of concepts, (2) problems of validity, and (3) the multitude of psychological, social and physiological factors given, we all the same find it necessary to make such studies, since these are the kinds of data we have, and since a retrospective technique is crucial in clinical evaluation work.

Clinical work and more stringent research will meet in our obligation to keep going the continuous process of defining and redefining the concepts we use for the purposes of causal explanation and treatment.

Frode Larsen, MD, Psykiatrisk Seksjon, Aker sykehus, *Oslo 5* (Norway)

Proc. 11th Eur. Conf. Psychosom. Res., Heidelberg 1976
Psychother. Psychosom. *28:* 127–132 (1977)

'Pensée opératoire' in Obesity

B. Waysfeld, M. Le Barzic, P. Aimez and B. Guy-Grand

Clinique Médicale de l'Hôtel-Dieu, Paris

Numerous attempts to determine a specific psychological profile in obesity have been unsuccessful: obese people were found no more neurotic, anxious, or depressed than control groups (1, 2).

This lack of difference between obese and normal people is a very disappointing fact from a theoretical and therapeutical point of view. However, the hypothesis that this heterogeneous population could include different entities has not held the attention of authors.

As clinicians dealing with obese subjects, our attention was drawn by the frequency of psychosomatic personality traits as defined by the psychoanalytic parisian school and mainly characterized by the presence of 'pensée opératoire' (3).

Thus, we were interested in examining this point in more details in order to answer the following questions: Are the obese subjects concerned with the psychosomatic phenomenon? If such, what are its clinical and biological correlation to obesity? Eventually, could it lead to an approach to the physiopathology of obesity?

Our clinical material consisted of 56 obese inpatient females studied at the beginning of a weight-loss program by the means of usual clinical investigation, psychiatric interview and projective tests (Rorschach and MMPI).

The distribution of the psychological structure is shown in table I. The most striking difference with a control group of non-obese females is the high incidence of psychosomatic structures among obese people confirming our first clinical idea. The other structures are distributed in a somewhat similar manner in obese groups and control groups except for the trend to find less neurotics among obese people.

The diagnosis of the psychosomatic structures was assessed both by the psychiatric interview and by the conclusions of the Rorschach test. All the patients who were diagnosed as 'psychosomatics' fulfilled the criteria shown in table II: popular responses and good shapes are more numerous than in control groups, which contrasts with the few coloured and movements responses.

Since the mental process of the psychosomatic is so far from the neurotic, clinical and biological differences were supposed to exist between these two groups. Thus, 14 neurotics have been compared in several respects to 12 psychosomatic patients.

Table III shows that the two groups are very similar in mean age, duration of obesity, age of onset, overweight, maximum weight, heredity and even adipose tissue cellularity. However, table IV shows that, as it could be expected, they are quite different from a psychological point of view.

Apart from the main traits characteristic of psychosomatic structure, 'pensée opératoire' was present in all the psychosomatic patients; they were much less able to relate dreams, and when they could the dream content was usually poor and stereotyped without any symbolic meaning and any fantasy production related to unconscious conflicts.

It could be interesting to note that 5 among 14 neurotics fulfilled the criteria for 'pensée opératoire' and this number must draw the attention; however, in these neurotics, as in the others, the dreams were frequent and with high symbolic content.

About the alimentary behaviour, table V shows that the psychosomatic patients usually have a rather low daily caloric intake, 66% eat less than 2,000 calories a day, which represents the mean daily caloric intake of the parisian female population. On the other hand, most neurotics are frankly hyperphagic. This could be related to the higher frequency of qualitative abnormalities of alimentary compulsions, bulimias, which are twice as frequent in neurotics than in psychosomatics. Overall, striking differences were found concerning the kind of latent demand underlying the overt demand which is always for weight loss (4).

As can be seen in table VI, in neurotic patients the latent demand was always classified as ambiguous or displaced. This means that in listening to the patients' discourse, it is possible to hear that what is asked for is, in fact, a psychological or environmental change. According to the greater or lesser relationship of this latent demand to the overt one, it was termed ambiguous or displaced.

It seems to us particularly important to take into account the latent demand of patients consulting for somatic symptoms. In these neurotic

Table I. Distribution of the psychological structures in obese and control females

Structure	Obese, %	Controls, %
Neurotic	25	35
Psychosomatic	22	8
Psychotic	11	12
'Anaclitic'	25	27
Unclassable	17	18

Table II. Theoretical summary scores of a psychosomatic subject

P	5
F + %	75
F %	70
A %	60
C + Fc + cF	1
M	1
(c) + F (c) + (c) F	1
FM + Ms	1

Table III. Non-significant parameters

	Mean age, years	Dura- tion, years	Age at onset, years	Over- weight, %	Max- imum weight	Direct heredity unilateral	bilateral	Cellularity 3.10^{10}
Psychosomatics (n = 12)	32.5 +3.6	13.5 ±2.6	18.4 ±2.8	62.7 ±8.1	96.6 ±5.7	9	3	4 (n = 8)
Neurotics (n = 14)	35.4 ±3.3	17.0 ±2.4	18.5 ±2.6	60 ±7.5	93.2 ±5.2	11	2	6 (n = 8)

Table IV.

	'Pensée opératoire'	Usual dream activity	Stereotyped dreams
Psychosomatics (n = 12)	12	5	4
Neurotics (n = 14)	5	13	0
p	0.001	0.01	0.05

Table V. Significant differences

	Daily caloric intake <2,000 kcal, %	Qualitative abnormalities of all behaviour, %
Psychosomatics (n = 12)	66	42
Neurotics (n = 14)	7	85
p	0.01	0.02

Table VI. Kind of demand

Demand	Neurotics (n = 14)		Psychosomatics (n = 12)	
Ambiguous	8		2	
Displaced	6	14	0	2
Stereotyped	0		7	
Somatic	0	0	3	10
Dynamic phase	12		4	

Table VII. Neurotic and psychosomatic constellation in obesity

	Neurotics	Psychosomatics	
Ambiguous Demand Deplaced Dynamic phase Daily caloric intake (2,000 cal/24 h)	6	0	
	0	4	Stereotyped Demand Somatic Static phase Daily caloric intake (2,000 cal/24 h)
p	0.01	0.01	

patients, this demand reflects the displacement of the primary conflict into the alimentary field, which could be considered as a great capacity to elaborate on a mental level.

In psychosomatic patients on the contrary, most of the demands were classified as stereotyped or somatic. That is to say either actually somatic, coming from themselves or induced by the medical pressure, or stereotyped when familial or social intolerance propels women otherwise not overly embarrassed by their obese body, into the medical office.

In summary, ambiguous or displaced demands appear to be almost specific to the neurotic patients, and the somatic and stereotyped demands seem typical of psychosomatic patients.

Similarly, it is important to note that the moment of consultation corresponds to different obesity phases for each group. The majority of neurotics come for consultation in the dynamic phase, the main symptom being the qualitative abnormality of alimentary behaviour, which is the equivalent of a psychological symptom.

On the other hand, 66% of the psychosomatic patients come for consultation in the static or descending phase: they are astonished by an already marked obesity which has neither apparent symbolic meaning, nor a relation to possible unconscious conflicts. They experience it as a pure somatic disease for which they ask medical scientific help.

In conclusion, if authors have not made the differences between obese and normal people evident, this is perhaps due to the fact that obese people have been considered as a homogeneous group and that a specific conflict has been the prevalent idea in instigating this research.

The reference to the psychological structure and what's more, to the manner in which conflicts are managed at a mental level, allow us to separate the obese women into at least two groups in which differences can easily be noted by the practitionner or the nutritionist. At the end of such a study, a clinical constellation proper to neurotic patients and perhaps specific to them can be proposed.

Among neurotic patients, 6 patients show together a daily caloric intake of more than 2,000, an ambiguous or displaced demand which was asked during the dynamic phase. None of the psychosomatics fulfilled these criteria (table VII).

This constellation, from our point of view, is a simple approach for diagnosing the psychological structure during the clinical phase which, without any doubt, carries therapeutical implications.

If psychotherapy is the chosen treatment of the neurotic patients, the relevancy of its application is reduced by the lack of real psychological demand and also by the traits of the typical obese people.

Whatever the organic basis on which obesity relies, the presence of a neurotic structure will lead to the exploitation of the fat body and abnormalities in alimentary behaviour into the neurotic system. This is perhaps possible because of a pregenital failure which hinders the neurotic symptomatology and obstructs the symbolisation of conflicts.

This observation affirms our first feeling that both during interviews and tests, we are dealing with acting out structures close to character neurosis. We were struck by the high score in the MMPI P scale which reflects the trend toward acting out and the frequency of eczema, in the past history (30% of neurotic patients).

Let us remember that 5 neurotic obese patients out of 14 showed 'pensée opératoire'.

In summary, large differences between the two groups of obese women studied have been demonstrated; particularly, it has been possible to show the prevalence of 'pensée opératoire' among the psychosomatic groups. However, we have the feeling that this separation between the two groups must not be too strictly defined.

Some neurotic obese females exhibit pregenital traits, a trend toward acting out and even in some cases 'pensée opératoire'; they share all these characteristics with the psychosomatic obese, as if neurotic symptomatology could not achieve the full expression of the underlying conflicts by itself.

These facts explain perhaps the difficulties which have been observed in undergoing and pursuing a classical psychotherapy, even in the neurotic obese females, and should auggest new technical management (5).

References

1 *Atkinson, M.R. and Ringuette, L.E.:* A survey of biographical and psychological features in extraordinary fatness. Psychosom. Med. *29:* 121 (1967).

2 *Guy-Grand, B.; Aimez, P.; Le Barzic, M. et Sitt, Y.:* Facteurs de personnalité; comportement alimentaire et régulation pondérale. 2e Congr. régulation du bilan d'énergie chez l'homme, Genève 1975, p. 84.

3 *Marty, P. et M'Uzan, M. de:* La pensée opératoire. Revue fr. Psychanal. *27:* 345 (1963).

4 *Waysfeld, B.; Aimez, P.; Le Barzic, M. et Guy-Grand, B.:* La demande thérapeutique de la femme obèse. 5e Congr. Int. méd. psychosom., Paris 1976.

5 *Sifneos, P.E.:* Problems of psychotherapy of patients with alexithymic characteristics and physical disease. Psychother. Psychosom. *26:* 65–70 (1975).

B. Waysfeld, MD, Clinique médicale de l'Hôtel-Dieu, 1, place du Parvis-Notre-Dame, *F-75181 Paris Cédex 04* (France)

Proc. 11th Eur. Conf. Psychosom. Res., Heidelberg 1976
Psychother. Psychosom. *28:* 133–140 (1977)

Alexithymia

I. The Communication of Physical Symptoms

John G. Flannery

Department of Psychiatry, Toronto General Hospital, Toronto, Ont.

Although it has been known for a long time that patients with psycho-somatic disorders have difficulty in putting their feelings into words, and tend to experience physical disturbances rather than emotional, it was only when a number of allied impressions were condensed into one brilliantly expressive word – alexithymia – by *Sifneos,* that this difficulty could be more clearly defined and examined (3). These allied impressions comprise a characteristic deficit in the ability to form fantasies, and to think about interpersonal relationships, along with a tendency to think only in a literal, utilitarian way ('La Pensée Opératoire') (4). Thus, alexithymia is now a working concept as well as an impression, and the findings of the present study suggest that it may be a useful clinical sign of at least a predisposition to serious psychoso-matic distress.

If alexithymic patients have difficulty in experiencing and expressing emotion, how do they fare when describing pathological body states – symptoms – to their physicians? The present study tries to provide an answer to that question. 22 alexithymic patients and their records were studied. These 22 patients were all referred to the Psychiatric Consultation Service of the Toronto General Hospital, between January 1975 and June 1976. Each patient was seen for at least two 1-hour diagnostic interviews, one of them with the author who is also a practising psychoanalyst.

Before a patient was considered alexithymic, these criteria had to be met: (1) All eight alexithymic questions in the Psychosomatic Questionnaire of the Beth Israel Hospital Psychiatric Service (5) had to be answered appropriately. (2) A minimum of 2 h diagnostic work, one of them with the author. (3) Unanimous agreement of the presence of alexithymia between both interviewers. (4) Patients with an imperfect vocabulary; who were reticent in replies, or habitually laconic in speech; who were either definitely untruthful or suspected of being untruthful; or who had an interest in presenting themselves as 'normal' as possible, were excluded from consideration. There are two exceptions to this last proviso, patients (G) and (J) had end-stage renal failure as a result of prolonged phenacetin abuse. Both tended to give confused accounts of drug ingestion, but they had been known for years to the renal team, psychiatrists, and social workers, and there could be no doubt of their alexithymia.

The commonest differential diagnoses considered were: hysterical neurosis with conversion symptoms; latent schizophrenia with somatic delusions; neurotic depression with depressive somatic equivalents; somatic diseases, unexplained.

On clinical and historical grounds each of these could be clearly ruled out. This is made easier with this sample because the Toronto General Hospital is a diagnostic referral centre for an area of about 6 million people. All of these patients had been extensively investigated, both before and during their stay in hospital, and there were ample records of previous admissions and contacts with physicians. These records were carefully reviewed. Once alexithymia was recognized, and this often took more than one interview, it was found to be a stable character trait. It can be altered during psychotherapy (this is described in part II) but not for long. As a trait, it appears that a given patient either has alexithymia or he does not; nor are there degrees of alexithymia. It does not seem meaningful to say that one patient is more alexithymic than another. The age, sex, current and previous diagnoses are described in the accompanying tables.

How such patients came to be referred to the Psychiatric Consultation Service is significant. Three of them (B), (D), and (F) referred themselves. The treating physician opposed the referral of (F) on the grounds that it was not necessary. Patients (A) and (E) were previously referred to other psychiatrists. The senior psychiatrist and psychiatric resident who saw patient (A), diagnosed her as emotionally normal; the psychiatrist who saw (E) professed surprise that she had been referred at all. The referral of patient (N) was at first vehemently opposed by the surgeon who had treated her for pancreatitis. Patient (V) was referred because he had seemed unaccountably normal in his emotional state, considering his advanced liver disease and cachexia. This referral was considered unnecessary by the medical resident treating him.

With these exceptions, all the other patients were referred because of the very loose fit the investigating physicians could make between the physical symptoms and the objective findings. In other words they were referred by default of an adequate explanation for their physical distress. Apart from reporting 'depression', or 'hysteria', occasionally, the medical team could not describe definite psychiatric signs and symptoms or exceptional ward behaviour in these patients. Given the implications of the alexithymic state, this is pretty much what would be expected. As might also be expected, all these patients were referred relatively late in their medical career, and a non-organic cause for their distress seems only to have been considered after considerable and fruitless investigation and therapy. The diagnoses (table I) show 8 (32%) with classical psychosomatic diseases, hypertension (4 patients), thyrotoxicosis (1 patient), asthma (1 patient), peptic ulcer (2 patients). It is relevant to point out that in over 1,000 consultations, none has been referred on the grounds of having a classical psychosomatic disease; it appears that present-day physicians do not regard Alexander's 'Holy Seven' as psychosomatic disorders, or at least that the psychiatric aspect warrants referral. This probably represents advances in the knowledge of pathogenesis and therapy of these conditions. Some diagnoses indicate an organic disorder as well as an unexplained symptom, e.g., patients (O) and (P) both complained of chest and abdominal pain, and patient (O) also had low back pain. Each patient was discovered to have mitral valve prolapse, confirmed by echocardiography, but although this is known to be associated in some patients with chest pain (2) the degree of prolapse in neither patient was commensurate with the frequency and intensity of the pain. Nor do the diagnoses indicate what part repeated investigation has played in the history of the symptoms – patient (A) was discharged with abdominal pain, not yet diagnosed, but in the years previous to this she had had a caesarean section, cholecystectomy, vagotomy, sphincterotomy (Oddi), accessory splenectomy, and gastro-jejunostomy (roux en y).

Undiagnosed pain, often at multiple sites, is the most frequent symptom, occurring as a present diagnosis in 15 (68%), and as a previous diagnosis in 9 (41%). Those patients who abused analgesics had chronic pain; the two alcoholic patients said alcohol made them feel better.

At psychiatric examination no formal diagnosis in terms of psychopathology or history suggestive of interpersonal disturbance could be made. The diagnosis returned to the referring physician was that of a psychophysiological reaction, involving one or more systems. Even those patients who had themselves sought psychiatric help, presented to the psychiatrist the same history of physical complaints as they had to the referring physician. Psychological data, as contrasted with physiological, is quite scarce. Two

Table I. Alexithymic patients (n = 22)

Patient	Age	Sex	Current diagnosis	Past diagnosis
(A)	31	F	abdominal pain[1]	abdominal pain[1]
(B)	27	M	diffuse pain[1] essential hypertension	gross obesity, hypertension
(C)	31	F	hypertension, digit spasm	thyrotoxicosis
(D)	31	F	abdominal pain[1]	abdominal pain[1]
(E)	42	F	extrasystoles, headaches[1]	extrasystoles, headaches[1]
(F)	28	M	hypertension, colitis	hypertension, colitis
(G)	44	F	headache[1], phenacetin nephropathy	headache[1]
(H)	47	F	obesity, low back pain[1]	asthma
(I)	24	F	atonic bladder, abdominal pain[1]	anorexia nervosa
(J)	41	F	headache[1], phenacetin nephropathy	duodenal ulcer
(K)	32	F	hypophagia, amenorrhoea	scoliosis
(L)	46	F	abdominal pain[1]	diffuse pain[1]
(M)	25	F	abdominal pain[1] headache[1]	necrotizing pancreatitis
(N)	26	F	headache[1]	low back pain[1]
(O)	38	F	chest[1] and abdominal pain[1] prolapsed mitral valve	low back pain[1] duodenal ulcer
(P)	45	F	diffuse pain[1] mitral valve prolapse	diffuse pain[1]
(Q)	31	F	hypertension	adrenal hyper- plasia
(R)	50	M	hemi-anesthesia[1] and Ekbom's syndrome	diabetes
(S)	48	F	diffuse pain[1]	alcoholism, duodenal ulcer
(T)	32	F	diffuse pain[1]	anorexia nervosa
(U)	23	F	ureteral stones, adipsia	
(V)	62	M	liver disease	alcoholism

[1] Not yet diagnosed.

types of response were met in reply to a question designed to challenge emotion, e.g. 'What did you feel when you knew your father was dead?' reply: 'Oh, I think I got a migraine headache' (indicating a symptom as a reaction to the bad news), or 'Well, I had to cope with my little brother' (indicating action rather than feeling). One patient (K) complained bitterly that she was becoming depressed; when asked 'What does your depression feel like?' answer: 'I keep thinking of things, then I can't think of things I should be doing'.

After one interview it was possible to elicit from almost all of these patients either a diffuse feeling of distress which was poorly articulated and seemed to partake of both physical and mental qualities; or a remarkable absence of distress where it would have been expected to occur, or a combination of both of these. At the base of the distress, or the failure to experience distress, seems to be an alteration in the experience of the body, including the functions of ingestion and excretion. *Bruch* (1) has described the same phenomenon in patients with eating disorders. It is this altered body experience that most commonly confuses physicians. Examples: patient (I) had been enuretic until the age of 14, then she developed acute retention but without distress. Catheterization was painful, and after that she required repeated catheterization for these episodes. Each time she would be encouraged to drink lots of water in order to minimize the risk of infection. After some time it was discovered that she was drinking up to 5 litres a day, and the bladder had expanded and become atonic. She was referred to endocrinology on the grounds of possible diabetes insipidus, and then for a psychiatric consultation. The history showed that while at present she was obese, her weight had been less than 40 kg 2 years previously and she had energetically travelled all over Europe looking 'like death'. This suggests anorexia nervosa. Her experience of her body mass, the distended viscus and the rate of fluid and food intake were all normal to her, so normal that she had not been able to scrutinize them sufficiently to protect her own health. Patient (K) was referred by an endocrinologist after investigation of amenorrhoea and weight loss. Following a caesarean section she had been constipated and had become extremely aware of the slightest sensation of rectal fullness. She would eat little and try to evacuate her bowel almost immediately after eating. Her weight dropped from 72.5 to 47.8 kg, she looked cachectic, yet continued to feel well and be active, concerned only with avoiding the uncomfortable rectal sensation, and quite oblivious of the change in body form. Patient (B) was of average height, and at the age of 14 his weight had rapidly increased to 109.2 kg. He was not in the slightest concerned and felt comfortable. His weight became normal at 95.0 kg in his 20s, but he then developed multiple painful sensations in the head, thorax and abdomen, accompanied by essential hypertension.

In reviewing the recorded histories, it appears that the physician tries to rationalize these complaints, concentrating on one physiological system (usually the one he specializes in), to discern a symptom complex and make a diagnosis. For example patient (N) presented with chronic low back pain following the birth of her first child. The notes revealed that she was a 'poor historian', and there were no definite clinical findings. A myelogram did suggest some disc protrusion at L-5, and she had a discotomy. 10 years later she reappeared at this hospital, referred for treatment of intractable headache. This time she admitted she never had a day without some pain somewhere, since puberty, and that her back hurt as much as it ever did. Patient (L) was referred by a cardiologist who had investigated her stabbing chest pain; he had been referred her by a gastroenterologist treating her nausea. She was also seeing a gynaecologist for metrorrhagia. The history revealed a constant low-grade diffuse discomfort, including all the above symptoms as well as alterated sensation in the gums and lips, easy fatigue, poor sleep, and a constant feeling of fullness in the right ear.

The question arises as to how far the 'significant others' of the alexithymic person perceive them as emotionally different. Of the twenty patients, ten spouses were interviewed for a minimum of one hour. Two of these (G) and (N), were embittered and arranging divorce, but this was because of the spouses' continued ill-health and personal incompatibility. Three other spouses of (A), (E) and (P), were impatient and showed anger at the partners' failure to respond to treatment, and yet the marriages were stable enough. Of the two alcoholics, patient (S) had a very disturbed marriage; while the second marriage of patient (V) – after he stopped drinking – was stable. The spouses of patients (K), (L), (R), (T), and (V), were contentedly married and reasonably supportive. In addition it seemed likely that patients (B), (C), (D), (F), (N), (Q), and (F) had happy marriages. It did not appear that any of the spouses other than those who were bitterly dissatisfied, saw the patients as qualitatively different in their emotional lives or emotional expressiveness, from other people. The spouses tended to hold the view the physicians first held: that there was organic pathology somewhere. Sexual dysfunction – frigidity – although never offered as a symptom, was relatively a minor problem in marriages of (A), (D), (E), (L), and (N). Thus alexithymia is not a character trait that spouses seem to notice much or care about, and is certainly not incompatible with stable and apparently satisfying marital relationships, although the prolonged psychosomatic distress that can be associated with it is.

It would seem then that alexithymic patients are likely to convince their physicians and their spouses that either they have organic illness which has not been detected, or the organic illness they do have should account for their symptoms. Such patients are as incoherent about body states as about emotional ones. They are also compliant, eager for a physical diagnosis, and for the most part impress their physicians as psychologically normal. Thus, they are referred late, or perhaps not at all, over-investigated and over-treated. If, as these findings suggest, alexithymia is linked not to psychosomatic disease per se, but to a predisposition to a variety of puzzling disorders that are referable to altered body experience, it should be possible to reduce the morbidity of these disorders. This means examining the assumption that a symptom represents a deviation from a presumed resting and 'normal' state, whereas it may be for some patients an attempt to put a more constant and generalized state of distress into focus and into words. This state of discomfort is related to the experience of the body, visceral tension and the functions of ingestion and excretion. Part of the morbidity that might be reduced by early detection of alexithymic people – before they are ill – is emotional: the reciprocal mystification, frustration and eventual fatigue that comes from fruitless medical investigation, and part is physical for these patients risk the loss of healthy tissue at surgery, not to mention the hazards of investigations, particularly those employing invasive techniques.

From an economic point of view it makes sense also to detect alexithymic patients early. Most of these had taken up a lot of medical and hospital time in the years before referral, and most of their symptoms, particularly the pain syndromes, were unchanged – (A), (D), (E), (M), (G), (I), (J), (L), (M), (N), (O), (P), (S), (T). Patient (A) had had a heroic series of surgical procedures for abdominal pain without relief; patient (B) had repeated ureteral surgery for impacted calculi until it was discovered that she 'naturally' drank only minute quantities of fluid a day. Conversely repeated cystoplication had failed for patient (I) because she 'naturally' drank large quantities of water and so on. Conventional history taking, medical and psychiatric, would not have picked up what was wrong with these patients, but an awareness of their alexithymia could have alerted their physicians early to the disturbance in body experience that might interfere with efforts to help them.

In summary, a study of 20 patients with alexithymia showed they appeared to experience the body, including ingestion and excretion processes in a way that it is difficult for them to describe, but which their physicians tend to mistake for undetected organic pathology. Even when organic disease is uncovered, it either responds paradoxically to treatment or proves insufficient to account for the severity of the symptoms. If physicians could be made aware of the possible implications of alexithymia it might at least minimize the iatrogenic contribution and reduce the evident waste of medical resources that continued unexplained symptoms create.

References

1   *Bruch, H.:* Conceptual confusion in eating disorders. J. Nerv. ment. Dis. *133:* 46–54 (1961).
2   *Hancock, E.W. and Cohn, K.:* The syndrome associated with midsystolic click and late systolic murmur. Am. J. Med. *61:* 183–196 (1966).
3   *Sifneos, P.E.:* The prevalence of 'alexithymic' characteristics in psychosomatic patients. Psychother. Psychosom. *22:* 255–262 (1973).
4   *Marty, P. et M'Uzan, M. de:* Revue fr. Psychoanal. *27:* suppl., p. 1345 (1963).
5   *Sifneos, P.E.* op. cit.

Dr. *John G. Flannery,* Room 111, Burnside Wing, Toronto General Hospital, 101 College Street, *Toronto, Ont. M5G 1L7* (Canada)

Proc. 11th Eur. Conf. Psychosom. Res., Heidelberg 1976
Psychother. Psychosom. *28:* 141–147 (1977)

Alexithymia and the Counter-Transference

Graeme J. Taylor[1]

The characteristic features of alexithymic patients are an impoverished fantasy life, poor dream recall, an inability to express feelings with words and a utilitarian mode of thinking which is concerned with conscious psychic processes and has no appreciable relationship with unconscious fantasies. These patients are frequently experienced by their doctors as dull, boring and frustrating. *Stephanos'* (1975a, 1975b) 'psychosomatic phenomenon' refers to similar phenomenological observations of many psychosomatic patients and the characteristic mode of thinking 'la pensée opératoire' was first described by *Marty and de M'Uzan* (1963). A 'psychosomatic character pattern' has been proposed (*Marty et al.,* 1963; *Stephanos,* 1975a, b) which is structurally distinct from that of neurotic patients. *Nemiah and Sifneos* (1970a) and *Nemiah* (1973, 1975) have challenged the traditional concept of denial which was previously invoked to explain the clinical behaviour of psychosomatic patients. They express the opinion that 'what appears as denial of emotion, is in fact an absence of feelings' (*Sifneos,* 1974). They conclude that since alexithymic patients are unable to produce fantasies or to establish an emotional interaction with their therapist, psychodynamic psychotherapy is contraindicated (*Sifneos,* 1973, 1974, 1975).

Whereas *Stephanos* (1975b) and the Paris group (*de M'Uzan,* 1974; *McDougall,* 1974) attempt to trace the genesis of alexithymic characteristics to faults in the earliest object relationship of the infant, the Boston group have previously emphasized neurophysiological rather than psychological explanations. There is also controversy over the phenomenological obser-

---

[1] Head, Consultation-Liaison Service, Mount Sinai Hospital, Toronto, Ont., Assistant Professor of Psychiatry, University of Toronto.

vations of the Paris and Boston groups. *Engel* (1972) and *Musaph* (1974) have independently claimed that many of their psychosomatic patients express affect freely and have rich creative fantasy lives.

Without disputing the presence of alexithymia in many psychosomatic and other physically ill patients, I would like to challenge some of the conclusions which have resulted from its identification, in particular the implications for psychotherapy. Following the lead of *Musaph* (1974) I will examine transactions within the doctor-patient relationship with particular attention to counter-transference phenomena.

Sandler (1976) recently indicated that 'the term "counter-transference" has a great many meanings, just as the term "transference" has'. It has been argued that counter-transference simply means transference on the part of the analyst and is therefore a hindrance which must be eliminated. However, I will employ the term counter-transference as defined by *Heimann* (1950, 1960). She suggested that the prefix 'counter' implies additional factors and she used the term counter-transference to cover 'all feelings which the analyst experiences towards his patient'. She stressed the positive value of counter-transference and viewed it as 'an instrument of research into the patient's unconscious'. *Heimann* assumed 'that the analyst's unconscious understands that of his patient. This rapport on the deep level comes to the surface in the form of feelings which the analyst notices in response to his patient, in his counter-transference'. She states 'this is the most dynamic way in which his patient's voice reaches him'. *Heimann's* (1950) contribution was to show clearly that the reaction of the analyst may be the first useful clue to what is going on in the patient. During the analytic work the emotions roused in the therapist are often 'much nearer to the heart of the matter than his reasoning, or, to put it in other words, his unconscious perception of the patient's unconscious is more acute and in advance of his conscious perception of the situation... The counter-transference is not only part and parcel of the analytic relationship, but it is the patient's *creation,* it is a part of the patient's personality'.

Similar views have been expressed by *Bion* (1955) and *Money-Kyrle* (1956) who consider that by way of a pre-verbal or archaic kind of communication... some patients succeed in imposing a fantasy and its corresponding affect upon their analyst in order to deny it in themselves. At first sight the therapist experiences these as being his own response to something, not recognizing that they have been made by the patient. The effort involved is in differentiating the patient's contribution from one's own. By using *Melanie Klein*'s theory of projective identification the therapist can analyse his coun-

ter-transference and then develop appropriate interventions and interpretations. Various negative counter-responses to projective identification
have been described by *Money-Kyrle* (1956). For example 'the analyst may
reproject the patient as something not understood, or foreign, in the external
world'. Projective identifications from the alexithymic patient may therefore
be reprojected as statements that he is a mechanical kind of being with a
neurophysiological defect. The affects of dullness, boredom and frustration
which the patient evokes appear to facilitate this reprojection and serve as
rationalisations for the conclusions that he is blocked up by an impregnable
wall and is unsuitable for psychodynamic psychotherapy. In my opinion
access may be gained to the patient's inner life by considering the feelings of
dullness, boredom and frustration as counter-transference experiences.

Grotjahn (1942) and *Fliess* (1961) have discussed the affects of dullness
and boredom which they indicate may evoke a stage of ego disintegration and
ego reconstruction. 'Dullness is an ego danger because it is a stage of ego
starvation. The dull situation offers no opportunity to apply the cognitive or
motor abilities of the ego so that the ego is put into a desperate situation of
unemployment, faces a mental death and the result is a certain disintegration'
(*Grotjahn,* 1942). To terminate the sense of dullness the therapist may fall
asleep and actually enter a stage of dreaming or else he indulges in a stage of
pre-conscious fantasy periodically interrupted by the demands of the treatment situation. The state of ego starvation is uncomfortable and the usual
response is to react with rather aggressive fantasies. The phrases *deadly dull*
and *bored to death* allude to the violent murderous fantasies which may arise.

With the alexithymic patient the therapist enters into a relationship
expecting to be *fed* interesting fantasies and feelings only to encounter increasing frustration, dullness and boredom. If the therapist relaxes ego
control he may experience oral-sadistic and oral-erotic fantasies which, as
Fliess (1961) indicates, parallel the infant's response to the trauma of weaning.
Fliess has also referred to an implied 'sucking-biting conflict' in the situation
of boredom.

These feelings and fantasies may be regarded as counter-transference
phenomena which are evoked by the patient's projective identifications.
Analysis of the counter-transference therefore provides 'secret access'
(*Little,* 1966) into the patient's inner world which the patient is still unable to
consciously perceive. According to *Grinberg* (1962) *Hanna Segal* has suggested that violent projective identifications made by patients presumably result
from infantile experiences during which the child was subject to violent
projective identifications on the part of the parents. As the doctor-patient

relationship parallels the mother-infant relationship there is an unconscious recreation of early feelings and fantasies associated with introjective and projective manoeuvres. By *sustaining* and *analysing* the counter-transference, the therapist can develop appropriate therapeutic strategies and interpretations which render the relationship with the alexithymic patient anything but sterile.

I would suggest that in the alexithymic patient, feelings are neither denied nor absent but rather deeply buried and felt as highly dangerous and ego disruptive. Via his counter-transference responses the therapist gathers information about the primitive internalized object relationships of the patient. The doctor-patient transactions may then be conceptualized in terms of introjective-projective relatedness and by fostering the development of a psychotic transference intense feelings, fantasies and dreams are released.

To illustrate these concepts I will briefly describe the case of a 28-year-old married Jewish female with a 4 year history of psychophysiological symptoms which included periodic abdominal cramps, muscular weakness, low grade fevers and skin rashes. Despite exhaustive medical investigations the patient was convinced that her illness was entirely organic. She could not conceive of any relationship between illness exacerbations and numerous stresses in her life. Her 2-year-old daughter had developed feeding difficulties, there was threat of a marital separation and indecision over living with the patient's parents in Canada or returning to Israel. Her mother had chronic ulcerative colitis and a malignant laryngeal tumor had been excised from her father. The patient was typically alexithymic. She was unable to express feelings and her only fantasy was that she would eventually die from her illness. Although she was college educated she in fact claimed that she had a *dull* mind and would quickly *bore* me. She also insisted that she had 'a barren fantasy life' and that I would only find emptiness behind her physical symptoms.

As my attempts to link her physical symptoms with inner feelings and life events proved futile I experienced increasing frustration which was at first a physically disagreeable sensation. It soon became associated with aggressive feelings and fantasies towards the patient. At other times her repetitive and monotonous communications generated boredom which when indulged led to a slight dissociation and my drifting off into mixed sadistic and erotic fantasies. Sometimes I experienced intense feelings of despair and hopelessness which persisted beyond the therapy hour and often into the weekend. Using Klein's theory of projective identification I regarded these counter-transference responses as split-off parts of the patient which she was unconsciously projecting into me. I had become aware of these before she had – she remained conscious only of the physical symptoms.

Psychotherapeutic strategies included: (1) Frequent interpretations that she was afraid of being overwhelmed by powerful aggressive impulses and intense despair. (2) Repeated indication of the absence of angry feelings and thoughts and requests that she bring aggressively laden fantasies or dreams to the sessions. (3) Attempts to direct descriptive language away from the soma to the psyche, e.g., when she referred to 'violent stomach cramps' I requested that she bring me 'violent' dreams. (4) Conceptualizing the doctor-patient transactions in terms of introjective-projective relatedness. For example her rejection of my interpretation linking symptoms to life events was further interpreted as a failure to swallow, digest and metabolize the good 'food' I was offering. I indicated her distortion that my interpretations were bad, harmful or even poisonous.

Through these manoeuvres access to childhood memories and feelings was gained and the patient began to recall dreams and express feelings and fantasies which were associated with the therapeutic relationship. Many of these reflected my own earlier counter-transference feelings and fantasies. During childhood there had been intense struggles with her mother over food, and she recalled feeling intense rage and threatening to kill her mother on one occasion. Her mother had responded by inducing guilt for many years and calling her the 'bad seed'. This was based upon a news report of a schoolgirl who had murdered three adults at that time. She recalled being frightened by attending school bomb drills and developing nausea and abdominal cramps which allowed her to stay home. At this stage in the therapy she developed an intense dislike for her mother's voice which she felt set off vibrations throughout her own body. When I left on a vacation she felt sad and developed a stomach ache which she associated with my departure. Once when she was feeling physically well she had a fantasy on the way to my office of a young girl enjoying licking an ice cream.

Her dreams included: (1) Being eaten by a spider which grew larger as she grew smaller. (2) She was in danger of being shot in the stomach as the Americans and Israelies formed a stronger alliance. (3) Emerging from a wedding ceremony and the ground was strewn with faeces. She also had a fantasy of being married to me. (4) Seeing the patients on the psychiatric ward with their bodies mutilated. (5) A dream of me poking out my tongue. (6) A dream of me returning from a war with an arm shot off. (7) She was being trained by a former psychiatrist for guerilla warfare and later the psychiatrist was shooting at her. (8) She was chased by an ugly man who stabbed and raped her. There was blood in her mouth.

It is clear from this clinical material that as access was gained to the patient's inner world of feelings and fantasies a psychotic transference emerged, and as *Sperling* (1955) has stated this is 'a major factor responsible for the reluctance to use psychoanalytic therapy in the treatment of such cases...'

In conclusion I have proposed an approach to the alexithymic patient which relies heavily on object-relations theory and requires intensive analysis of unconscious transactions in the doctor-patient relationship. Creative use of the counter-transference permits access to the patient's archaic inner world and the emergence within the transference of the primitive internalized object relations which contribute significantly to the genesis of psychosomatic illness.

References

Bion, W.R.: Language and the schizophrenic; in *Klein, Heimann and Money-Kyrle* New directions in psychoanalysis, chapt. 9 (Basic Books, New York 1955).

Engel, G.: Discussion in physiology, emotion and psychosomatic illness. Ciba Foundation Symp. No. 8, p. 27 (Elsevier, Amsterdam 1972).

Fliess, R.: Boredom, in Ego and body ego, pp. 191–194 (Int. Univ. Press, New York 1961).

Grinberg, L.: On a specific aspect of counter-transference due to the patient's projective identification. Int. J. Psychoanal. *43:* 436–440 (1962).

Grotjahn, M.: The process of awakening. Psa. Rev. *1942:* 29.

Heimann, P.: On counter-transference. Int. J. Psycho-anal. *31:* 81–84 (1950).

Heimann, P.: Counter-transference. Br. J. med. Psychol. *33:* 9–15 (1960).

Little, M.: Transference in borderline states. Int. J. Psychoanal. *47:* 476–485 (1966).

Marty, P.; M'Uzan, M. de et David, C.: L'investigation psychosomatique (Presses Univ. de France, Paris 1963).

Marty, P. and M'Uzan, M. de: La 'pensée opératoire'. Rev. fr. Psychoanal. *27:* suppl. pp. 1345–1356 (1963).

McDougall, J.: The psychosoma and the psychoanalytic process. Int. Rev. Psychoanal. *1:* 437–459 (1974).

Money-Kyrle, R.E.: Normal counter-transference and some of its deviations. Int. J. Psychoanal. *37:* 360–366 (1956).

Musaph, H.: The role of aggression in somatic symptom formation. Int. J. psychiat. Med. *1974:* 449–460.

M'Uzan, M. de: Psychodynamic mechanisms in psychosomatic symptom formation. Psychother. Psychosom. *23:* 103–110 (1974).

Nemiah, J.C.: Psychology and psychosomatic illness. Reflections on theory and research methodology. Psychother. Psychosom. *22:* 106–111 (1973).

Nemiah, J.C.: Denial revisited. Reflections on psychosomatic theory. Psychother. Psychosom. *26:* 140–147 (1975).

Nemiah, J.C. and *Sifneos, P.E.:* Psychosomatic illness. A problem in communication. Psychother. Psychosom. *18:* 154–160 (1970a).

Nemiah, J.C. and Sifneos, P.E.: Affect and fantasy in patients with psychosomatic disorders; in *Hill* Modern trends in psychosomatic medicine, vol. 2, pp. 26–34 (Butterworth, London 1970b).

Sandler, J.: Counter-transference and role-responsiveness. Int. Rev. Psychoanal. *3:* 43–47 (1976).

Sifneos, P.E.: The prevalence of 'alexithymic' characteristics in psychosomatic patients. Psychother. Psychosom. *22:* 255–262 (1973).

Sifneos, P.E.: A reconsideration of psychodynamic mechanisms in psychosomatic symptom formation in view of recent clinical observations. Psychother. Psychosom. *24:* 151–155 (1974).

Sifneos, P.E.: Problems of psychotherapy of patients with alexithymic characteristics and physical disease. Psychother. Psychosom. *26:* 65–70 (1975).

Sperling, M.: Psychosis and psychosomatic illness. Int. J. Psychoanal. *36:* 320–327 (1955).

Stephanos, S.: The object relations of the psychosomatic patient. Br. J. med. Psychol. *48:* 257–266 (1975a).

Stephanos, S.: A concept of analytical treatment for patients with psychosomatic disorders. Psychother. Psychosom. *26:* 178–187 (1975b).

Graeme J. Taylor, M.B., Department of Psychiatry, Mount Sinai Hospital, 600 University Ave., *Toronto, Ontario M5G 1X5* (Canada)

Proc. 11th Eur. Conf. Psychosom. Res., Heidelberg 1976
Psychother. Psychosom. *28:* 148–155 (1977)

Alexithymia in Twelve Commissurotomized Patients

Klaus D. Hoppe and Joseph E. Bogen

University of California at Los Angeles, Hacker Clinic, and University of Southern California, Ross-Loos Medical Group, Los Angeles, Calif.

It is a common feature of psychosomatic patients that they have unusual difficulty giving verbal expression to their hopes, fears and fantasies. This behavioral deficit was called alexithymia by *Sifneos* (1973, 1975) and was examined also by *Nemiah* (1976); it is still, as those authors admit, not yet fully formulated, and not uniform in appearance. For example, *Freyberger* and his co-workers (*Drees et al.,* 1976) have described mixed and semiforms of alexithymia. There is a discrepancy between clinical reports that describe such patients as not experiencing feelings in their bodies (*Nemiah,* 1972) and those reports that they express hypochondriacal details of their bodies (*Drees et al.,* 1976). In addition, it may be asked: How dependent on socio-cultural factors is alexithymia, and how closely is a diminished capacity of symbolization connected with it? We present here some data on the nature and possible significance of alexithymia.

Patients

Following the studies of *Sperry* and co-workers (*Sperry,* 1967) on brain bisection in animals, a small number of humans who suffered from intractable epileptic seizures had complete cerebral commissurotomy, i.e., the two cerebral hemispheres were surgically disconnected by sectioning the corpus callosum and the anterior commissure. Therapeutically, cerebral commissurotomy has largely been successful (*Bogen et al.,* 1969; *Wilson et al.,* 1975).

From the psychological point of view, the commissurotomy patients appear normal in ordinary social situations; but a wide variety of deficits in interhemispheric transfer (the 'split-brain syndrome') can be elicited using special testing procedures (*Sperry et al.,* 1969). Among other findings, it has been possible to confirm that the two cerebral hemispheres serve different functions. In right-handed people, the left hemisphere has been found to be

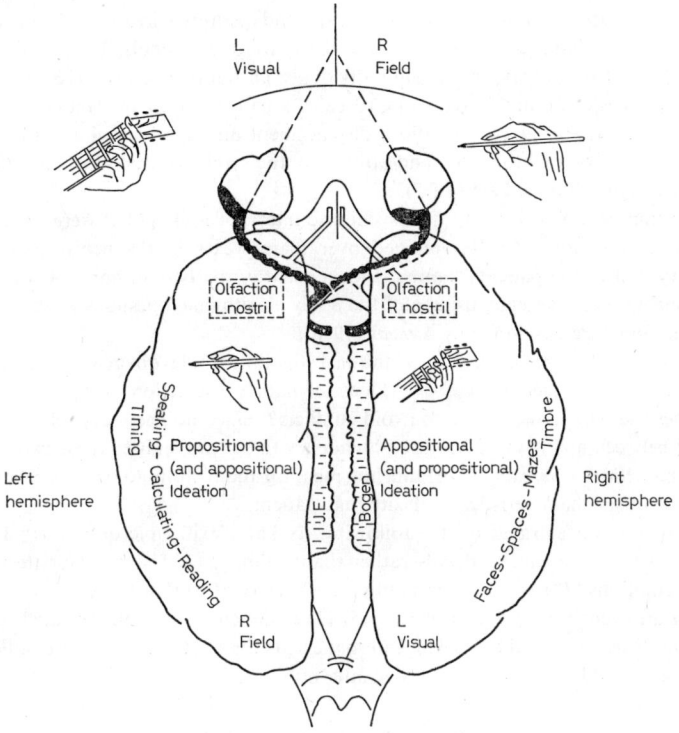

Fig. 1. A schematic outline of the brain as seen from above, to indicate the lateral specialization of the cerebral hemispheres, based on evidence from cases of lateralized lesions and from testing of patients with cerebral commissurotomy.

verbal, logical and analytic, while the right hemisphere specializes in holistic perception of configurations or gestalts (*Levy et al.,* 1972) (fig. 1).

If as much as half of the cerebral activity of a split-brain subject is no longer available for verbal report, such patients might be expected to manifest at least some aspects of alexithymia.

Method

In the course of a systematic long-term evaluation of the split-brain patients, they were seen for both neurologic and psychiatric evaluations. The neurologic status has previously been reported (*Bogen and Vogel,* 1975). The psychiatric evaluation, still in progress, has included intensive interviewing of the patients and of their relatives. The interviews followed partly *Deutsch's* technique of associative anamnesis (*Deutsch and Murphy,* 1955). All interviews were taped.

Particular attention was paid to the quantity and quality of dreams and fantasies prior to and after commissurotomy, as well as the ability to form symbols. The examinations of five females and seven male split-brain individuals, all but one of them right-handed and between the ages of 21 and 50 years old, revealed a paucity of dreams, fantasies and symbols. The dreams lacked condensation, displacement and symbolizations; the fantasies were unimaginative, tied to reality and utilitarian, the symbolization was concretistic, discursive and rigid (*Hoppe,* 1975, 1977).

The impressions gained by the psychiatric interviewer (K.D.H.) were quite distinct from the observations (J.E.B) obtained over many years in the neurosurgical office, laboratory and in the patients' homes. Independently, the two authors rated the twelve commissurotomized patients, using 6 of the 8 key alexithymic questions of the psychosomatic questionnaire developed by *Sifneos* (1973).

Two questions seemed not to fit the investigation of alexithymia which means the inability to *verbalize* feelings; namely, 'Does the patient use action to express emotions?' and, 'Does the patient use action to avoid conflicts?' Since no necessary relation need be obtained between ability to verbalize and tendency to act, we omitted these two questions concerning actions. *Nemiah* (1976) did not mention these shifts to actions in his recent delineation of six characteristics of alexithymic patients.

Thus, we concentrated on the following six key alexithymic questions: 'Does the patient: (1) Describe endless details rather than feelings? (2) Use appropriate words to describe emotions? (3) Have a rich fantasy life? (4) Tend to describe circumstances surrounding an event rather than feelings? (5) Have difficulty to communicate? (6) Is the thought content associated more with external events than with fantasies or emotions?' In our rating, we added 'somewhat' to 'yes' and 'no'.

Results

In spite of a very different viewpoint – *J.E.B.* examining and knowing his patients for years as a neurosurgeon, *K.D.H.* relying on one or two intensive psychiatric interviews – the rating was rather concordant regarding five questions (fig. 2).

One question: 'Does the patient have difficulty to communicate?' was interpreted in a different way. *J.E.B.* supposed the communication to be of facts, *K.D.H.* of feelings. A clarification of this question appears desirable, if it is to be of further use.

In addition to the pictorial representation (fig. 2), the results can be scored numerically. The six questions were answered in an alexithymic direction for a 'yes' score of 41 *(J.E.B)* or of 58 *(K.D.H.)* for a 'somewhat' score of 23 *(J.E.B.)* and of 10 *(K.D.H.),* respectively – whereas the 'no' score was rated with 8 *(J.E.B.)* and 4 *(K.D.H)*.

Another way to present the data is to add up the scores and obtain a mean for the group. 'Yes' and 'somewhat' scores represent a positive result

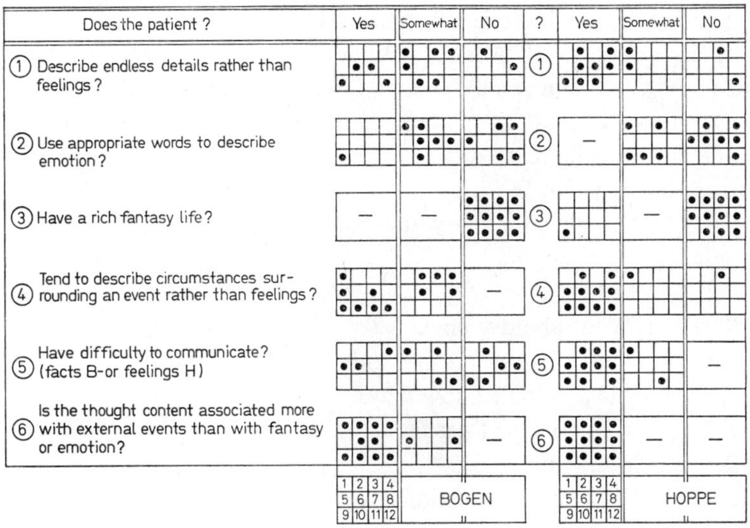

Does the patient ?	Yes	Somewhat	No	?		Yes	Somewhat	No
① Describe endless details rather than feelings ?					①			
② Use appropriate words to describe emotion?					②	—		
③ Have a rich fantasy life?	—	—			③		—	
④ Tend to describe circumstances surrounding an event rather than feelings?				—	④			
⑤ Have difficulty to communicate? (facts B- or feelings H)					⑤			—
⑥ Is the thought content associated more with external events than with fantasy or emotion?				—	⑥		—	—

1 2 3 4		1 2 3 4	
5 6 7 8	BOGEN	5 6 7 8	HOPPE
9 10 11 12		9 10 11 12	

Fig. 2.

concerning alexithymia and can be combined. The results read therefore: 64 positive to 8 negative scores *(Bogen);* 68 positive to 4 negative scores *(Hoppe).*

In other words: the mean positive alexithymic score in commissurotomized patients is 5.66 *(K.D.H.),* or 5.33 *(J.E.B.),* whereas *Sifneos* found only a mean positive score of 5.12 and his student found 4.84, in their psychosomatic groups. Since we found a mean ratio of 5 positive answers out of 6 whereas *Sifneos* found a mean ratio of 5 positive answers out of 8, we can conclude that our commissurotomized patients tended to show definitely more alexithymic characteristics than the psychosomatic group of *Sifneos.*

Examples

To illuminate our findings, we give a brief example of alexithymia in a commissurotomized patient. *K.D.H.* asked a 30-year-old man: 'How do you feel about the separation from your wife?' The patient answered: 'It's hard to explain.' Question: 'How do you feel about it?' Answer: 'I don't like it.' Question: 'You don't like the separation?' Answer: 'No, because I like my kids to have a mother to support them.'

A little later the interviewer tried again: 'How do you feel about your wife leaving you in 1973?' Answer: 'What I feel is hard to explain.' Question: 'Hard to explain? You cannot really tell me how you feel?' Answer: 'I cannot.' Question: 'Are you sometimes thinking of your wife?' Answer: 'No.'

The same patient reacted to the attempt at free association and a guided daydream in the following way:

K.D.H.: 'Go ahead, close your eyes and tell me what's going through your mind?'

Patient: 'My kids.'

K.D.H.: 'What about your kids?'

Patient: 'I just think about my kids, like I'm scared I'm going to lose them or something, I don't know why.'

K.D.H.: 'Can you see their faces?'

Patient: 'Yes, I can.'

K.D.H.: 'What are they doing?'

Patient: 'Right now, I just picture them as they are.'

K.D.H.: 'What are they doing?'

Patient: 'I just see their faces, but I don't know what they are doing.'

K.D.H.: 'What about their faces?'

Patient: 'I'm seeing that they're cleaned up and healthy, I know that, and that's about all I can tell you.'

K.D.H.: 'Nothing else?'

Patient: 'No.'

K.D.H.: 'Okay. Now close your eyes, continue this and imagine you are in a meadow. You are going to the woods and there is a beautiful meadow and you are in the meadow. What can you see now?'

Patient: 'A meadow?'

K.D.H.: 'A meadow.'

Patient: 'What's a meadow – the middle?'

K.D.H.: 'No, a meadow, I mean a kind of – I mean playing in the grass and so on. You are going to the woods, to a forest and there is a meadow. Now you know what I mean?'

Patient: 'Yes.'

K.D.H.: 'Now, you are on the meadow, what are you doing?'

Patient: 'Just walking along and playing, skipping along – trying not to have any worries in my mind, that's about it.'

K.D.H.: 'Can you see anything?'

Patient: 'No.'

K.D.H.: 'Can you hear anything?'

Patient: 'No.'

K.D.H.: 'Can you touch anything?'

Patient: 'No.'

K.D.H.: 'Can you smell anything?'

Patient: 'Yes, it smells good, that's about it.'

K.D.H.: 'The air smells good. How does the air smell?'

Patient: 'Clear.'

K.D.H.: 'Clear? And what else?'

Patient: 'No smog.'

K.D.H.: 'No smog, mm, mm.'

Patient: 'It's green – the grass smells real green, I can smell that.'

K.D.H.: 'Can you see anything?'

Patient: 'No, I'm just walking alone, that's all.'

K.D.H.: 'Walking alone and there is nobody else around?'

Patient: 'No, which I would like to be with my kids.'

K.D.H.: 'Oh, you have your kids with you?'

Patient: 'Yes.'

K.D.H.: 'And what are you doing with your kids now on the meadow?'

Patient: 'Playing along with them.'

K.D.H.: 'What are you playing?'

Patient: 'We run for awhile and then we stop, then we get some rest and then we run a bit more.'

K.D.H.: 'Running, ah, hah. What are you playing with your kids?'

Patient: 'Let's see. We play tag with one another until they get tired.'

Discussion

Based on his observations of the twelve commissurotomized patients, *Hoppe* (1975, 1977) developed two hypotheses. The first one consists of fitting his findings into the psychoanalytic theory. He postulated that the impoverishment of dreams, fantasies, and symbolization might be due to an interruption of a preconscious stream between the two hemispheres. This in turn causes a separation of word-presentations from thing-presentations. Furthermore, he assumed the predominance of a feedback-free primary process or organization in the right hemisphere.

His second hypothesis focused on the similarity between commissurotomized and psychosomatically ill patients with regard to their observed operational thinking (pensée opératoire). The findings of *Marty and de M'Uzan,* (1963), *Mitscherlich* (1969), *Bräutigam* (1975), *Freyberger and* co-workers in Germany (1976), as well as *Nemiah and Sifneos* (1970) in Harvard were matched by observations on 200 survivors of severe Nazi persecution (*Hoppe*, 1962, 1971). All of them suffered from psychosomatic reactions or disorders (*Hoppe*, 1968), dreamed exclusively about details of their persecution in concentration camps or hiding places and had difficulties in expressing their feelings. In survivors of severe persecution, the sense of an empty and meaningless life (*Venzlaff*, 1963) is combined with a paucity of symbols and fantasies, as well as a loss of security in interpersonal relationships (*von Baeyer et al.*, 1964).

The similarity of operational thinking in psychosomatically ill patients and split-brain people led *Hoppe* (1975, 1977) to hypothesize a 'functional commissurotomy' in cases of severe psychosomatic disturbances. Such a functional commissurotomy might anchor in psychophysiological terms the model of biphasic defense (*de Boor and Mitscherlich*, 1973). According to this model, psychosomatic patients at first suffer from a neurotic conflict. In the second phase of defense, they regress further to the psychosomatic level and exhibit a resomatization of affect (*Schur*, 1955).

Following *Hoppe*'s hypothesis, the first phase of a neurotic process engages both hemispheres with defenses being mainly intrahemispherical. The second phase of defense mechanisms involves the transcallosal interhemispheric system (i.e., functional commissurotomy), thus blocking certain emotions and gestalt perceptions of the right hemisphere from being verbalized by the left hemisphere. Instead, these emotions are hypercathected in the right hemisphere, leading to a resomatization of affect.

Whatever the fate of the foregoing speculations, it seems clear that the commissurotomized patients are quite alexithymic, thus validating the usefulness of this concept and possibly even suggesting a physiologic basis.

References

Baeyer, W. von; Haefner, H. und Kisker, K.: Psychiatrie der Verfolgten (Springer, Berlin 1964).

Bogen, J.E.; Sperry, R.W., and Vogel, P.J.: Commissural section and the propagation of seizures; in *Jasper, Ward and Pope* Basic mechanisms of the epilepsies (Little, Brown, Boston 1969).

Bogen, J.E. and Vogel, P.J.: Neurologic status in the long-term following cerebral commissurotomy; in *Schott and Michel* Clinical disconnection syndromes (Hôpital Neurol., Lyon 1975).

Boor, C. de und Mitscherlich, A.: Verstehende Psychosomatik: ein Stiefkind der Medizin. Psyche *27:* 1–20 (1973).

Bräutigam, W. und Christian, P.: Psychosomatische Medizin. Ein kurzgefasstes Lehrbuch für Studenten und Ärzte (Thieme, Stuttgart 1975).

Deutsch, F. and Murphy, W.F.: The clinical interview (International Universities Press, New York 1955).

Drees, A.; Arnold, M.A.; Freyberger, H.; Otte, H. und Ritter, J.: Das Alexithymiekonzept in der Psychosomatik. Therapiewoche *26:* 1067–1077 (1976).

Hoppe, K.D.: Verfolgung, Aggression und Depression. Psyche *16:* 521–537 (1962).

Hoppe, K.D.: Psychosomatische Reaktionen und Erkrankungen bei Überlebenden schwerer Verfolgung. Psyche *22:* 464–477 (1968).

Hoppe, K.D.: Chronic reactive aggression in survivors of severe persecution. Comp. Psychiat. *12:* 230–237 (1971).

Hoppe, K.D.: Die Trennung der Gehirnhälften – ihre Bedeutung für die Psychoanalyse. Psyche *29:* 919–940 (1975).

Hoppe, K.D.: Split-brains and psychoanalysis. Psychoanal. Q. *46:* 220–244 (1977).

Levy, J.; Trevarthen, C., and Sperry, R.W.: Perception of bilateral chimeric figures following hemispheric deconnexion. Brain *95:* 61–68 (1972).

Marty, P. et de M'Uzan, D.C.: L'Investigation psychosomatique. (Presses Univ. de France, Paris 1963).

Mitscherlich, A.: Krankheit als Konflikt; Studien zur psychosomatischen Medizin, 2 (Suhrkamp, Frankfurt/M 1969).

Nemiah, J.C.: Emotions and physiology. An Introduction; in Physiology, emotion and psychosomatic illness. Ciba Foundation Symposium 8, pp. 15–29 (North Holland, Amsterdam 1972).

Nemiah, J.C.: Value of free association doubted for some patients, pp. 12–13 Psychiatric News, August 6 1976.

Nemiah, J.C. and Sifneos, P.E.: Affect and fantasy in patients with psychosomatic disorders; in *Hill* Modern trends in psychosomatic medicine. 2, pp. 26–34 (Appleton-Century-Crofts, New York 1970).

Schur, M.: Comments on the metapsychology of somatization; in The psychoanalytic study of the child, vol. X, pp. 119–164 (International Universities Press, New York 1955).

Sifneos, P.E.: The prevalence of 'alexithymic' characteristics in psychosomatic patients. Psychother. Psychosom. *22:* 255–262 (1973).

Sifneos, P.E.: Problems of psychotherapy of patients with alexithymic characteristics and physical disease. Psychother. Psychosom. *26:* 65–70 (1975).

Sperry, R.W.: Split-brain approach to learning problems; in *Quarton, Melnechuck and Schmitt* The neurosciences: A study program (University Press, New York 1967).

Sperry, R.W.; Gazzaniga, M.S., and Bogen, J.E.: Interhemispheric relationships. The neocortical commissures; syndromes of hemispheric disconnection. Handbook of clinical neurology, vol. 4, pp. 275–290 (North Holland, Amsterdam 1969).

Venzlaff, U.: Erlebnishintergrund und Dynamik seelischer Verfolgungsschäden; in *Paul und Herberg* Psychische Spätschäden nach politischer Verfolgung (Karger, Basel 1963).

Wilson, D.H.; Culver, C.; Waddington, M., and Gazzaniga, M.: Disconnection of the cerebral hemispheres. Neurology, Minneap. *25:* 1149–1153 (1975).

Klaus D. Hoppe MD, 160 Lasky Drive, *Beverly Hills, CA 90212* (USA)

Proc. 11th Eur. Conf. Psychosom. Res., Heidelberg 1976
Psychother. Psychosom. *28:* 156–166 (1977)

A Pragmatic Approach to the Concept of Alexithymia[1]

R. Pierloot and J. Vinck

Department of Psychopathology, University Hospital 'St. Rafaël', Leuven

Marty and de M'Uzan (1963) first described a way of mental functioning characterized by what they call operatory thinking, absence of fantasy life and stereotyped perception of other people. These ideas have been further elaborated by *Marty et al.* (1963) and in a later contribution by *de M'Uzan* (1974). Analogical findings have been reported by *Nemiah and Sifneos* (1970a). Difficulties to communicate with some patients suffering from psychosomatic disorders, they attributed to a difficulty of expressing emotions appropriately and a poor fantasy life encountered in these patients (*Sifneos,* 1967). Using the term 'alexithymia', *Sifneos* (1973) wanted to stress the inability to find appropriate words to describe feelings. *Musaph* (1974a) stressed the importance of the therapist's attitude in the judgment of this phenomenon. Finally, the elaboration of the Psychosomatic Questionnaire of the Beth Israel Psychiatric Service offered the possibility of 'rating' the alexithymia characteristics.

We can approach the pragmatic value of the concept under three headings, representing the three aspects of our study:

(1) The explanation of the phenomenon, which can be conceptualized on different levels: the level of intrapsychic conflicts and defenses; the level of deficient mental functioning in the area of verbalizing feelings and fantasies; the level of neurophysiological connections between the limbic system and the neocortex (*Nemiah and Sifneos,* 1970b). Our study has been directed on connections between alexithymia and some aspects of social and mental functioning, which could contribute to an explanation of the phenomenon.

[1] Study supported by a grant of the Belgian National Fund for Scientific Research.

(2) The link between this communication pattern and the occurrence of psychosomatic symptoms. A difficulty resides in the term 'psychosomatic symptom'. Some authors want to reserve this term for a limited number of syndromes. The basis, however, for this limitation is not always clear. Absence of relationship between the symptom and any physiological activity, proposed as a criterium by *de M'Uzan* (1974), is difficult to manage (*Musaph,* 1974b). It is likely that in the genesis of somatization processes, different psychological mechanisms interfere. One of these mechanisms may find its expression in the alexithymic communication style. A certain deficiency in the capacity for differentiated paternal and maternal symbol formation, we could demonstrate in a group of patients suffering from different psychosomatic disorders could possibly refer to the same mechanism (*Hoornaert and Pierloot,* 1976). In the actual state of our knowledge it seems justified to assume that the appearance of a more pronounced alexithymia in a given person involves a greater chance of detecting also some somatization processes.

(3) Psychodynamic psychotherapy, based on transference and interpretation, has a poor outcome where the alexithymia communication pattern prevails. This statement does not apply to other forms of psychotherapy.

Studied Group and Methodology

Our study was carried out at the Psychiatric Out-patients department of the University Hospital 'St. Rafaël', Leuven. It is part of a larger research design on prognostic criteria for short-term psychodynamic psychotherapy (*Malan,* 1963) and systematic desensitization (*Wolpe,* 1969) in, as much as possible, unselected patients.

As only criteria for selection have been retained, on the one hand the presence of important anxiety manifestations, on the other the absence of severe disturbances presenting an obstacle to the mentioned forms of therapy. A score of 35 or more on the Taylor Manifest Anxiety Scale (TMAS; *Taylor,* 1953) has been fixed as an indication of important anxiety manifestations. This scale can be considered as a reliable measure for trait anxiety and also includes such aspects as somatic anxiety equivalents. The limit of 35 has been fixed on basis of the distribution of TMAS scores in the general population of the out-patients department. Too disturbed patients have been automatically eliminated because they were referred to other settings of therapy.

During the period from November 1973 through May 1975, the TMAS has been administered to every new patient. Of the 93 patients obtaining a score of 35 or higher, 39 have been eliminated for different reasons (necessity of admission in a psychiatric hospital, refuse of therapy, etc.). The remaining 54 patients went through the pretherapy evaluation and, except for one patient included in this study who dropped out before this point, were referred to one of the mentioned forms of therapy. The choice of the therapy form was decided entirely by chance. The therapies, restricted to 20 sessions, were per-

Table I. Demographic characteristics of the studied group

	Number[1]	Mean	SD
Age	50	34.29	12.46
Intelligence (extrapolated WAIS verbal IQs)	48	96.42	19.50
Educational level[2]	48	3.40	1.78
Professional level[3]	48	2.33	1.15

[1] For some patients data relevant to one of these characteristics are lacking.
[2] In 9 categories, 1 meaning no degree completed and 9 meaning studies at academic level completed.
[3] In 6 categories, 1 meaning lowest and 6 meaning highest level.

formed, under supervision, by residents in training. For 4 of these 54 patients alexithymia ratings are lacking.

Demographic characteristics of the group of 50 patients, available for our study, consisting of 31 female and 19 male patients, are shown in table I. Considering these mean characteristics we may conclude that our group is relatively representative of a population of young adults with average intelligence, some professional training or high school education, and with professions in the lower middle class.

The pretherapy evaluation contained, besides the alexithymia rating with the Beth Israel Psychosomatic Questionnaire, a number of psychological tests (WAIS vocabulary (*Stinissen et al.,* 1970), MMPI, STAI (*Spielberger et al.,* 1970, etc.), rating scales (Psychiatric Status Schedule (*Spitzer et al.,* 1970), Check-list of Worries, etc.) and topics of subjective appraisal by the interviewer. This offers the opportunity of checking up correlations between the rating for alexithymia and other data of the evaluation.

A portion of 29 patients dropped out in the very beginning of the therapy (12 of the short-term psychodynamic therapy group, 17 of the systematic desensitization group). The relation between drop out, considered as a therapeutic failure, and alexithymia has been studied.

In the patients who completed therapy, the subjective appraisal of several aspects regarding the outcome of the therapy was rated on a 10-point scale. This instrument is constructed at the Counseling Center of the KUL[2] on the basis of a study by *Nichols and Beck* (1960), and includes judgments on symptomatic improvement, insight, happiness, general appreciation of therapy, etc. Patients filled out this scale at the end of therapy and after a follow-up period of at least 3 months. For the therapists we dispose only of their

[2] The authors gratefully acknowledge the permission of Dr. *C. Lietaer* to use this scale.

appreciation at the end of the therapy. Besides this subjective appraisal, pre-post-follow-up gain scores are calculated for the STAI, PSS and number of worries. The relation between the ratings for alexithymia and some aspects of the outcome has been looked after.

Results

Connections between Alexithymia and some Demographic and Mental Characteristics

Age. The Spearman rho correlation coefficient (*Siegel,* 1956) of 0.2004 between age and alexithymia is not significantly different from zero.

Sex. As shown in table II, there exists no significant difference between the mean alexithymia ratings of the female and the male subgroups; the point biserial correlation (*Edwards,* 1967) of 0.2057 is low.

Intelligence, education and socioeconomic level. When considering the concept of alexithymia, one does not see marked reasons to assume that persons with a predominance of alexithymic characteristics should be more or less intelligent or should have other educational or socioeconomic backgrounds than people in general. Because of their specific communication problems it could be expected, however, that they make an unfavorable *impression* in interpersonal contacts, especially when personal and emotional problems are discussed.

Disposing for each patient of objective data and of estimations of the interviewer on these characteristics, we are in a position to examine these expectations. Table III shows the correlations between alexithymia ratings and both the objective and subjective rating for intelligence, educational level and socioeconomic background.

Table II. Relation between alexithymia ratings and sex

	Female (n = 31)		Male (n = 19)		p
	mean	SD	mean	SD	
Alexithymia ratings	4.83	2.20	5.30	1.89	NS

NS = Not significant; Mann-Whitney U test (*Siegel,* 1956).

Table III. Correlation coefficients between alexithymia ratings and intelligence, educational level and socioeconomic level measured by objective criteria and estimated by rater

	Objective (Pearson correlation coefficients, n = 48)	Estimated (point biserial correlation coefficients, n = 50)
General intelligence	–	−0.3087[1]
Verbal intelligence	−0.1026	−0.5003[2]
Educational level	−0.1253	−0.0299
Socioeconomic level	−0.2484	−0.2067

[1] $p < 0.05$, two-tailed; [2] $p < 0.01$, two-tailed.

Two conclusions can be drawn from these data: first, all correlations are negative, indicating that a more pronounced presence of alexithymic characteristics tends to be accompanied by lower levels of intelligence, education and socioeconomic status, but this relationship is weak; second, as far as intelligence is concerned, alexithymia is linked significantly with an impression of lower intelligence. The alexithymic communication style entails that patients are judged as less intelligent than they really are.

The Relation between Alexithymia and the Occurrence of Somatization

The occurrence of a stronger tendency toward somatization of conflicts and emotions is crucial to the concept of alexithymia. We dispose of several criteria of somatization which can be used to test the validity of this aspect of the concept. On one hand we can compare the mean alexithymia score of groups with and without somatic symptoms; on the other hand we can look for correlations between the alexithymia rating and the results on some standard scales of somatization.

As shown in table IV, the group with somatic symptoms is rated significantly higher on alexithymia than the group without somatic symptoms. The point biserial correlation of 0.2231 between alexithymia and presence or absence of somatic complaints is approaching statistical significance ($0.05 < p < 0.10$, one-sided).

The correlations between the alexithymia ratings and the results on other scales referring to somatization tendencies are represented in table V.

Table IV. Mean alexithymia ratings for groups with and without somatic symptoms at intake

Somatic symptoms					p^1
present (n = 35)			not present (n = 15)		
mean	SD		mean	SD	
5.36	2.10		4.14	1.79	<0.05

[1] Mann-Whitney U test, two-tailed.

Table V. Spearman Rank correlations between alexithymia and scales of somatization (n = 48)

Scale of somatization	Spearman Rank correlation	p (one-sided)
Hypochondriasis scale MMPI	−0.0932	NS
Somatic complaints scale PSS	0.2352	=0.05
Percentage of somatic worries	0.3809	<0.005

There exists a significant positive correlation between alexithymia and the score on the Somatic Complaints subscale of the Psychiatric Status Schedule. With the hypochondriasis scale of the MMPI correlation is almost of a zero order. In the checklist of worries, presented to the patients, 15 of the 100 items referred to somatic symptoms (e.g., pain, breathlessness, tiredness, etc.). The percentage of somatic complaints in the total number of worries, checked by the patient, has been considered as an index of somatization. The correlation between this index and the alexithymia ratings is highly significant.

It can be concluded that these results offer fairly consistent support to the hypothesis of a relation between alexithymia and somatization in the expected direction.

Relation between Alexithymia and the Outcome of Therapy

The presence of alexithymic characteristics is supposed to offer serious impediments to the normal course of psychodynamic therapy. For other forms of psychotherapy, there are no reasons to expect the same influence; so we expect alexithymia ratings to be unrelated to the course and outcome of our systematic desensitization therapies.

To test these assumptions we could look at the drop out rates in both forms of therapy, considering a drop out as a therapeutic failure or as an indication of an incompatibility experienced by the patient between the requirements of the therapy and his communication style. We could also examine the relation between alexithymia ratings and some aspects of outcome for the completed therapies.

Drop out. The results concerning the relation between alexithymia and drop out in both therapy forms are summarized in table VI.

When both sets of variables are intercorrelated it is apparent that we find a statistically significant relation in the expected sense for the psychodynamic therapy group while both variables are unrelated in the systematic desensitization group. Patients with more alexithymia characteristics are more likely to drop out from psychodynamic therapies, but in systematic desensitization they persist as well as those without alexithymia characteristics. The differ-

Table VI. Relations between alexithymia ratings and drop out versus completion of therapy

a Mean alexithymia ratings in drop out and completed therapy groups

		Number	Mean	SD	p[1]
Psychodynamic therapy	drop out	12	5.75	1.66	0.09
	completed	9	4.11	2.76	one sided
Systematic desensitization	drop out	17	4.88	2.12	NS
	completed	11	5.00	1.73	

b Point biserial correlation coefficients between alexithymia ratings and drop out versus completed therapy status (n = 49)

Psychodynamic therapy	−0.3628[2]
Systematic desensitization	0.0301

[1] Mann-Whitney U test.
[2] p = 0.05, one-sided.

ences between the mean alexithymia ratings of the different subgroups, although only approaching statistical significance, point in the same direction: in the psychodynamic therapy group we find a clear difference between both groups in the expected direction, i.e., with the drop outs scoring higher than those who complete their therapy, while in the systematic desensitization group the very small difference even goes in the opposite direction.

Outcome of the completed therapies. In our study we relied upon two main categories of outcome criteria: first, the subjective appraisal of patient and therapist, who expressed their appreciation on a series of 10-point scales, as described above, and, secondly, upon pre-post, post-follow-up and pre-follow-up difference scores or gain scores on the State-Trait-Anxiety Index, forms State and Trait, on a checklist of worries and on several scales of the Psychiatric Status Schedule: the Anxiety scale, the Denial of Illness scale, the Subjective distress scale, the Total score scale and the Summary role scale.

For the systematic desensitization group, correlations between the alexithymia ratings and the different outcome scores all approach the zero order. This result corresponds to our expectations. For the psychodynamic therapy group, however, the findings are quite divergent.

On nearly all the categories of subjective appraisal the ratings correlate positively with alexithymia, which means that the presence of alexithymic characteristics tends to be associated with greater success of psychodynamic therapy. This is most clearly so in the relation between the alexithymia ratings and the appraisal of symptomatic improvement: here we find the only statistically significant Pearson correlations: 0.7078 ($p < 0.05$, two-sided) with the therapists judgment and 0.6079 ($p = 0.082$, two-sided) with the patients judgment at the post-tests. The only exceptions to this trend of a positive relation are the very slight negative Pearson correlations with the judgments concerning gain in insight (–0.0495 for the patients iudgment at the follow-up evaluation and –0.2007 for the therapist judgment at the post-therapy evaluation).

In general, the correlations between the several gain scores in psychodynamic therapy and the alexithymia ratings are low. The only one approaching statistical significance is a Pearson correlation of –0.6417 ($0.10 < p < 0.05$, two-sided) between alexithymia and the pre-post difference score of the Summary role scale of the PSS, indicating a trend toward a greater improvement in role functioning for those with lower alexithymia ratings.

If we take into account only the more striking connections, we notice that in the results of psychodynamic psychotherapy, more pronounced alexithymia characteristics are associated with more symptomatic improvement and with less improvement in general role functioning. For all the other aspects of outcome, correlations are too low to justify any conclusion.

Comment and Conclusions

Our studied group, composed on the basis of only two criteria – the presence of sufficiently pronounced anxiety manifestations and the absence of severe psychiatric disturbances – can be considered, with regard to alexithymia, as unselected. For this group, by checking up on the correlations between alexithymia ratings and different other variables, we have tried to contribute to the solution of three problems: the explanation of the phenomenon of alexithymia; the relation between alexithymia and psychosomatic symptom formation, and the relation between alexithymia and the prognosis of different forms of therapy.

It seems obvious that persons with more pronounced alexithymic characteristics are judged as less intelligent. Still, the negative correlations between alexithymia and the objective features of intelligence, education and socioeconomic status are too weak to provide any arguments to the explanation of alexithymia in the framework of a more generalized mental deficiency.

Our findings offer serious arguments to the hypothesis that more pronounced alexithymia goes together with a stronger tendency to somatization. Three of the four indices of somatization (presence of somatic symptoms, somatic complaints subscale of the PSS and the percentage of somatic worries) show significant positive connections with alexithymia.

The expectation that alexithymia would not effect the results of a behaviour therapy form, such as systematic desensitization, is confirmed as well by the percentages of drop out as by the outcome ratings of the completed therapies.

Drop out percentages also confirm the assumed negative influence of alexithymia on psychodynamic psychotherapy. The outcome ratings of the completed psychodynamic therapies, however, are rather puzzling. Symptomatic improvement is connected with more pronounced alexithymia, role performance improvement with less-pronounced alexithymia. Trying to explain these divergent data, several possibilities should be considered. First we must take into account that the subgroup of the completed psychodynamic therapies is already a selection of patients with lower alexithymia ratings, because the higher rated group of drop outs is eliminated. It could be that alexithymia ratings under a certain level are not reliable or unimportant. On the other hand, it is possible that the completing of the psychodynamic therapy proves that patient and therapist have been able to engage in a relationship overcoming the alexithymic impediments. That would mean that the phenomenon in itself is not irreversible. A third possibility remains that alexithymia affects different aspects of outcome in psychodynamic therapy in a different way. On the basis of our data we are not able to opt for one of these explanations; further and more on these problems oriented research is needed.

In general, we may conclude that our findings are in favor of the pragmatic value of the concept of alexithymia, as a form of communication which on the one hand enhances the possibilities of somatic symptom formation, and on the other promotes drop out in psychodynamic therapy, while not affecting behavior therapy. For the explanation of the phenomenon itself, our data offer no clear arguments.

References

Edwards, A.L.: Statistical methods (Holt Rinehart & Winston, New York 1967).

Hoornaert, F. and Pierloot, R.: Parental symbolism in the doctor image of psychosomatic and neurotic patients. J. psychosom. Res. *20:* 247–253 (1976).

Malan, D.H.: A study of brief psychotherapy (Tavistock, London 1963).

Marty, P. et M'Uzan, M. de: La pensée opératoire. Revue fr. Psychanal. *27:* 1345–1354 (1963).

Marty, P.; M'Uzan, M. de et David, C.: L'investigation psychosomatique (PUF, Paris 1963).

Musaph, H.: The role of aggression in somatic symptom formation. Int. J. Psychiat. Med. *5:* 449–460 (1974a).

Musaph, H.: Discussion of the paper of de M'Uzan. Psychother. Psychosom. *23:* 110 (1974b).

M'Uzan, M. de: Psychodynamic mechanisms in psychosomatic symptom formation. Psychother. Psychosom. *23:* 103–110 (1974).

Nemiah, J. and Sifneos, P.: Affect and fantasy in patients with psychosomatic disorders; in *Hill* Modern trends in psychosomatic medicine, pp. 26–40 (Butterworths, London 1970a).

Nemiah, J. and Sifneos, P.: Psychosomatic illness. A problem of communication. Psychother. Psychosom. *18:* 154–160 (1970b).

Nichols, R.C. and Beck, K.W.: Factors in psychotherapy research. J. Consult. Psychol. *24:* 388–399 (1960).

Siegel, S.: Non parametric statistics for the behavioral sciences (McGraw Hill, New York 1956).

Sifneos, P.: Clinical observations on some patients suffering from a variety of psycho-somatic diseases; in Acta medica psychosomatica, pp. 452–458 (SJMP, Rome 1967).

Sifneos, P.: The prevalence of 'alexithymic', characteristics in psychosomatic patients. Psychother. Psychosom. *22:* 255–262 (1973).

Spielberger, C.D.; Gorsuch, R.L., and Lushene, R.E.: STAI manual (Consulting Psychologists Press, Palo Alto 1970).

Spitzer, R.L.; Endicott, J.; Fleiss, J.L., and Cohen, J.: The psychiatric status schedule. Archs gen. Psychiat. *23:* 41–55 (1970).

Stinissen, J.; Willems, P.J.; Coetsier, P. en Hulsman, W.L.L.: Handleiding bij de Nederlandstalige bewerking van de Wechsler Adult Intelligence Scale (Swets en Zeitlinger, Amsterdam 1970).

Taylor, J.: A personality scale of manifest anxiety. J. abnorm. soc. Psychol. *48:* 246–250 (1953).

Wolpe, J.: The practice of behavior therapy (Pergamon, New York 1969).

Prof. Dr. med. *R. Pierloot,* Universitaire St-Jozef kliniek voor Psychiatrie, Leuvenbaan 68, *B-3070 Kortenberg* (Belgium)

Proc. 11th Eur. Conf. Psychosom. Res., Heidelberg 1976
Psychother. Psychosom. *28:* 167–171 (1977)

A Comparison of the Oxygen Consumption of Normal and Alexithymic Subjects in Response to Affect-Provoking Thoughts

John C. Nemiah[1], Peter E. Sifneos[2] and Roberta Apfel-Savitz[3]

Department of Psychiatry of the Beth Israel Hospital, Harvard Medical School, Boston, Mass.

Introduction

As we have pointed out in other communications (3, 4), many patients with certain psychosomatic disorders manifest alexithymic characteristics – that is, they are unable to express affects in words and do not have fantasies associated with affects, their thought content being characterized by a preoccupation with the minute details of their external environment and actions – the so-called 'pensée opératoire'.

We have postulated that the alexithymic phenomena result from a disruption in the processes that normally follow as a response to an affect-provoking event or situation. Under ordinary circumstances, such an event leads, on the one hand, to a cognitive perception of the external elements involved, and, on the other, to an arousal of the somatic components of affect (emotion). The latter in its turn undergoes a psychic elaboration consisting of the subjective experience of the affect (feeling), the linking of the experience with affective words descriptive of it, the production of fantasies expressive of the affect, and the arousal of a network of related associations and memories. In the alexithymic individual the channels leading to the mental elements of psychic elaboration are blocked (or absent), and the affect-provoking event

[1] Psychiatrist-in-Chief, Beth Israel Hospital, and Professor of Psychiatry, Harvard Medical School.

[2] Associate Director, Psychiatric Service, Beth Israel Hospital, and Professor of Psychiatry at the Beth Israel Hospital, Harvard Medical School.

[3] Assistant Psychiatrist, Beth Israel Hospital and Clinical Instructor in Psychiatry, Harvard Medical School.

produces only the somatic, emotional component of affect in a specific and possibly intensified fashion that results ultimately in a localized bodily lesion as the manifestation of a psychosomatic disorder.

In individuals with a normally functioning affective system the channels of communication are reciprocal – that is, activity in the somatic component arouses psychic elaboration, and activity in the psychic component arouses a somatic response. Witness, for example, the autonomic arousal that occurs in phobic patients forced to think of the phobic situation. In alexithymic individuals, however, one would predict from the postulated blocks and discontinuities in the affective system that arousal of the psychic elements would produce little or no response in the somatic components of the system. To test this prediction we have carried out a pilot study, the results of which are presented here.

Experimental Procedure

We chose oxygen consumption as our measure of somatic function on the basis of the work of *Clynes* (2), who showed that oxygen consumption was increased when individuals thought of affective words such as 'anger' or 'fear'.

A total of 14 subjects were examined. Seven of these were normal controls without a history of psychosomatic disorders or evidence of alexithymic characteristics. The remaining seven subjects were patients, all showing alexithymic characteristics and with somatic illnesses as noted in table I. For each subject, the presence or absence of alexithymia was determined through a standard interview and 'Alexithymia Questionnaire' (4).

Each of the subjects, after an explanation of the study and instructions in a simple relaxation technique (1), was seated in a comfortable chair, with EKG electrodes attached and a face mask positioned to permit comfortable breathing. During the experiment the contents of the expired air were continuously analyzed by a specially constructed machine (Prophet 34) that gave a direct and continuous measure of its oxygen content. In this setting,

Table I. Diagnosis and alexithymia in patient group

Patient, No.	Alexithymia	Illness
1	+	hypertension
2	+	peptic ulcer, asthma
3	+	epilepsy
4	+	peptic ulcer
5	+	ulcerative colitis
6	+	thyrotoxicosis
7	+	eye spasms

each individual was required to perform sequentially three different types of tasks: (1) relaxation (R): performing the relaxation technique in which they had been instructed earlier; (2) calculation (C): subtracting in their heads 7 from 300; (3) affective thoughts (AT): each was instructed to think in turn (a) 'sad thoughts', (b) 'angry thoughts', (c) 'happy thoughts' and (d) 'frightening thoughts'. Each such task lasted 2 min in the following sequence: R-C-R-AT (sad) -R-C-R-AT (angry) -R-C-R-AT (happy) -R-C-R-AT (frightening) -R, the whole process occupying 34 min. Blood pressure was taken at the beginning and the end of the experiment, and heart rate was monitored throughout.

Results

From the continuous measurement of the expired air, the total volume of oxygen consumed was calculated in every subject for each of the 2-min periods allotted to the various tasks described above, Next, the average figure was calculated for each subject for all of the R, C, and AT periods. Finally, the difference was calculated between the average of the AT periods and the average of the R periods, and between the average of the C periods and the average of the R periods. These differences for each individual (in cm³ of oxygen consumed/min) are shown in figure 1.

From an inspection of figure 1, it is immediately apparent that all of the normal controls, save one, consumed more oxygen while thinking affective

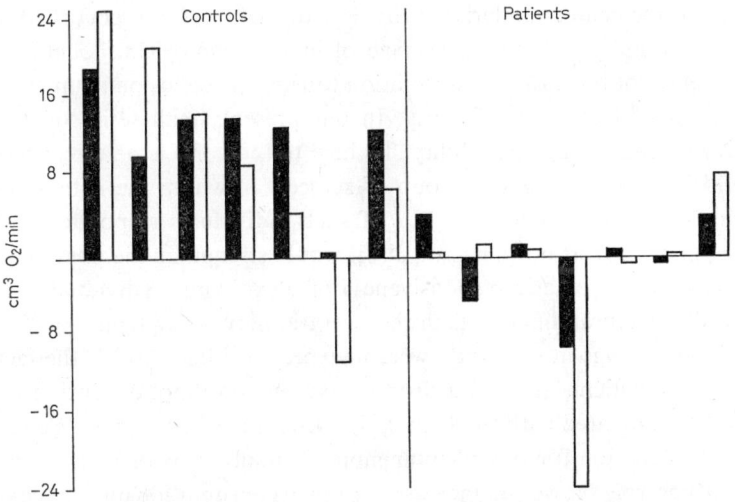

Fig. 1. Changes in oxygen consumption from baseline relaxation during periods of affective thoughts (■) and calculations (□).

thoughts than when employing the relaxation technique. By contrast, in the patients there was little or no increase during the AT period, and, in fact, two patients showed a *decrease* in oxygen consumption while thinking affective thoughts. The consumption of oxygen during the period of calculation showed a similar pattern. The difference between the group of subjects and group of patients in oxygen consumption change for the AT and C periods was significant at the 0.01 level of probability for each (Wilcoxon Two-Sample Test).

Discussion

What is of most interest in this study is the finding that as a whole the normal controls showed a greater somatic responsiveness to affective thoughts than did the patients. This confirms our initial prediction, and gives further evidence for the hypothesis that in alexithymic individuals there is a significant discontinuity between the somatic component of affect (emotion) and the psychic component of affect (feeling and fantasy) such that the one cannot effect the other.

Our findings do not, however, help us to determine the nature of that discontinuity. Two hypothetical models are possible: (1) the discontinuity might be the result of a lack of adequate neuronal connections between the centers responsible for the somatic response (limbic system and hypothalamus) and the centers underlying the psychic elaboration (neocortex), or (2) the discontinuity might be conceived of in a psychological model invoking the defenses of repression and isolation causing an exclusion from conscious awareness of feeling and fantasy. In our present small series of subjects, either explanation is a possibility. To help to settle the issue the experiment should be repeated using a group of subjects in whom the defense of isolation is present to a high degree. If such individuals responded with the same pattern as our normal controls, it would strengthen the possibility that the diminished somatic responsiveness of alexithymic individuals was the result of structural differences in their central nervous system.

Two findings in our study were unexpected. First of all is the fact that two of our patients showed a drop in oxygen consumption during the AT period as compared with the R period, one to a marked degree. We have no ready explanation for this phenomenon. Secondly, it is of interest that the normal controls showed an increase in oxygen consumption during the period of calculations in marked contrast to the patients. This is perhaps because the controls were able to experience anxiety when confronted with this intellectual task. Indeed, one normal subject (A.G.) reported after the experiment that performing mathematical calculations always made him anxious. Again, it should be noted that two individuals showed a marked drop in oxygen consumption during the calculation period. Here, too, we have no explanation for this finding, although it is interesting to note that the only control who showed this pattern of response (D.S.) was also the only control who showed no increase in oxygen consumption during the AT period.

Finally, we should emphasize once more that this is a pilot study undertaken to see whether there was any merit at all in our initial prediction from our working hypothesis. We believe that our findings in this small group of individuals tentatively confirm our prediction and give us sufficient reason for repeating the experiment on a larger population to help to answer the many hypothetical and etiological questions inherent in the concept of alexithymia. Even in the limited study we have reported here, we feel there is another small piece added to the jig-saw puzzle that along with other findings such as those on the genetic aspects of alexithymia and its relation to hypnotizability, give further evidence that alexithymia is a valid phenomenon worthy of further exploration and definition.

Acknowledgements

We should like to express our sincere appreciation to Dr. *Hebert Benson* for making his laboratory facilities available to us, to Miss *Jamie Kotch* and Miss *Kasey Crassweller* for their invaluable technical assistance, and to Dr. *Richard Brodie* for carrying out the necessary statistical calculations.

References

1   *Beary, J.F. and Benson, H.:* A simple psychophysiologic technique which elicits the hypometabolic changes of the relaxation response. Psychosom. Med. *36:* 115–120 (1974).

2   *Clynes, M.:* Sentics. Biocybernetics of emotion communication. Ann. N.Y. Acad. Sci. *220:* 55–131 (1973).

3   *Nemiah, J.C. and Sifneos, P.E.:* Affect and fantasy in patients with psychosomatic illness; in *Hill* Modern Trends in Psychosomatic Medicine (Butterworth, London 1970).

4   *Sifneos, P.E.:* The prevalence of 'alexithymic' characteristics in psychosomatic patients. Psychother. Psychosom. *23:* 255–262 (1973).

Prof. *John C. Nemiah,* Department of Psychiatry, Harward Medical School, Beth Israel Hospital, 330 Brookline Avenue, *Boston, MA 02215* (USA)

Proc. 11th Eur. Conf. Psychosom. Res., Heidelberg 1976
Psychother. Psychosom. *28:* 172–178 (1977)

The Relationship between Hypnotizability and Alexithymia[1]

*Fred H. Frankel, Roberta Apfel-Savitz, John C. Nemiah and
Peter E. Sifneos*[2]

Department of Psychiatry, Beth Israel Hospital and Harvard Medical School,
Boston, Mass.

The subject matter of this presentation utilizes a concept of hypnosis
that is, while not yet universally accepted, at least gaining ground rapidly.
We refer to the recognition of the importance of the subjective experience of
an altered perception, or of an altered sense of awareness in hypnotized
subjects (1). Feelings of relaxation, the motivation to be hypnotized, emotional involvement in the procedure, deep trust, and a readiness to respond to
persuasive comments, while generally necessarily associated with hypnosis,
are not the cardinal characteristics of the event. It is, indeed, the additional
element of a distorted or altered perception that seems to justify the use of
a separate concept, namely, that of hypnosis; we could, otherwise, consider
the whole phenomenon as a manifestation of an intense transference.

Although the precise mental mechanism involved in hypnosis is uncertain, it is a process where images and fantasies can become so vivid and real
as to be confused with the world outside, where incongruities cease to be
troublesome, and where logic becomes superfluous. For example: imagine,
for a moment, what might be taking place when you redistribute your
attention to focus it specifically on the sensations in your fingers, hand and
forearm, encouraging the feeling of lightness to permeate the limb, and then
permitting it to float into an upright position where it remains suspended
comfortably, and weightless.

It is readily apparent that this behavior just described largely depends on
allowing free rein to the imagination, and a minimum of logic.

[1] Supported in part by grant MH 25101 from the National Institute of Mental Health.

[2] The authors thank *Herbert Benson,* MD, for permission to use data gathered in the
study 'Therapy of Anxiety'.

Recent studies (2- 4) have stressed the importance of *absorption, imaginative involvement,* and *mental imagery* in a person's response to a hypnotic induction procedure. The association between this imaginative ability and hypnotizability is recognized. *Absorption* is interpreted as a disposition for having episodes of 'total' attention that fully engage one's perceptual, imaginative and ideational resources. This kind of attentional functioning is believed to result in a heightened sense of the reality of the object attended to, imperviousness to distracting events, and an altered sense of reality in general, including an empathically altered sense of self. In the study by *Tellegen and Atkinson* (2), absorption was consistently correlated with hypnotizability. This kind of attentional functioning depends upon rich fantasies that can endure, that become indistinguishable from reality, and that withstand the demands of logic.

Let us quote items directly from the questionnaire on which the trait of absorption was rated. Positive answers indicate the presence of the trait:

'The sound of a voice can be so fascinating to me that I can just go on listening to it.

While acting in a play, I have sometimes really felt the emotions of the character and have "become" him (her) for the time being, forgetting as it were, both myself and the audience.

If I wish, I can imagine (or daydream) some things so vividly that they hold my attention in the way a good movie or story does.

I can tell a story with elaborations to make it sound better, and then have the elaboration seem as real to me as the actual incident, or almost so.

I am sometimes able to forget about my present self and get absorbed in a fantasy that I am someone else.'

Compare such comments with the descriptions that fit the alexithymic responses, where the emphasis is on elaborate descriptions of trivial environmental details, on an absence of differentiated feelings, and on a commitment to action rather than to thought (5).

It can come as no surprise then that the relationship between the two types of responses attracted some attention in a department intent on trying to understand more about both hypnotizability and alexithymia. Before proceeding to an examination of the comparison, however, let us comment on a few other important aspects of hypnosis and hypnotizability.

A most important advance in the study of hypnosis has been the development of standardized and reliable measures of individual differences in hypnotic responsivity. Scales have been developed that measure, directly, a subject's responses to a series of specific suggestions. As a result, the nature of hypnosis has become clearer. Among the several parameters that have been uncovered, we now know that an individual's responsiveness to hypnosis tends to be relatively stable (6), and that there is evidence to suggest that hypnotizability is the product of both a genetic predisposition and subsequent environmental influences (7). It is also worth noting that whereas hypnotizability has, in the past, been considered by some to represent a weakness or lack of steadfastness in subjects who are responsive, we now know, from the thousands of college students who have been tested, that among that population the ability to enter hypnosis is normally distributed; indeed individuals able to respond to hypnosis are likely to be somewhat better adjusted and more normal and outgoing than those who show a lower level of response (6).

We will now return to the relationship between alexithymia and hypnotizability. We were interested in learning whether the presence of alexithymia would hinder responses to hypnotizing procedures. The method involved a comparison of the hypnotic responsivity of alexithymic patients with the responses of others who did not fall into the alexithymic category. From our descriptions of the differences between hypnosis and alexithymia, we expected the alexithymic subjects to be less hypnotizable.

Method

The 32 subjects investigated were all patients referred to a study for the treatment of anxiety (8). Routinely they were evaluated psychiatrically, and in addition to the rating of their anxiety, they were tested for responsivity to hypnosis on three separate occasions. Although the findings that we are presenting here emerge, in the main, from the investigative steps of that ongoing unrelated project, they are merely incidental to that study, and independent of its goals. Nevertheless that study provided us with an ideal opportunity for collecting the necessary data.

The alexithymic ratings were based on the Psychosomatic Questionnaire of the Beth Israel Hospital Psychiatric Service, completed by the examiner at the end of the psychiatric interview, before the hypnotizability scales were administered. The hypnotizability scales could not, therefore, have influenced the ratings. The questionnaire has 17 questions about patient's behavior, and 6 related to the interviewer's reactions.

The hypnotizability ratings were based on the administration of three scales, divided between two interviews on different days. The precaution of including more than one assessment was introduced because, although an individual's overall responsivity tends to be stable, fluctuations can occur from day to day as a result of the circumstances in which the tests are administered, and because of minor indispositions in the subject.

Of the three scales, one is a widely standardized and validated test that has been in use since 1962 and has been administered to many thousands of subjects. It is the Harvard

Group Scale (HGS) (9) which involves a self-rating by the subject, and is a modification of the individual rating scale known as the Stanford Hypnotic Susceptibility Scale A (SHSS: A) (10). The ratings range from 0 to 12. It should be noted that the scores on this scale are considered by top calibre investigators to be as reliable as those achieved on the widely recognized intelligence tests.

In order to corroborate the Harvard Group Scale rating, we also administered the Hypnotic Induction Profile (HIP) (11), and then a recently assembled six-item test including the subject's own ratings of the vividness and reality of a hypnotic dream, and of his experience of age-regression. Other investigators have found the scores on the Hypnotic Induction Profile to correlate quite highly with those of the SHSS. The HIP contains fewer items than the SHSS, and measures fewer aspects of the hypnotic experience.

Subjects

Of the 32 subjects examined, 25 scored consistently on all three scales. In other words, their experiences and observed behavior left little doubt that they were either highly hypnotizable, average, or poor responders. The remaining seven subjects were excluded from this study because of the incongruity of their scores. Among the seven excluded were five subjects who differed in the self-rating of their hypnotic experience on the HGS from their observed behavior. In other words, their behavior reflected a more, or less impressive response than actually experienced, or reported. Their *true* experience of hypnosis is therefore difficult to rate. Such discrepancies do occur in a small percentage of subjects tested on the HGS; the reasons are not always clear. We chose not to include them because of the confusing nature of their responses, and because of the difficulty in assessing their true levels, even though their scores on the other two scales were unquestioned.

Findings

Among the 25 subjects included in the study, we considered those who scored 4 or below on the HGS to be poor responders, and those who scored 7 and up to be good. In other words, we arbitrarily excluded the two subjects who scored 5 and 6 on the 12-point scale, as falling in an ambiguous zone. Ideally, we would have preferred to consider as low, all those who scored 4 and below, and as high, all those who scored 8 and above, excluding from the study all of those in the average range who scored 5, 6 or 7. This clear-cut distinction was not possible because of the limited numbers available for analysis. A large proportion of those tested scored 7 (6 of the 25). However, as a score of 7 on the HGS reflects a distinct ability to respond and make use of fantasy, we had little question about including them among those who responded well; their scores on the other 2 scales corroborated the HGS rating.

Among the remaining 23 subjects, we found 12 highs, and 11 lows. Of the 12 highs, 1 was rated alexithymic (8%), and 11 (92%) were considered not to be. Of the 11 poorly hypnotizable subjects, 8 (73%) were considered to be alexithymic, and 3 (27%) were not.

Of those 9 with alexyithymic characteristics, 1 (11%) was highly hypnotizable, while of 14 without alexithymic characteristics, 11 (79%) were quite hypnotizable. The average (arithmetic mean) hypnotizability rating on the HGS of the 9 alexithymic patients was 2.7. The average hypnotizability rating of the 14 nonalexithymic patients was 6.9.

Using the chi square with Yates correction for small numbers (X^2y) the p level is <0.01.

Discussion

This is not presented as a methodologically tight demonstration of an inverse relationship between two characteristics of personality. Furthermore, the alexithymic ratings were carried out by only one of us *(R.A.S.)*. They were not confirmed by a second rater. The findings strongly suggest, however, that what is essential to hypnosis, namely, the ability to be totally attentive to and engaged with one's perceptual, imaginative and ideational resources, is that which is specifically diminished or lacking in the presence of alexithymia.

In the climate that prevailed 20 years ago, we would have been hard pressed in trying to define any kind of relationship between hypnotic and alexithymic behavior. For the past two decades, however, experimental findings in hypnosis research have led to an understanding of the event that has emphasized many of its important aspects. We know, for example, that hypnosis is not a unitary phenomenon, and that in addition to at least several recognizable factors in hypnotic responsivity, we must also acknowledge the varying depths of the different dimensions involved (12). We understand that in addition to the essential and varying ability to distort perception by means of engaging the attention in imaginative fantasy, hypnotizable subjects are willing, to a varying extent, to become emotionally involved in the experience, and seem, also, to relate to the hypnotist with a varying degree of trust associated with near magical expectations. Hypnotic behavior is also marked by an ability to tolerate illogic in a most dramatic way, and can often be associated with memory changes, namely, either hypermnesia or amnesia.

We mention these aspects of hypnotic responsivity, because they have attracted the attention of serious investigators in recent years. Although the

studies are not exhaustive, and further inquiry is indicated, we must spe-
culate on the relevance of these characteristics of hypnosis to a greater understanding of the fascinating concept of alexithymia, if the latter is indeed the
obverse of hypnotizability.

Will we, for instance, be able to define any special characteristics of the
trust and expectations that alexithymic patients exhibit; might we expect
them to have less access to the memories of relevant events in their lives; and
how would such factors influence the nature of psychotherapy? Might their
preoccupation with action be predicated in any way on their inability to
tolerate illogic and their need to protect themselves with the logical consistency of reality? What might be the relevance of a possible genetic predisposition in both hypnotizability and alexithymia?

We raise these questions in the hope that further work on the understanding of alexithymia will pay attention to them, in the same way that work
in hypnosis must, enabling us ultimately to clarify both types of human
behavior.

We have, perhaps, given too free a rein to our own imagination in this
discourse. (We are, we imagine, relatively hypnotizable and not obviously
alexithymic.) Our first step, however, must be to measure the hypnotizability rating of more patients considered to be alexithymic, thereby refining
and enriching as we proceed, both the concepts of hypnosis and alexithymia.

References

1   *Orne, M.T.:* The nature of hypnosis. Artifact and essence. J. abnorm. soc. Psychol.
    58: 277–299 (1959).
2   *Tellegen, A. and Atkinson, Y.:* Openness to absorbing and self-altering experiences
    ('absorption'), a trait related to hypnotic susceptibility. J. abnorm. Psychol. *83:*
    268–277 (1974).
3   *Hilgard, J.R.:* Personality and hypnosis. A study of imaginative involvement (Uni-
    versity of Chicago Press, Chicago 1970).
4   *Sheehan, P.W.:* Hypnosis and the manifestation of 'imagination'; in *Fromm and Shor*
    Hypnosis: research developments and perspectives (Aldine Atherton, Chicago 1972).
5   *Sifneos, P.E.:* Problems of psychotherapy of patients with alexithymic characteristics
    and physical disease. Psychother. Psychosom. *26:* 65–70 (1975).
6   *Hilgard, E.R.:* Hypnotic susceptibility (Harcourt, Brace & World, New York 1965).
7   *Morgan, A.H.:* The heritability of hypnotic susceptibility in twins. J. abnorm. Psychol.
    82: 55–61 (1973).
8   *Benson, H.:* Therapy of anxiety. A new psychophysiologic approach (study in process).
9   *Shor, R.E. and Orne, E.C.:* The Harvard group scale of hypnotic susceptibility.
    Form A (Consulting Psychologists Press, Palo Alto 1962).

10 *Weitzenhoffer, A.M. and Hilgard, E.R.:* Stanford hypnotic susceptibility scale. Forms A and B (Consulting Psychologists Press, Palo Alto 1959).
11 *Spiegel, H. and Bridger, A.A.:* Manual for hypnotic induction profile. Eye-roll levitation method (Soni Medica, New York 1970).
12 *Shor, R.E.:* Three dimensions of hypnotic depth. Int. J. clin. exp. Hypnosis *10:* 23–38 (1962).

Fred H. Frankel, MBChB, DPM, Harvard Medical School, Beth Israel Hospital, Department of Psychiatry, 330 Brookline Avenue, *Boston MA 02215* (USA)

Proc. 11th Eur. Conf. Psychosom. Res., Heidelberg 1976
Psychother. Psychosom. *28:* 179–186 (1977)

Psychopathology and 'Pseudo-Normality' in Ulcerative Colitis

Murray Jackson [1]

Ulcerative colitis is a serious disease of bad prognosis and unknown cause. There is evidence that its incidence is increasing (as is the case with Crohn's disease) and that immunological mechanisms are central in its pathogenesis. The fact that some 50% of ulcerative colitis patients have circulating antibodies to milk protein in their blood suggests that the earliest physical and mental transactions between mother and suckling infant need to be considered in research by paediatricians concerned with the investigation of the establishment of patterns of immunity in earliest life, and I will refer to some of these transactions in my paper.

The subject of psychopathology in ulcerative colitis is a controversial one. Personal experience of 20 cases seen in psychosomatic liaison work and a comparable number encountered in a supervisory capacity, has convinced me that psychological factors are more common in the aetiology of this disorder than is generally recognised. I wish to draw attention to the concept of 'pseudo-normality' and employ some current psychoanalytic theory to help explain this neglect. I also wish to comment on the status of the concept of 'alexithymia' the term coined by *Sifneos* (1967) to draw attention to a type of hidden psychopathology that may be common to most, if not all, psychosomatic disorders.

Many experienced physicians believe that subjects of ulcerative colitis are psychologically normal, or simply showing the effects of having to live with such a devastating disorder. The obvious somatopsychic consequences of the disorder are not in dispute, whereas the role of causal factors is still

[1] Consultant Psychiatrist and Psychotherapist, The Bethlem Royal and Maudsley Hospital, and Kings College Hospital, London.

very much so. Despite pioneer work by *Engel* (1955) and subsequent extensive surveys of therapeutic work by many other experienced physicians, there is no general agreement at all about the aetiological role of psychological factors. Some physicians still believe that pure psychogenesis is being claimed, despite *Engel's* clarification of the contributory status of such factors, which are neither necessary nor sufficient (*Engel* 1967).

The studies of *Feldman et al.* (1967) are widely regarded by physicians as convincing evidence of the irrelevance of psychological factors in the genesis of ulcerative colitis. It seems to me to be a remarkable phenomenon that so much psychopathology can pass unnoticed by experienced physicians. The concept of 'pseudo-normality' may help explain this and I will enlarge on it shortly. My own clinical experience is derived from a highly biased selection of cases, mostly inpatients with serious disease not responding quickly to treatment. An unbiased selection of cases would no doubt reveal a whole spectrum of psychopathology, from minimal to extreme, but I believe that the lessons to be learned from the serious psychopathology that was usual in my cases have general and important significance. In this series of cases significant life stresses were always present before disease onset. The acknowledgement by the patient of the significance of these stresses was usually minimal and often absent. This phenomenon could be explained by the concept of denial which could be seen as a spectrum ranging from an unwillingness to face conflict which could be easily overcome, right through to an intractable absence of connection of important life events and emotions.

The first of the series was a 4-year-old girl, encountered 25 years ago. She was dangerously ill, requiring blood transfusions and not responding to treatment. She was generally regarded as a quiet and normal child although simple psychotherapy gradually uncovered feelings of the most intense sort. Over a period of 12 months she became able to express these feelings and the ulcerative colitis disappeared. She remained well for 15 years, then had a period of severe asthma from which she soon recovered, and has had no further illness. This child was neither delinquent, neurotic nor psychotic, but had the most severe emotional conflicts which at first she was quite unable to verbalise. The relief she experienced when she slowly became able to give expression to her feelings was so dramatic that I have never since doubted the crucial *causal* importance of psychological conflict in these disorders. This patient showed at first the lack of capacity for verbal communication of affects and apparent impairment of fantasy formation, which is the defect described by *Sifneos* (1967) and designated by the neologism 'alexithymia' (no words for feelings). It is certainly not always so easy to remove such inhibitions, a fact that has led *Nemiah and Sifneos* (1970) to suggest that the defect may be at times irreversible, the result of a maturational failure of appropriate physiological structures in the brain. The majority of my series of cases showed this alexithymic characteristic, and all showed psychopathology that I considered to be of major aetiological significance. The following features were common:

(1) Psychotic characteristics – paranoid traits and hypochondriasis.

(2) Agoraphobia and in a few cases severe spider-phobia, long antedating illness onset.

(3) Marked symbiotic dependency on a key figure, with extreme sensitivity to loss or separation.

(4) Severe environmental trauma in infancy and childhood – separations, maternal death, depression or severe illness were commonly encountered.

(5) Co-existent or consecutive psychosomatic symptoms (asthma, migraine, alimentary, gynaecological, etc.).

(6) Precipitating stress almost invariable – object loss, severe frustration or entrapment, occasional very gradual decompensation.

(7) Major pathology in family relationships.

(8) Marked deficiency of impulse control – 'bottling up' or 'exploding'. (A feature observed by *Greer* (1975) in a precise study of the attributes of women with rapidly progressing breast cancer.)

(9) The use of denial as a predominant method of coping.

(10) Severe defect in the capacity to tolerate psychic pain, particularly that of depression.

(11) Severe difficulty in reflecting in any meaningful way on their own experience and behaviour.

(12) Inability to report dreams or fantasies.

The repeated impression has been of a major impairment of the capacity of knowing about, recognising, and containing certain sorts of feelings. This defect was not always obvious at once, and I believe that it is extremely common, as *Sifneos* (1967) contends, and that it may at times require an interview in depth, or engagement in psychotherapy to reveal it.

The fact of significant psychopathology existing in a person who may at first sight seem to be effective and mature, has led to more than one observer to employ the term 'pseudo-normal'. It is the use made by the French psychoanalyst *McDougall* (1974) that seems to me to be particularly valuable. In discussing aspects of character that she has encountered in various psychosomatic disorders she uses the term to describe an apparently normal person who, on closer inspection, reveals evidence of impoverishment in emotional life, an adequate or even an outstanding performance in individual or educational pursuits (which she calls a super-adaptation to external reality) (compare *Brown's* (1971) concept of the 'super-stable' personality) but revealing a shallowness which is not always easy to detect and is difficult to describe. She uses the concept of 'pensée opératoire' (the precursor of the alexithymia concept) originally formulated by *Marty and de M'Uzan* (1963) to investigate this phenomenon. She points out that this deficit may result from a specific sort of failure in the mother-infant relationship which leads to arrest of development of the capacity for fantasy. Referring to the researches in infant observation of French workers she points out that fantasy may be regarded as a function that develops in order to allow representation of the absent mother, and thus to ease the experience of separation and transition to sleep. These researches extend the original work of Spitz which showed how the mother-child relationship may hinder the development of normal autoerotism. A mother who is 'addictive' or 'restrictive' may be preventing this necessary maturation with the consequence that fantasy life in general is impoverished and the capacity for creating fantasy to deal with infantile and current present day anxiety is damaged. *McDougall* (1974) sees this early environmental failure as a likely basis for 'pseudo-normality' and also as a general factor predisposing to the development of psychosomatic disorders in general at a later date. She points out how the work of *Winnicott* (1953) on transitional phenomena, and *Bion* (1962) on the origins of the capacity for fantasy, can help the understanding of this area.

Current psychoanalytic theory of object-relationships, developed by Klein and Fairbairn, allows a deeper understanding of the psychopathology of certain psychosomatic disorders, particularly of those bodily systems connected to the external world by way of systems and apertures as described by *Kubie* (1953). In many such disorders it can be seen that psycho-social stress has precipitated the regression to a level where symbol formation breaks down and schizoid mechanisms predominate. The life stress is commonly one which brings the threat of depression, and the regression represents a retreat from the intolerable pain. At this regressed level the subject is unable to contain painful emotions, and uses primitive methods to get rid of them and the associated mental content. If projective methods are possible, psychotic, phobic or paranoid symptoms may appear, whereas acting out may give rise to behavioural disorders or delinquency. Hypochondriacal symptoms may appear as a defence against psychosis, as shown by *Rosenfeld* (1965). Neurotic mechanisms, which require more mature symbolic capacity (conversion, displacement, fantasy) are inoperative. Under these circumstances a massive physiological activation may occur, representing a regressive resomatization of affect or in object-relation terms a regression to an undifferentiated psycho-biological state where fantasy is inoperative because no containing object was originally available in the form of an effective mother, or a transitional object.

These processes may help to answer the question I raised at the beginning 'How is is that so much important psychopathology apparently goes undetected'? In the case of ulcerative colitis the Feldman studies have failed to detect it. In the case of asthma, the work of *Zealley et al.* (1970) has shown conclusively that properly selected asthmatic subjects have no greater incidence of neurosis than normal.

The explanation I am suggesting is that the psychopathology is not neurotic at all and may be hidden, and that the attack of psychosomatic symptoms may itself be the representation of the missing psychopathology.

I wish to conclude by some miscellaneous comments, speculations and tentative conclusions:

(1) Significant psychopathology of a causal nature certainly exists in ulcerative colitis and is much more common than is generally realised. A truly representative sample could be expected to show a spectrum of such psychopathology. It may be very difficult to detect, and the concept of 'pseudo-normality' helps to make this understandable. The psychopathology involves the use of primitive defence mechanisms of splitting and projective identification (psychotic mechanisms in Kleinian usage) and is associated with an impairment of the capacity to find and express certain feelings in words. Thus, 'alexithymia' appears in a spectrum of varying degrees of severity or obviousness. Efforts that are currently being made to identify alexithymic characteristics by the use of interviews, questionnaires, and projective tests, should have an important place to play in investigation of the psychopathology of ulcerative colitis.

(2) All the psychopathology which can be observed in ulcerative colitis can also be seen in schizoid or narcissistic personalities who do not suffer from colitis, and so the subject of organ choice will have to be illuminated by our theories.

(3) In order to understand the genesis of the alexithymia we must consider (a) The family and cultural context in which development takes place (*Wolff*, 1973). (b) The process by which an infant normally acquires the capacity for fantasy and how this may be impaired through failure in the mother-infant relationship. The work of *Bion* (1962), and *McDougall's* (1974) illuminating comments serve as an introduction to this area. (c) The

acquisition of speech, with its discharge, communication and symbolic aspects and how the sign and symbol functions of words may fail to develop adequately. Alexithymia implies that transformations allowing for the proper use of words has failed and that certain emotions are thus expressed in somatic ways. A split in the self may take place where one part of the self uses words adequately, and another does not. Some moods can be communicated effectively and others cannot. The work of Piaget and psycholinguistics is of relevance in this area. (d) The organ and system vulnerability of the preverbal child who reaches the state of speech acquisiton. This is the problem of 'target organ' and amongst the multiple determinants both biological and psychological that may be involved, the disputed concept of psycho-physiological fixation (with subsequent regression) is helpful. When speech fails to express impulses (the associated capacity for fantasy having already been impaired to varying degrees) pre-existent discharge processes are activated, which are likely to affect particularly the skin or aperture systems.

(4) To call these somatizations 'discharge processes' is to use language which is not yet truly psychological. Object-relations theory can help conceptualize the idea that an organ or sphincter may behave like a person in a state of conflict between impulses to take in and impulses to push out, exclude, or get rid of, concrete objects which are (in the language we are using) elements of thought not yet transformed into thought. *Rey* (1975) has given vivid clinical illustrations of this failure of transformation. Primitive experiences – raw sensations and perceptions, are not yet transformed into forms susceptible of representation by fantasy and symbol. By analogy we might say that the colon treats ideas in the process of formation like antigens. Such reflections may throw light on the psychological significance of *spasm* of a sphincter or viscus and make it psychologically meaningful in terms of confusion of impulses. An infant who had failed to negotiate these oral conflicts might displace them on to bowel function during the phase of the acquisition of speech. The bowel could then be conceived of as functioning like an excited and angry mouth, which could become a permanent vulnerability if speech then fails to acquire its normal function during the anal phase of development. Certain types of stammering might arise in a comparable way. *Knapp* (1969) has explored the physiology of these processes in terms of 'purging' and 'curbing' mechanisms in asthma, and *Szentivanyi's* (1968) concept of 'biochemical lesion' could be seen as an attempt to conceptualize the physiological aspects of these processes. One would expect such conflicts also to find expression in inhibition of muscular co-ordination in general.

(5) Object relations theory can help explain how these processes can go on in a personality that may appear, or even be, normal. Splitting is a normal phenomenon in development of basic mental organisations, one which makes it possible for the ego to develop in a healthy way because of functional independence from psychopathology which may be potentially severe (*Gallwey*, 1976). By contrast the classical linear model of mental development with fixation points occuring along a longitudinal path leads to the idea that psychopathology is inevitably global and easily detectable by the expert eye.

(6) The foregoing considerations have implications for treatment in ulcerative colitis and other psychosomatic disorders. In order to exert a therapeutic influence, in the direction of insight and personality develop-ment, we need to be armed with adequate theories and a *setting* appropriate to our purposes. Formal psychoanalysis provides such a setting, but the difficulty in engaging these patients in the search for insight may be formi-dable, considering the discipline and sacrifices that may be presented by for-mal psychoanalysis. Attempts to modify the setting are currently being reported and include the following: (a) Group therapy both with formal and modified methods. (b) The provision of skilled in-patient therapy in a specially organized milieu as reported by *Stephanos* (1975) *Wittich* (1975) and others. (c) Co-operation with physicians and surgeons of an intense sort, such as appears to have been achieved by the Parisian group (*Bonfils and de M'Uzan* 1974), and in the psychosomatic centres in West Germany.

I think that these developments in theory and practice bring hope for the psychotherapy of ulcerative colitis and psychosomatic disorders in general, and for the further understanding and alleviation of the alexithymia defect.

References

Bion, W.R.: Learning from experience (Heinemann, London 1962).

Bonfils, S. and M'Uzan, M. de: Irritable bowel syndrome vs. ulcerative colitis. Psycho-functional disturbance vs. psychosomatic disease. J. psychosom. Res. *18:* 291–296 (1974).

Brown, D.G.: Psychiatric treatment of eczema. A controlled study. Br. med. J. *ii:* 729–734 (1971).

Engel, G.L.: Studies of ulcerative colitis. Am. J. Med. *19:* 231 (1955).

Engel, G.L.: Psychological factors and ulcerative colitis. Br. med. J. *iii:* 56 (1967).

Feldman, F. et al.: Psychiatric studies of a consecutive series of 34 patients with ulcerative colitis. Br. med. J. *iii:* 14–17 (1967).

Gallwey, P.L.G.: Transference utilization in aim restricted psychotherapies. Brit. J. Med. Psychol. (in press).

Greer, S.: Psychological attributes of women who develop breast cancer. J. psychosom. Res. *19:* 147–153 (1975).

Knapp, P.H.: The asthmatic and his environment. J. nerv. ment. Dis. *149:* 135–150 (1969).

Kubie, L.S.: The central representation of the symbolic process in relation to psychosomatic disorders. Psychosom. Med. *15:* 1–7 (1953).

Marty, P. and M'Uzan, M. de: La pensée opératoire. Revue fr. Psychanal. *27:* 1345 (1963).

McDougall, J.: The psychosoma and the psychoanalytic process. Int. Rev. psychoanal. *1:* 437 (1974).

Nemiah, J.C. and Sifneos, P.E.: Affect and fantasy in patients with psychosomatic disorders; in *Hill* Modern trends in psychosomatic medicine, vol. 2, pp. 26–34 (Butterworths, London 1970).

Rey, J.H.: Liberté et processus de pensée psychotique. Vie méd. Can. fr. *4:* 1046–1060 (1975).

Rosenfeld, H.: The psychopathology of hypochondriasis. Psychotic states. A psychoanalytical approach, pp. 180–199 (Hogarth, London 1965).

Sifneos, P.E.: Clinical observations on some patients suffering from a variety of psychosomatic disorders. Acta med. psychosom. Proc. 7th Eur. Conf. psychosom. Res., Rome 1967.

Stephanos, S.: The object relations of the psychosomatic patient. Br. J. med. Psychol. *48:* 257–266 (1975).

Szentivanyi, A.: The beta adrenergic theory of the atopic abnormality in bronchial asthma. J. Allergy *42:* 203–232 (1968).

Winnicott, D.W.: Transitional objects and transitional phenomena. Int. J. Psychoanal. *34:* 2 (1953).

Wittich, G.H.: Therapy in psychosomatic hospitals. Paper presented at 3rd Congr. Int. College Psychosomatic Medicine, Rome 1975.

Wolff, H.H.: Psychotherapy. Its place in psychosomatic management. Psychother. psychosom. *22:* 233–249 (1973).

Zealley, A.K.; Aitken, R.C.B., and Rosenthal, S.V.: Asthma. A psychophysiological investigation. Proc. R. Soc. Med. *64:* 825–829 (1970).

Murray A. Jackson, MB.FRCP, Consultant Psychiatrist, Department of Psychological Medicine, King's College Hospital, Denmark Hill, *London SE5 9RS* (England)

Proc. 11th Eur. Conf. Psychosom. Res., Heidelberg 1976
Psychother. Psychosom. *28:* 187–192 (1977)

Personality Features of Patients with Ulcerative Colitis

R. Liedtke, H. Freyberger and S. Zepf

Medizinische Hochschule Hannover, Abteilung für Psychosomatik
(Direktor: Prof. Dr. *H. Freyberger*), Hannover

Since *Murray* (14) referred to certain outstanding traits of patients with unspecific ulcerative colitis in 1930, a great many other researchers have sought for specification of the personality features of these patients. This research has produced findings which are partly in agreement, partly at variance with and to a certain extent contradictory to each other. In the majority of cases these investigations have been based on methods – such as the biographical anamnesis or the psychiatric interview – which seldom allow sufficient comparison and reproduction or even allow none at all. Our own investigation was an attempt to determine personality features of patients with ulcerative colitis via a comparison with 'healthy' control persons, using a clearly-defined psychological test procedure, the MMPI Saarbrücken.

30 colitis patients (group I) whose diagnoses were confirmed by recto-sigmoidoscopy and/or by X-ray were compared with 30 controls (group II). Group I was composed of former inpatients of the medical university clinics and medical clinics of the municipal hospital in Kiel. For the statistical comparison the 'matched pairs' procedure was used. Each colitis patient was matched to a control person with a combination of six social attributes – age, sex, family status, education, professional status and income. Persons were not taken for controls if they had had psychotherapy or if they had had a psychosomatic illness diagnosed. The social features of the patients and controls cannot be reported here in detail (12). It need only be mentioned that 18 of the 36 male and the 24 female testees were between 31 and 35 years old, 20 persons were between 36 and 45, and 22 test persons were between 18 and 30.

One-third of the patients had become ill with colitis between the 21st and 25th year of life, most of them between their 26th and 45th year of life. The duration of illness lay between 2 and 10 years for 21 patients. None of the patients was in hospital at the time of investigation and none had had psychiatric treatment during the course of his illness. The controls were acquaintances of persons we selected on the grounds of their social status.

The evaluation of the MMPI was carried out for the 14 standard scales, 4 validity and 10 clinical scales (17). Table I summarizes the results of the comparison. The colitis patients differ from the controls as regards significantly higher ratings on the scales hypochondriasis, depression, paranoia and social introversion. On the other scales there are no significant differences.

The significance of hypochondrial features in our study can be compared with only a few analogous results of other research works (6, 8). For the most part colitis patients are only occasionally classified as hypochondrical in the literature. But if hypochondrical traits are regarded as significant, the authors accentuate that apart from observing his intestinal function accurately, the

Table I. Statistical comparison of the raw score values of patients and controls for the 14 standard scales of the MMPI
(significance calculated according to the Wilcoxon matched-pairs signed-ranks test, one-tailed test for the scales D, Pa, Si, two-tailed test for the scales ?, L, F, K, Hs, Hy, Pd, Mf, Pt, Sc, Ma)

Scale	Colitis group	Direction of difference	Control group	n	t	p
?	I	=	II	22	90.0	>0.05
L	I	=	II	24	101.5	>0.05
F	I	=	II	27	149.0	>0.05
K	I	=	II	29	208.5	>0.05
(Hs) hypochondriasis	I	>	II	26	89.5	<0.05
(D) depression	I	>	II	28	96.5	<0.01
(Hy) hysteria	I	=	II	29	160.5	>0.05
(Pd) psychopathic deviation	I	=	II	28	143.0	>0.05
(Mf) masculinity femininity	I	=	II	29	198.5	>0.05
(Pa) paranoia	I	>	II	27	103.0	<0.05
(Pt) psychasthenia	I	=	II	29	186.5	>0.05
(Sc) schizophrenia	I	=	II	29	202.5	>0.05
(Ma) Hypomania	I	=	II	28	151.5	>0.05
(Si) Social introversion	I	>	II	30	126.5	<0.05

patient also registers the slightest deviations in his general somatic condition (6, 9). Supposing that the MMPI really measures hypochondrical features according to our own results, these seem after all to be more often present in colitis patients than was noted in the literature hitherto.

The significantly higher scores of the colitis patients on the depression scale can be viewed as a substantiation of the observations of a great many authors (1, 3, 6, 9). The depression scale of the MMPI covers various depressive syndromes. The construction of the scale is based on the responses of patients who were either diagnosed as reactive or as endogenous depressives (17).

In accordance with several observations made in the literature there can be no doubt that in colitis patients psychotic as well as nonpsychotic depressions are found. Judging from our investigation there are more grounds for the assumption of depressive disorders in most of these patients, but of course it cannot be decided whether these disorders have a psychotic, neurotic or nonpsychotic quality.

The result on the paranoia scale corroborates the assumption that paranoid mechanisms are not seldom observed in patients with ulcerative colitis – especially in the course of psychotic developments (2, 5, 11, 19). For the group of patients whose responses were taken for the construction of the scale, sensitivity was a typical feature in addition to suspicion and ideas of persecution (17). In this connection it must be mentioned that numerous researchers accentuate a sensitivity, a tendency to emotional vulnerability in colitis patients (5, 7, 15, 19). Even if this sensitivity is not mentioned mainly with direct regard to paranoid disorders, nevertheless this agreement in the description of these patients affords a preliminary possibility of substantiating the assumption of a tendency to paranoid mechanisms.

The results of one american study (13) are to some extent contradictory to our findings on the introversion scale. In this study the colitis patients did not differ from controls in terms of living alone (question for living alone 5 years or more) or in terms of joining formal social groups (question for membership of sport clubs, etc.). In all probability the reason for this contradiction is that the questions chosen are too coarsely meshed to be able to include finer deviations of social contact behavior. Otherwise, our own test results on this scale are on the whole similar with the reports of other authors (16, 19).

It has sometimes been argued against the personality traits of colitis patients described in the literature and also against the features objectified in our study that these characteristics could mainly be the result of reactions to the chronic and serious intestinal disease (4, 10). To take this argument into consideration the colitis group was divided into 3 subgroups (I_1, I_2, I_3, table II) with different durations of illness and these subgroups were compared with regard to the MMPI scales which had produced significant differences. The classification into different illness intervals for each of the 3 subgroups followed from the number of patients necessary for statistical reasons in each class. Table III summarizes the results of the comparison as regards this dependency on the duration of illness. Thus, the significantly higher ratings of the colitis patients can be regarded as independent of the length of illness.

We finally would like to go into some of the results on the psychasthenia scale. On this scale – measuring phobic and compulsive features (17) – the colitis patients did not obtain significantly higher ratings. To some degree this result is surprising because a great many studies have produced sufficient evidence that compulsive traits are significant for patients with ulcerative

Table II. Grouping of patients according to duration of illness

Duration of illness in years	Group
0.5–2.5	I_1 (n = 9)
3–5	I_2 (n = 10)
Over 5	I_3 (n = 11)

Table III. Statistical comparison of patients with different duration of illness for the scales hypochondriasis, depression, paranoia, social introversion
(significance calculated according to the Kruskal-Wallis one-way analysis of variance, two-tailed test – corr. f. ties)

Scale	Patients with short duration of illness	Direction of difference	Patients with medium duration of illness	Direction of difference	Patients with long duration of illness	h	p
Hypochondriasis	group I_1	=	group I_2	=	group I_3	0.72	>0.05
Depression	group I_1	=	group I_2	=	group I_3	2.02	>0.05
Paranoia	group I_1	=	group I_2	=	group I_3	1.89	>0.05
Introversion	group I_1	=	group I_2	=	group I_3	1.52	>0.05

colitis (2, 3, 5, 15, 16). But despite the fact that a general presence or even dominance of compulsive features is frequently reported, by way of comparison a compulsive-obsessive neurosis with marked compulsive symptoms is seldom diagnosed in colitis patients (3, 5). Similarly, phobias or phobic symptoms are also seldom reported (11, 18, 19). It is possible that because of the secondary importance of phobic symptoms (5) and compulsive features not developing into a compulsion neurosis, the psychasthenia scale is not able to reveal significant differences between the patient and control group.

The results on the other clinical scales for which no differences could be attained are essentially in agreement with the literature.

Finally, it can be stated that our investigation supports the thesis that patients with ulcerative colitis have a tendency to hypochondria, depression, paranoia and social introversion.

References

1   *Daniels, G.E.:* Psychiatric factors in ulcerative colitis. Gastroenterology *10:* 59–62 (1948).

2   *Boor, C. de:* Die Colitis ulcerosa als psychosomatisches Syndrom. Psyche *18:* 107–119 (1964).

3   *M'Uzan, M. de; Bonfils, S. et Lambling, A.:* Etude psychosomatique de 18 cas de rectocolite hémorragique. Sem. Hôp. Paris *34:* 922–928 (1958).

4   *Tombal, F.T. de:* Ulcerative colitis. Epidemiology and aetiology, course and prognosis. Brit. med. J. *1:* 649–650 (1971).

5   *Engel, G.L.:* Studies of ulcerative colitis. III. The nature of the psychologic processes. Am. J. Med. *19:* 231–256 (1955).

6   *Freyberger, H.:* Colitis ulcerosa. Psychosomatik und Psychotherapie; in *Krauspe, Müller-Wieland und Stelzner* Colitis ulcerosa und granulomatosa, p. 265ff. (Urban & Schwarzenberg, München 1972).

7   *Grace, W.J. and Wolff, H.G.:* Treatment of ulcerative colitis. J. Am. med. Ass. *146:* 981–987 (1951).

8   *Head, R.G.:* Experiences in the psychiatric treatment of ulcerative colitis. J. Louis med. Soc. *107:* 321–324 (1955).

9   *Jores, A.:* Psychopathologische Befunde bei Patienten mit Colitis ulcerosa. Ther. Umsch. *26:* 5–10 (1969).

10 *Judd, E.S.:* Surgical progress in the management of chronic ulcerative colitis. Surgery *60:* 783–789 (1966).

11 *Karush, A.; Daniels, G.E.; O'Connor, J.F., and Stern, L.O.:* The response to psychotherapy in chronic ulcerative colitis. I. Pretreatment factors. Psychosom. Med. *30:* 255–276 (1968).

12 *Liedtke, R.; Tschirch, L. und Zepf, S.:* Untersuchung mit dem MMPI Saarbrücken von Patienten mit einer Colitis ulcerosa. Medsche Klin. *71:* 807–813 (1976).

13 *Monk, M.; Mendeloff, A.I.; Siegel, C.I., and Lilienfeld, A.:* An epidemiological study of ulcerative colitis and regional enteritis among adults in Baltimore. III. Psychological and possible stress-precipitating factors. J. chron. Dis. *22:* 565–578 (1970).

14 *Murray, C.D.:* Psychogenic factors in the etiology of ulcerative colitis and bloody diarrhea. Am. J. med. Sci. *180:* 239–248 (1930).

15 *Paulley, J.W.:* Ulcerative colitis. A study of 173 cases. Gastroenterology *16:* 566–576 (1950).

16 *Prugh, D.G.:* The influence of emotional factors on the clinical course of ulcerative colitis in children. Gastroenterology *18:* 339–354 (1951).

17 *Spreen, O.:* MMPI Saarbrücken. Handbuch zur deutschen Ausgabe des Minnesota Multiphasic; in *Hathaway and McKinley* Personality inventory (Huber, Bern 1963).

18 *Weinstock, H.I.:* Hospital psychotherapy in severe ulcerative colitis. Archs gen. Psychiat. *4:* 509–512 (1961).

19 *Wijsenbeek, H.; Maoz, B.; Nitzan, I., and Gill, R.:* Ulcerative colitis. Psychiatric and psychological study of 22 patients. Psychiat. Neurol. Neurochir. *71:* 409–420 (1968).

Dr. *R. Liedtke,* Medizinische Hochschule Hannover, Abteilung für Psychosomatik, Karl-Wiechert-Allee 9, *D-3000 Hannover 61* (FRG)

Proc. 11th Eur. Conf. Psychosom. Res., Heidelberg 1976
Psychother. Psychosom. *28:* 193–198 (1977)

Is 'Alexithymia' but a Social Phenomenon?

An Empirical Investigation in Psychosomatic Patients

R. Borens, E. Grosse-Schulte, W. Jaensch and K.-H. Kortemme[1]

Psychotherapeutische Abteilung, Psychosomatische Klinik Kinzigtal, Gengenbach

When in the 1960s the work of the French school around *Marty, M'Uzan* and *David* and that of the Boston school around *Sifneos* and *Nemiah* about particularities in psychosomatic patients were known, more and more vivid discussions arouse, centring around the problem: Do psychosomatic patients differ qualitatively and structurally from neurotic patients? It is finally the discussion of this main problem that brought us together here in Heidelberg.

As our discipline is not a merely scientific one, the concepts of 'phénomène psychosomatique' and 'alexithymia', are not mere scientific concepts. It seems that the discussion of these concepts cannot be made in a wholly matter-of-fact and scientific way; too many emotions, resistances, problems of transference and countertransference are involved in the discussion as well as in the formation of these concepts. Our paper as well cannot be a strictly scientific and statistic one, but rather a first approach to this subject, settling nevertheless on an empirical study.

The following are some preliminary remarks about the concepts of 'phénomène psychosomatique' and 'alexithymia'.

Reading through the 'Investigations psychosomatiques' I was astonished by the setting of the described interviews: the patient is sitting in front of quite a number of students; all the interventions – in the 'Investigations Psychosomatiques' as well as in the interviews, published by *Sifneos* and *Nemiah* – made by the interviewers are questions: no other interventions are made.

[1] Mr. *W. Jaensch* made the psychological testings, while Dr. *E. Grosse-Schulte* and Dr. *K.-H. Kortemme* made the clinical interviews.

Very little is known about the social provenience of these patients; from the little information one can conclude that they belong mostly to the lower classes. It seems also strange and questionable to me that all the descriptions were formulated in negative words; lack of fantasy, lack of emotions, lack of contact. I think, it was this negative view of things, which led to the formation of the concept of 'alexithymia' and which can be found as well in the negative definition of the concept of 'phénomène psychosomatique'. I conclude from this fact that the approach of the patients was made in a given frame of concepts which prevented an individual and adequate approach and made it impossible to the patients to speak their own language.

To draw extensive conclusions from a first interview seems to me rather rash and biassed, looking at the fact that this setting favours largely the neurotic patients and is disadvantageous for psychosomatic patients. The initial situation in the first interview is quite a different one for these two groups of patients: the psychosomatic patients went through a real 'Odyssee' of medical visits and almost all of them are damaged iatrogenely by number-less examinations and remarks on the somatic origin of their illnesses. One can imagine how surprising and troubling the first-interview-situation must be for the psychosomatic patients and how much more his ego would have to perform, in order to make him behave like a neurotic patient.

Last but not least we want to draw attention to the view of *Schneider,* who says: 'After the inquiry period one has to admit that the psychosomatic patient possesses the same abilities for fantasy work as the normal human being...'

Our observations and the inquiry following these observations are as follows. They were made during our clinical and therapeutic work in a 230-bed psychosomatic hospital. In this hospital patients with purely psychoso-matic illnesses like peptic ulcer, colitis ulcerosa and so on, patients with functional troubles as well as neurotic patients are in the care of 25 doctors and clinical psychologists. From the 230 beds, 160 are on general wards and 70 beds on private wards where mostly patients from the upper classes and higher income brackets are hospitalized. In both wards the doctor-patient ratio is the same.

On the general wards there are chiefly manual workers, and craftsmen, on the private ward there are mainly members of independent professions, higher employees and businessmen. I want to stress these social facts for the reason that very little is known about the social standing of the patients in the studies I told you about formerly. Our patients who come from different social classes do not differ in the way they are sent to our hospital, neither in the history of their illness nor in the diagnoses, nor – and this seems to me a crucial point – in their 'psychosomatic carreer'. Most came almost by accident, having finally met after numerous visits to GPs, surgeons and so on, a doctor with a psychological understanding, who drew their attention to a possible psychological background of the disease and the possibility to be treated in a psychosomatic clinic.

When they come to us they are generally poorly informed about what is going on, their fear is enormous and even more enormous is their apprehension of the word 'psycho'. At the first contact with these patients we have made the observation that they are extremely fixed on their symptoms and diseases whatever their diagnosis is. Very often they are unable to introduce themselves in another way than by their symptoms; the tensions arising during the interviews cannot be perceived and verbally elaborated, but are expressed by body-movements and body-sensations. Emotions cannot be perceived or at least cannot be told. But we made the observation that these phenomena occur not only with our psychosomatic patients but also in the interviews with functionally disturbed and neurotic patients. *It was a most astonishing observation to find these particularities rather, if not only, with patients from the general wards, but very seldom with private patients.*

So we concluded that the difficulties to perceive and handle emotions and conflicts were not specific for the psychosomatic patient but correlated with the certain social class the patient originates from.

To test these observations and hypotheses, we started an empirical clinical study, which is not yet finished, so the following is to be seen as a *pilot study*.

Until now we have examined 23 patients with psychosomatic diseases like peptic ulcer, anorexia nervosa and colitis ulcerosa, which we could divide in two subgroups:

Group I with 13 patients, including workers, lower-level employees and housewives, all of them brought up in a lower social class environment with a very limited education and an income of less than DM 1,500.– per month.

Group II with 10 patients, including students, business-men, employees with higher functions, all of them brought up in an upper class family environment with a much better schooling and an income largely over 2,000.– DM per month.

In the first days after admission to our hospital, these 23 patients were interviewed by two experienced, analytically trained doctors of our staff, who did not know the work hypothesis. Further, they were tested by a psychologist with the WIP (a reduced form of the Wechsler Intelligence Scales for Adults), the Giessen test, the Rorschach and the ORT. The statements of the projective tests were not interpreted but evaluated quantitatively.

In subgroup I we found an average IQ of 97, and in subgroup II an average IQ of 111.4.

The ORT

This technique is a projective thematic test based on the analytical theory, made by 3 series of 4 pictures. From the ORT we gave the 4 pictures from the B-series, representing situations with 1, 2 and 3 persons and a group situation. The patient was instructed to tell a story for each picture. We divided the statements into 3 categories: category 1: a mere description of the picture; category 2: a description of an action; category 3: a description of an interaction.

An example for category 1. I see a room, the door is open, somebody is coming home. I see a bed, a vitrine, that's all I have to say.

An example for category 2. Yes, I see again 3 persons. One who is standing near the door, I suppose that it is the mother, waiting for the daughter, the daughter is accompanied by her boyfriend.

An example for category 3. She is alone and in front of her I see quite a lot of men, a real bunch of men. Perhaps she is too shy to walk by, afraid to be adressed by them; but she might also wait for someone, want to join the group, a mixed group that just met there, but she does not dare to join them. It is difficult for me to see whether she wants to stay alone or not. The group is watching her, perhaps they are curious, perhaps they are hostile or simply indifferent, I can't tell.

In subgroup I there were 8 persons with answers of category 1 and only 2 persons with answers of category 3. In subgroup II there were 2 persons with answers of category 1 and 6 persons with answers of category 3.

For a more detailed analysis of the verbal behaviour all adjectives and verbs were counted. In subgroup I we found an average of 1.9 adjectives and 9.1 verbs for the 4 pictures. In subgroup II we have an average of 5.1 adjectives and 17.8 verbs for the 4 pictures.

Rorschach

In the Rorschach technique we counted the answers and found an average of 17 in subgroup I, and in subgroup II an average of 19 answers; a not significant difference. Nor did the group differ in amplitude and extensivity of the answers. We counted the movement answers, as these answers stand for imagination and empathy, and found no significant differences between our 2 groups. The same is true for anatomy answers, which stand for preoccupation with body problems and point towards rationalization tendencies. The only significant difference we found concerned the human answers that stand for empathy and participation. Here we had an average of 1.9 human answers in subgroup I, and an average of 3.5 human answers in subgroup II.

Giessen Test

The GT is a personality questionnaire coping with analytically described personality traits. We tried to test the differences between the self-image of the patient and the image the interviewer gained from him.

The average deviation between self and foreign image is of 27.9 points in subgroup I, and 37.4 points in subgroup II. These differences result out of the dimensions 'social appeal' and 'permeability'. The fact that there are not other significant deviations in the self-judgements by the patients and the judgements by the interviewers, leads to the preliminary hypothesis that the therapist was able to perceive similar phenomena in both groups. Would it be rash to conclude that the patients in both groups, in spite of their different behavior, succeeded to communicate even using quite different means and that these communications were understood by the therapist on a subconscious level?

The Interviews

The interviews lasted 50 min and were made by analytically well-trained psychotherapists in an analytical setting. This setting as we understand it, is defined by the reserved behavior of the therapist, who tries to create a warm atmosphere where the patient can deploy himself and where a common comprehension of his problems and conflicts is favored.

After the interview, the interviewers commented on the following items: operatory thinking, uniformity of thoughts and words, self-reflexion, introspection, fantasy work, conflict perception and verbalization as well as silent behavior. Furthermore, the interviewers had to answer questions on a questionary about the way their patients handled the interpretations.

As to the results we found that subgroup I differs significantly from subgroup II in the factors 'operatory thinking, uniformity of thoughts and words'; subgroup I presenting twice as many of these 'pensées opératoires' as subgroup II. The abilities of reflexion and fantasy, as well as the perception of conflicts and their verbalization are much higher in subgroup II.

As to the factor 'silence', we made the interesting observation that in the interviews of the upper-class group of patients there were only two longer periods of silence, silence which the therapist qualified as retentive and obstinate.

In the lower-class group we found longer and more frequent periods of a silence qualified as boring and dull.

In the handling of interpretations there were also great differences between the two groups.

Conclusions

Our *pilot study* allows a few conclusions. But before looking at them we want to emphasize that these conclusions base only on observations made in psychosomatic patients in their first interviews and in their first psychological testings. We found quite a number of divergent traits as to verbalization, access to feelings and fantasies and as to perception of conflicts. These preliminary results enable us to correlate these differences with the *social status, the social origin and the degree of sophistication of the psychosomatic patients.* There seems to be no correlation with diagnoses or psychodynamic structures. This confirms our everyday observations that the thing called 'alexithymia' or 'phénomène psychosomatique' by some people occurs more or less exclusively in patients of lower social classes. First findings of our further investigations in patients with functional and neurotic disorders together with the results of *Cremerius* (1975: 'Schichtenspezifische Schwierigkeiten bei der Anwendung der Psychoanalyse' [Stratum-specific difficulties in the use of psychoanalysis]) seem to permit us to state that the 'phénomène psychosomatique' is not a psychosomatic phenomenon but a social one.

In his above-mentioned paper, *Cremerius* made quite similar observations in psychotherapeutic work with low-class patients despite their diagnoses. He made the conditions of socialization responsible for it. These conditions hostile to the instincts, to the fantasy and to spontaneity lead to a strict superego, to a lack of fantasy and to an inability to perceive and verbalize emotions. In view of the present stage of our studies and the preliminary results, we feel we can fully agree with his interpretations.

Dr. *R. Borens,* Chefarzt der Psychotherapeutischen Abteilung, Psychosomatische Klinik Kinzigtal, *D–7614 Gengenbach* (FRG)

Theories

Proc. 11th Eur. Conf. Psychosom. Res., Heidelberg 1976
Psychother. Psychosom. *28:* 199–206 (1977)

Alexithymia

Theoretical Considerations

John C. Nemiah[1]

Department of Psychiatry of the Beth Israel Hospital, Harvard Medical School,
Boston, Mass.

It is my purpose in this paper to discuss the theoretical aspects of
alexithymia, and I shall do so by putting them in the context of the various
theoretical models and explanations for the processes of psychosomatic
symptom formation, to which alexithymia is closely related. With regard to
alexithymia, two facts stand out: Alexithymic individuals (1) have a marked
difficulty in expressing feelings in words, and (2) do not have fantasies
appropriate to or expressive of feelings, their thought content being dominated by the details of the events in their external environment *(pensée opératoire)* (9, 10). These characteristics are found in many patients with psychosomatic disorders, and our theoretical considerations should be aimed at
helping us to understand this relationship.

As a point of departure, let us consider for a moment the internal
processes that normally occur in response to an affect-provoking external
event. There are at least two sets of reactions put in motion: *perceptual-
cognitive* and *affective*. (1) There is, on the one hand, a conscious perception
and cognitive evaluation of the elements of the external event. (2) On the
other, the *somatic* components of affect (that is, *emotion*) are aroused. The
latter in turn undergo a *psychic* elaboration consisting of several elements:
(1) a refinement and delineation of the raw emotion into a variety of qualitatively different nuances that have the potential for conscious experience as
feelings, e.g., anger, fear, joy, sadness; (2) a linking of the feelings with
words descriptive of them; (3) the production of fantasies expressive of the
feelings, which at the same time determine the imagery of the fantasies, and

[1] Psychiatrist-in-Chief, Beth Israel Hospital and Professor of Psychiatry, Harvard
Medical School.

(4) the arousal of a network of memories and associations related to the feelings. In the normal course of events all, or most of these elements will appear in *conscious awareness* and will be expressed in an appropriate manner.

Disturbances in the affective component of the response to an external stimulus could occur at several points: (1) there could be a blocking of the pathways from the process of psychic elaboration to conscious awareness; (2) there could be an absence of defect in any or all of the elements of psychic elaboration, or (3) there could be a disruption or blocking of the pathways leading from the somatic, emotional component of affect to the area of its psychic elaboration. Such blocking or deficits in the system would lead to a short-circuiting and deflection of the transmission of the energies aroused by the external stimulus so that instead of being dissipated in normal affective expression they might result in an increase in activity of other elements in the system (the somatic emotional component, for example) or in other abnormal discharges manifested as somatic symptoms. Finally, it should be noted that these disruptions could be conceived of as resulting from *psychological* defenses and deficits, or from *physical* discontinuities in the neuronal structures and pathways forming the anatomical substrate of the psychological processes. Depending, then, on the concepts and language used to describe them, the theoretical models employed to explain the process of psychosomatic symptom formation would be either psychological or neuroanatomical. In the survey of theoretical models that follows, we shall group them under these two major categories, beginning with psychological theories.

Psychological Theories

Psychodynamic Models

Let us start with a review of psychodynamic models. Included here are theories that attempt to explain the production of psychosomatic symptoms as the result of conflict among currently operating psychological forces.

Conversion. The most venerable of these is the theory of *conversion*. As in the symptoms of conversion hysteria, the psychosomatic symptom is viewed as a symbolic representation of repressed fantasies arising from unacceptable drives and affects. Unlike hysteria, however, in which the drives are libidinal and oedipal in nature, in psychosomatic disorders the drives are generally pre-genital (oral and anal libido, and pre-oedipal aggression). *Deutsch* (3) and his colleagues particularly have extended the concept of conversion to include all of the organ systems and somatic functions. His formulations will be described in more detail below (cf. 'Developmental Models').

Specific dynamic conflict. Related to conversion, but with significant differences, is the concept of a specific dynamic conflict. Proposed by *Alexander* (1), this formulation invokes the repression of specific affects as the basic mechanism behind symptom formation. There is, however, no symbolic representation of the associated fantasies as in conversion symptoms. Instead, there occurs a chronic arousal of the autonomic processes that normally accompany affects, which, because of the repression of the affects, cannot be discharged in overt emotional expression. The chronicity of the arousal leads eventually to lesions in the organs supplied by the autonomic nervous system. In this model psychosomatic symptoms are viewed as the secondary result of repression, not as the product of converted psychic representations.

Denial. Finally, let us briefly consider the role of *denial.* The term 'denial' has come increasingly into use during the past decade to designate a defense against affect and fantasy found in patients with psychosomatic disorders. It is not exactly clear how it is to be distinguished operationally from repression, except that from the context in which it is used, it seems to be applied to patients who are unusually devoid of emotions and fantasies. In Alexander's theoretical formulation, repression is viewed as having a selective effect on specific individual emotions specifically related to the various psychosomatic disorders. Denial, on the other hand, although qualitatively similar to repression, constitutes quantitatively an extreme defensive measure applied globally to the totality of affective phenomena. Once the mechanism of denial has been set in operation, the subsequent processes leading to the appearance of psychosomatic symptoms are presumably the same as those proposed by Alexander that follow on repression.

A Deficit Model

Instead of viewing psychosomatic symptoms as the product of dynamic psychological conflicts, *Marty and de M'Uzan* (7) conceive of them as being the result of specific ego deficits, in particular an absence of the capacity for the formation of fantasy, and for experiencing feelings. In this model, as *McDougall* (8) writes, 'emphasis (is) laid upon urgent instinctual discharge which escapes psychic elaboration because of deficient representation and diminished affective response: in short, an impoverishment of the capacity to symbolize instinctual demands and their conflict with reality, and to elaborate fantasy, Instinctual energy, bypassing the psyche, thus affects soma directly, with catastrophic results. This particular theoretical approach to psychosomatic formations is in complete opposition to the theory of hysterical formation: the latter being the result of repressed fantasy elaborations while the former would result precisely from the lack of such psychic activity.'

Developmental Models

The models that we have reviewed thus far have dealt with fully-established mechanisms in the adult individual, and have been devised to explain emotional reactions in terms of psychological processes taking place in a mental apparatus that is the end-product of a long period of growth and development. Developmental models, on the other hand, attempt to provide an explanation for the structure of the adult mechanisms by delineating the early-life factors that have helped to shape and determine their form. Developmental models are not, then, fully explanatory in themselves, but are complementary to and add depth to those models that pertain to internal processes in the adult. We shall examine briefly two developmental models.

A psychoanalytic learning theory model. Deutsch (3) proposes that when an early childhood illness affecting an organ system coincides with a psychological conflict involving any one of the phases of growth and development, the function of that organ system and the psychological conflict become associatively linked in a stable and persisting complex. When external stimuli activate that conflict (now unconscious) in adult life, the function of the organ system associated with it is also affected, resulting in the symptoms of a psychosomatic disorder.

Pathogenic mother-infant-relationships. We have already noted that *Marty* and his colleagues, and in particular *McDougall*, attribute psychosomatic processes to ego defects in the realm of fantasy formation and the experiencing of affects. The source of these defects is traced to disturbances in the earliest mother-child relationships. A mother, according to *McDougall* (8), who either provides too much gratification of her infant's instincts, or unduly prohibits him from normal autoerotic gratification of these instincts, prevents him from developing a mental representation of the mother as a compensation for her temporary absence. This earliest image of the mother is the prototype of fantasy, and the failure to develop it irrevocably damages henceforth the capacity to form fantasy as a symbol and expression of instinctual drives.

Neuroanatomic Theories

In contrast to those theories involving psychological concepts are those that focus on brain structure and function. Like the psychological theories, they may be concerned with adult structures, or with the early developmental factors that have led to the formation of those structures.

Structural Models

Structural models propose that there is either an absence of or a defect in pathways between neuronal centers underlying affect, or an absence of or a defect in the neuronal centers themselves. With respect to the model proposed earlier concerning the normal and usual internal aspects of affective processes, we might postulate disturbances: (1) in the pathway between the center for psychic elaboration and that for consciousness; (2) in the pathway between the center underlying emotion and that for psychic elaboration, or (3) in the center for psychic elaboration itself. The first and third possibilities are of theoretical interest only, since our current knowledge of neuroanatomy gives us no clues as to the anatomical structures that underlie repression or the ego functions involved in psychic elaborations. On the other hand, there is perhaps more justification for considering the second possibility, since, as *MacLean* (6) long ago pointed out, the nature of psychosomatic processes suggests a disturbance in the connections between the limbic system and cortical centers. Possibly in the current investigations of the anatomy and physiology of the limbic system (and of limbic-cortical connections) there may be clues as to the structural mechanisms underlying psychosomatic processes and to the disturbances in them that lead to illness.

Developmental Models

In reviewing developmental models, as in our consideration of structural models, the lack of solid factual knowledge prevents us from leaving the realm of conjecture. Theoretically, one might conceive of a *developmental model* in terms of a defective post-natal development of neuronal structures resulting from a lack of adequate environmental input, such as has recently been demonstrated by *Borges and Berry* (2) to occur in rats deprived from birth of visual stimuli. One might, thus, consider inadequate maternal stimulation during infancy as a factor in the failure to develop connections between limbic and cortical structures. A *genetic model* could likewise explain neuroanatomical abnormalities on the basis of an inherited defect, and in this regard *Heiberg*'s (5) findings concerning alexithymia in twins are of great interest.

Model Applicable to Alexithymia

Thus far, we have been considering theoretical models for the processes involved in psychosomatic symptom formation. Each model provides a possible mechanism for such symptom formation, but not all are equally successful in accounting for the presence of alexithymic characteristics as well. *Alexander's* concept of a specific dynamic conflict, for example, provides a reasonable explanation for the appearance of somatic dysfunction as the result of a psychological conflict over a specific drive or affect. It does not, however, necessarily imply the global absence of affect and fantasy that characterizes the alexithymic individual. Only three of the models are sufficiently broad to include both alexithymia and psychosomatic symptom formation in their purview: (1) denial; (2) the deficit model, and (3) the structural model. Let us briefly consider each in turn.

Denial. With its implication of a massive, global inhibition of affects, the concept of denial provides a theoretical basis for alexithymia in conjunction with symptom formation. At the same time, viewed as a psychological defense, the notion of denial also allows theoretically for a reversal of the defensive process and for a consequent disappearance of alexithymic behavior and of somatic symptoms. It is, therefore, a possible and valid model for what has been called by *Freyberger* (4) and others secondary *alexithymia* – i.e., a condition manifested by some individuals with catastrophic physical illness and some patients with psychosomatic disorders who, with psychotherapy, are able to recover the affects and fantasies initially so strikingly absent.

Deficit model. In many alexithymic patients with psychosomatic illness, however, the alexithymic characteristics are irreversible, despite long, intensive and skillful depth psychotherapy. Such patients remain totally unable to experience either affect or fantasy. For such patients the *deficit model* appears more applicable, implying, as it does, not an *inhibition* of functions, but an *absence* of functions and the mental apparatuses underlying them. In bringing this concept to bear on psychosomatic processes, *Marty* and his colleagues have made an important contribution to our theoretical thinking about psychosomatic and alexithymic phenomena.

Structural model. It is, however, a weakness of the psychological deficit model that by staying within the psychoanalytic frame of reference, it employs constructs and hypotheses that are not readily testable. Instinctual energy, for example, cannot be measured nor can the pathways by which it directly affects the soma (as *McDougall* postulates) be determined. Nor can one determine the presence or absence of the postulated fantasies in infants at a time when they have no language with which to communicate them. It is just here that the structural model comes to the rescue, for by making possible the translation of intangible, unmeasurable psychoanalytic constructs into the concepts of neurochemical processes taking place in neuronal pathways and centers, it gives promise of providing us with a basis for understanding alexithymic behavior and psychosomatic symptom formation in terms of their neuroanatomical substrates.

Let me conclude with one point that cannot be too strongly emphasized. I have attempted to convey the variety and complexity of the theoretical models that pertain to psychosomatic phenomena. Each has been devised to explain specific clinical observations and each has its usefulness. Consider, for example, the fact that while many patients psychosomatic disorders show alexithymic characteristics, some do not. For the latter, *Alexander*'s psychological, dynamic concepts may provide the most useful and precise explanation, while the former can perhaps best be conceived of in terms of the models involving functional and structural deficits. What I am suggesting is that the term psychosomatic process does not necessarily refer to a unitary phenomenon. There are possibly a number of different constellations of internal events that lead over a final common pathway to produce a psychosomatic symptom. To utilize one explanatory model when the facts require it does not mean that we must ignore others when they may be more appropriate. On the contrary, we must beware of a premature closure in our conceptualizing and of focusing on one theoretical approach to the exclusion of others. Open-mindedness to new observations and flexibility in our theoretical thinking about them are essential if we are to make any progress in our understanding of psychosomatic phenomena.

References

1   *Alexander, F.:* Psychosomatic medicine (Norton, New York 1950).
2   *Borges, S. and Berry, M.:* Preferential orientation of the stellate cell dendrites in the visual cortex of the dark-reared rat. Brain Res. *112:* 141 (1976).
3   *Deutsch, F.:* On the mysterious leap from the mind ot the body. (International Universities Press, New York 1959).
4   *Freyberger, H.:* Psychosomatic aspects of an intensive care unit; in *Howells* Modern perspectives in the psychiatric aspect of surgery (Brunner/Mazel, New York, in press).
5   *Heiberg, A.:* Alexithymia. An inherited trait? 11th Eur. Conf. Psychosom. Res., Heidelberg 1976, pp. 14–17.

6   *MacLean, P.D.:* Psychosomatic disease and the 'visceral brain', Psychosom. Med. *1:* 338 (1949).
7   *Marty, P. and M'Uzan, M. de:* La pensée opératoire. Rev. fr. Psychoanal. *27:* suppl. p. 1845 (1963).
8   *McDougall, J.:* The psychosoma and the psychoanalytic process. Int. Rev. psychoanal. *1:* 437 (1974).
9   *Nemiah, J.C. and Sifneos, P.E.:* Affect and fantasy in patients with psychosomatic disorders; in *Hill* Modern trends in psychosomatic medicine, vol. 2 (Butterworths, London 1970).
10 *Sifneos, P.E.:* The prevalence of 'alexithymic' characteristics in psychosomatic patients; *in Freyberger* Topics of psychosomatic research (Karger, Basel 1972).

Prof. *John C. Nemiah,* Department of Psychiatry, Harvard Medical School, Beth Israel Hospital, 330 Brookline Avenue, *Boston, MA 02215* (USA)

Proc. 11th Eur. Conf. Psychosom. Res., Heidelberg 1976
Psychother. Psychosom. *28:* 207–220 (1977)

The Triune Brain in Conflict

Paul D. MacLean

Laboratory of Brain Evolution and Behavior, National Institute of Mental Health, Bethesda, Md.

It is evident that one can derive the *laws of thought* without taking the brain apart piece by piece and looking at the machinery. The situation is quite different with respect to other forms of mentation. In my research, I have attempted to learn whether a better knowledge of the brain's machinery would help to explain 'paleopsychic processes' and their expression as non-verbal behavior.

Emanations of the psyche, like other forms of information, have no material substance. In order to be communicated they must be translated into some kind of behavior. Human communicative behavior can be classified as verbal and nonverbal. Like *Bridgman* (1959), the physicist-philosopher, people usually assume that 'most human communication is verbal'. But many behavior scientists place a far greater emphasis on nonverbal communication in day-to-day human activities. Many forms of human nonverbal behavior show a parallel to behavioral patterns of animals. Since it is hardly appropriate to refer to nonverbal behavior of animals, we need another term for this kind of communication. The word 'prosematic', derived from the Greek (προ + σημα) and meaning rudimentary signalling, is appropriate for referring to any kind of nonverbal signal – vocal, bodily, or chemical (*MacLean,* 1975a). Prosematic behavior, like verbal behavior, has its semantics and syntax. Somewhat comparable to words, sentences, and paragraphs, prosematic behavior becomes meaningful in terms of its components, constructs, and sequences of constructs. Every species has its own typical modifiers of prosematic behavior for communication involved in self-preservation and the preservation of the species. Hence, I shall be referring to species-typical, prosematic behavior.

The relevance of work on animals to human affairs becomes evident when it is realized that the primate brain evolves and expands along the lines of three basic patterns that may be characterized as reptilian, paleo-mammalian and neomammalian. Figure 1 shows a schematic representation of the three evolutionary formations. Radically different in chemistry and structure, and in an evolutionary sense countless generations apart, we have so to speak a hierarchy of three brains in one, or what may be termed a *triune* brain (*MacLean* 1970, 1973c).

What this situation implies is that we are obliged to look at ourselves and the world through the eyes of three quite different mentalities. To compli-cate things further, there is evidence that the two older mentalities lack the necessary neural machinery for verbal communication. But to say that they lack the power of speech does not belittle their intelligence, nor does it relegate them to the realm of the 'unconscious'.

One might imagine that our brain represents an amalgamation of three biological computers, each with its own special intelligence, its own special subjective sense, its own sense of time and space, its own memory, motor and other functions. What seems notably lacking, is a commonly shared neural code for intersignalling in verbal terms. It is evident how misunder-standing generated by this situation might result in *intra*personal and *inter*-personal conflict.

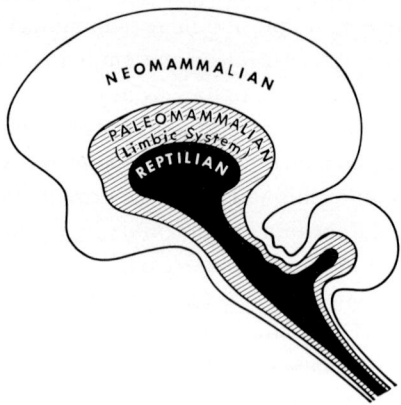

Fig. 1. In its evolution, the human forebrain expands in hierarchic fashion along the lines of three basic patterns that may be characterized as reptilian, paleomammalian, and neomammalian (from *MacLean*, 1967).

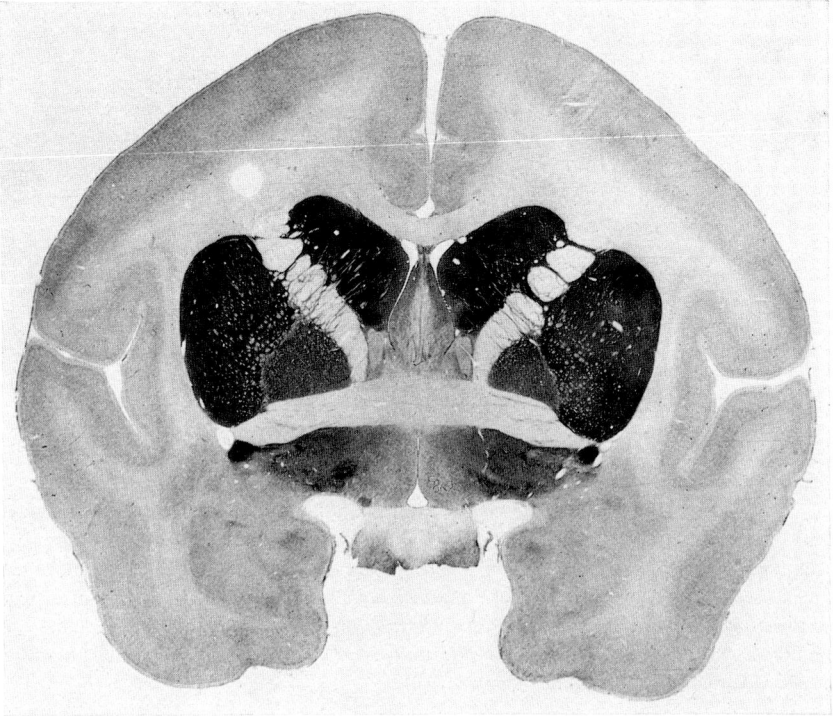

Fig. 2. This section from the brain of a squirrel monkey shows how the greater part of the R-complex is selectively colored (black areas) by a stain for cholinesterase (from *MacLean,* 1972).

The Reptilian Formation

Thanks to recent anatomical, physiological, and histochemical techniques, the three basic evolutionary formations of the forebrain stand out in clearer detail than ever before. Let us look at the large fist of ganglia in our forebrain which in their organization and chemistry reflect our reptilian ancestry. Included in this mass are the olfactostriatum, the corpus striatum, globus pallidus and satellite gray matter. Since there is no name that applies to all of these structures, I shall simply refer to them as the *R-complex*. The black areas in figure 2 show how a stain for cholinesterase sharply demarcates the R-complex in the monkey's brain. Figure 3 illustrates how the same stain distinguishes the R-complex in animals ranging from reptiles to man. In

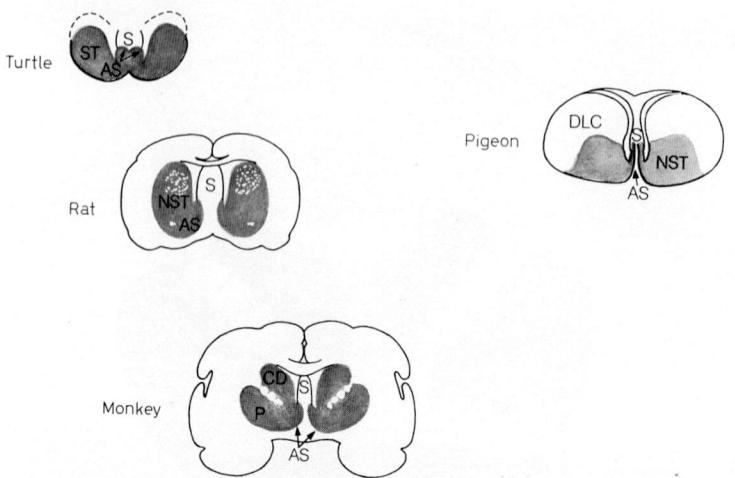

Fig. 3. Shaded areas indicate how a stain for cholinesterase distinguishes the greater part of the R-complex in animals ranging from reptiles to primates. With the fluorescent technique of *Falck and Hillarp* (1959), the same areas shown above would glow a bright green because of the high content of dopamine (*Juorio and Vogt, 1967*). The pallidal part of the striatal complex does not fluoresce. No existing reptiles represent the forerunners of mammals. Birds are an offshoot from the *Archosauria* – 'ruling reptiles' (from *MacLean, 1973b,* adapted from *Parent and Olivier, 1970*).

using the fluorescent technique of *Falck and Hillarp* (1959), it is striking to see the greater part of the R-complex glow a bright green because of large amounts of dopamine, a neural sap that seems to be necessary for setting into motion the total energies of the organism.

From an evolutionary standpoint, it is curious that ethologists have paid little attention to reptiles, focusing instead on fishes and birds. Some authorities believe that of existing reptiles, lizards would bear the closets resemblance to the mammal-like reptiles believed to be the forerunners of mammals. At all events, lizards and other reptiles provide illustrations of complex prototypical patterns of behavior commonly seen in mammals, including man. In table I, 24 such behaviors that may primarily involve self-preservation and the survival of the species are listed. First and foremost are all those activities that involve the establishment and defense of territory.

It requires no reminder that the will-to-power became the heart of *Nietzsche*'s (1883) philosophy. He regarded the will-to-power as the basic life force of the entire universe. 'Thus life taught me', he wrote. Nietzsche's writ-

Table I. Prototypical patterns of behavior

1	Selection and preparation of homesite
2	Establishment of territory
3	Trail making
4	'Marking' of territory
5	Showing place-preferences
6	Patrolling territory
7	Ritualistic display in defense of territory, commonly involving the use of coloration and adornments
8	Formalized intraspecific fighting in defense of territory
9	Triumphal display in successful defense
10	Assumption of distinctive postures and coloration in signaling surrender
11	Foraging
12	Hunting
13	Homing
14	Hoarding
15	Use of defecation posts
16	Formation of social groups
17	Establishment of social hierarchy by ritualistic display and other means
18	Greeting
19	'Grooming'
20	Courtship, with displays using coloration and adornments
21	Mating
22	Breeding and, in isolated instances, attending offspring
23	Flocking
24	Migration

ings on this subject may yet earn him recognition as a foremost ethologist and an authority on human reptilian behavior!

Regardless of interpretation, let me say that one will hardly find the will-to-power more dramatically expressed than in the behavior of some lizards. To see two rainbow male lizards *(Agama agama)* striving for dominance, is like returning to the days of King Arthur. These animals have beautiful colors, and like many lizards, use head bobbing and push-ups in territorial and courtship displays. In a contest, once the gauntlet is thrown down, the aggressive displays give way to violent combat, and the struggle is unrelenting. Twice we have seen dominant males humiliated in defeat. They lost their majestic colors, lapsed into a kind of depression, and died 2 weeks later.

As yet, hardly any experiments have been performed on reptiles in an attempt to identify forebrain structures involved in species-typical, prosematic forms of behavior. Recently, we have conducted pilot experiments in the green Anolis lizard that indicate that the R-complex is a requisite for the organized expression of the territorial display (*Greenberg et al.,* 1976).

In contrast to reptiles, the R-complex of mammals has been subjected to extensive investigation. It cannot be overemphasized, however, that 150 years of experimentation have revealed little specific information about its functions. The finding that large destructions of the mammalian R-complex may result in no impairment of movement, speaks against the traditional clinical view that it subserves purely motor function. As with reptiles, we are conducting experiments on mammals, testing the hypothesis that the R-complex plays a basic role in species-typical, prosematic behavior. Thus far, crucial findings have turned up in the work on squirrel monkeys *(Saimiri sciureus)*. Showing a remarkable parallel to reptiles, males of this species perform the same kind of display in courtship as in the show of aggression *(Ploog and MacLean,* 1963). In each situation, the male vocalizes, spreads one thigh and directs the erect phallus towards the other animal. The display is also used as a form of greeting. I have described one variety of squirrel monkey that will regularly perform a greeting display upon seeing its reflection in a mirror (*MacLean,* 1964). We refer to the mirror displaying animal on the left in figure 4 as the gothic-type because the ocular patch forms a peak over the eye like a gothic arch, whereas we call the other variety romans because the patch is round like a roman arch.

I have used the mirror display test as a means of learning what parts of the brain are involved in display rituals. In experiments involving more than 100 monkeys, I found that extensive removals of parts of the neomammalian and paleomammalian formations may have no effect or only a transitory effect on the display. Lesions, however, of pallidal part of the R-complex (*MacLean,* 1973a) or interruptions in its pathways (*MacLean,* 1975b) result in a profound alteration or elimination of the display.

These results are of great interest because of the demonstration for the first time in a mammal that the R-complex is involved in species-typical, prosematic, ritualistic behavior.

Since the mirror display also involves isopraxic factors, the results indicate that the R-complex is implicated in *natural* forms imitation. Isopraxic refers to behavior in which two or more individuals engage in the same kind of activity (*MacLean,* 1975a). In circular language, one might define a species as a group of animals that has genetically acquired the perfect ability to imitate itself (*MacLean,* 1975c). It cannot be overemphasized that isopraxis is basic to maintaining the identity of the species or social group.

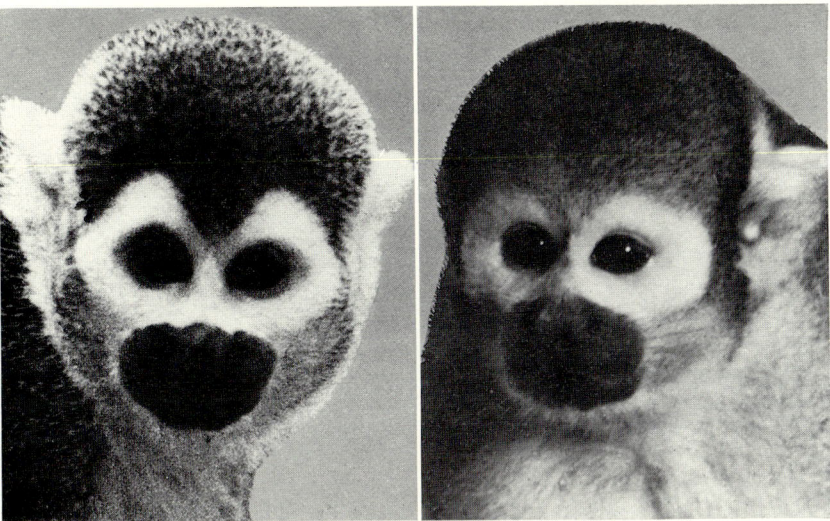

Fig. 4. Two varieties of squirrel monkeys referred to as 'gothic' and 'roman' because of the pointed and rounded shape of the ocular patch above the eye. Both varieties use the same type of display in the communal situation, but only the gothic type (left) will consistently display to its reflection in a mirror (from *MacLean*, 1964).

Isopraxis is one of a pentad of important interoperative behaviors seen in reptiles and higher forms (*MacLean*, 1975a). The four other behaviors may be denoted as perseverative, reenactment, tropistic (positive and negative), and deceptive. Without the defining them, I shall simply say that in human activities, they find expression in obsessive, compulsive behavior; personal day-to-day rituals and superstitious acts; slavish conformity to old ways of doing things; ceremonial reenactments; obeisance to precedent, as in legal and other matters; responding to partial representations, whether alive or inanimate; and all manner of deception.

The Paleomammalian Brain (Limbic System)

We go upstairs now to the next mentality! Reptiles have a perfect memory for what their ancestors have learned to do over millions of years, but there are behavioral indications that the reptilian brain is poorly equipped for learning to cope with new situations. The reptilian brain has only a

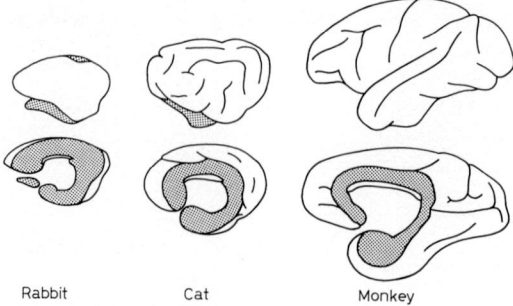

Rabbit   Cat   Monkey

Fig. 5. The limbic lobe of Broca (shaded) is found as a common denominator in the brains of all mammals. It contains the greater part of the cortex corresponding to that of the paleomammalian brain. The cortex of the neomammalian brain (shown in white) mushrooms late in evolution (after *MacLean*, 1954).

rudimentary cortex. In the lost transitional forms between reptiles and mammals, it is presumed that the primitive cortex ballooned out and became further differentiated. The primitive cortex provides the animal a better means of viewing the environment and learning to survive.

In all existing mammals, the old cortex is found in a large convolution which *Broca* (1878) called the limbic lobe because it surrounds the brain stem. Identified by the shading in figure 5, this lobe is a common denominator in the brains of all mammals. In 1952, I suggested the term limbic system as a designation for the limbic cortex and structures of the brain stem with which it has primary connections (*MacLean*, 1952). In the past 40 years, clinical and experimental studies have provided evidence that the limbic system derives information in terms of emotional feelings that guide behavior required for self-preservation and the preservation of the species.

Clinical findings provide the best evidence that the limbic system is involved in emotional experience and behavior. Epileptic discharges in or near the limbic cortex result in a wide variety of vivid emotional feelings, ranging from intense fear to ecstasy. It is one of the wonders of the brain that epileptic discharges arising in the limbic cortex tend to spread in, and be confined to, the limbic system. Elsewhere, I have referred to this condition as a *schizophysiology* (*MacLean,* 1954) and have suggested that the underlying factors may contribute to inexplicable conflicts between *what we feel* and *what we know.*

Except for the crocodilia and a few skink, reptiles show no interest in their young, which come into the world prepared to do everything that they have to do, except to procreate. The Big News with the evolution of mammals is the progressive attention and care that they give to their young. The evolution of this concern for other members of the species amounts to an evolution of conscience, and by implication, to conflicts that we associate with conscience.

Three Subdivisions of the Limbic System

The evolution of parental care seems to be correlated with the development of three subdivisions of the limbic system (fig. 6). The two older divisions are closely related to the olfactory apparatus. Experimental work has shown that the one connected with the amygdala (fig. 6, No. 1) is primarily concerned with feeding, fighting and self-protection; whereas the division just across the way in the septal region (No. 2) is concerned with genital and procreational functions.

The close relationship of oral and genital functions in this part of the brain is apparently due to the olfactory sense which dating far back in evolution plays a primary role in both feeding and mating. The findings are relevant to oral-sexual manifestations in feeding, mating, and aggressive and violent behavior (MacLean, 1973c).

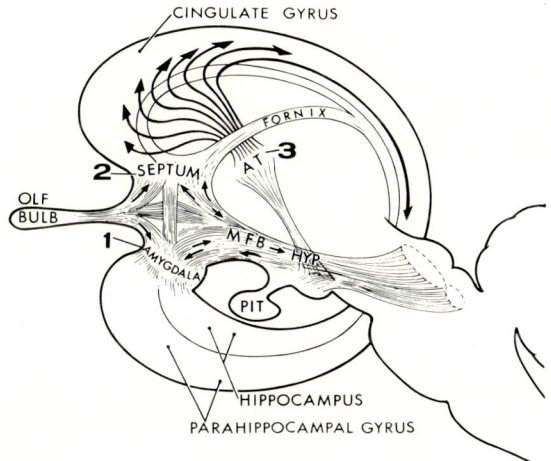

Fig. 6. Diagram of three main subdivisions of the limbic system and their major pathways. See text for summary of their respective functions. AT = Anterior thalamic nuclei; HYP = hypothalamus; MFB = medial forebrain bundle; PIT = pituitary; OLF = olfactory (after *MacLean*, 1958).

The major pathway to the third subdivision (fig. 6, No. 3) bypasses the olfactory apparatus. This division becomes progressively larger in higher primates and reaches its greatest development in the human brain. Experimental evidence suggests that the great development of this division reflects a shift in emphasis from olfactory to visual influences in sociosexual behavior. We will consider in a moment how this division ties in with the neomammalian brain, seeming to provide a neural substrate for empathy, compassion, and a far-seeing concern for the species.

The Basic Personality

But first, let me say a word about the substrate of the basic personality. In mammals, the major pathways to and from the reptilian and paleomammalian brains pass through the hypothalamus and subthalamic region. If the majority of these pathways are destroyed in monkeys, they are greatly incapacitated but with the careful nursing, recover the ability to feed themselves and to move around. They retain, of course, the great motor pathways from the neocortex to the lower brain stem and spinal cord. The most striking characteristic of these animals is that although they look like monkeys, they no longer behave like monkeys. Almost everything that one would characterize as species-typical behavior has disappeared. If one were to interpret these findings in the light of certain clinical case material, one might say that these large pathways of the repto-limbic formations provide the avenues to the basic personality. Here certainly would seem to be the pathways for the expression of prosematic behavior.

The Neomammalian Brain

Finally, we climb a second flight of stairs to the neomammalian brain. There are indications that the insistent signals from the inside world make it difficult for the organism to make cold, reasoned decisions required for survival. Nature designs the neocortex so that it receives information largely from the eyes, ears, and body wall. Compared with the limbic cortex (fig. 5), the neocortex is like an expanding numerator. It mushrooms late in evolution and culminates in human beings, providing a vast neural screen for the portrayal of symbolic language. In some higher primates the new cortex comes perilously close to operating like a giant, heartless computer. As though

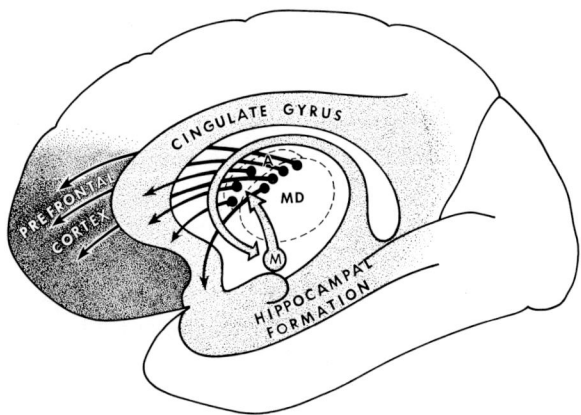

Fig. 7. This diagram indicates how the limbic system (light stipple) is anatomically related to the prefrontal cortex through the third pathway shown in the preceding figure. Recently, connections have been found between the visual system and the limbic cortex of the retrosplenial region, posterior hippocampal gyrus, and parahippocampal portion of the lingual gyrus. Through connections of these structures with the hippocampus, impulses of visual origin could be relayed to the hypothalamus by projections in the fornix (F). Such a neural substrate may help to explain how the cold light with which we see is transformed into the warm light which with we feel (*MacLean*, 1973c). M = Mammillary bodies of hypothalamus; MD = medial dorsal nucleus; A = anterior thalamic nuclei (from *MacLean*, 1967).

recognizing a genie had been let loose from the bottle – a veritable Franken-stein – nature creates an enlargement of that part of the neocortex known as the prefrontal area (fig. 7) – a development, one might say, that for the first time brings a sense of compassion into the world. In the progress from the Neanderthal to Cro-Magnon man, one sees the human forehead develop from a lowbrow to a highbrow. The prefrontal cortex is the only neocortex that looks inward to the inside world. This once speculative statement can now be said with conviction because recently we have shown in monkeys that more than 25% of the cells of the mediodorsal nucleus are activated by the vagus – the great visceral nerve (*Hallowitz and MacLean*, 1977). In figure 7, emphasis is given to the tie-in of prefrontal circuits with the great third subdivision of the limbic system that I mentioned a moment ago. Clinically, there is evidence that the prefrontal cortex by looking inward, so to speak, obtains the gut feeling required for identifying with another indi-vidual. This is the second Big News about the evolution of mammals. It is this new development that makes possible the insight required for the foresight to plan for the needs of others as well as the self – to use our knowledge to alleviate suffering everywhere.

In designing for the first time a creature that shows a concern for suffering of other living things, nature seems to have attempted a 180° turnabout from what had previously been a dog-eat-dog world. But this added dimension has ironically increased the suffering that we feel when torn by conflict between our own selfish concerns and our concern for others.

Prefatory to some concluding remarks, I will use a metaphor to summarize what has been said up to this point: In the field of literature, it is recognized that there is an irreducible number of basic plots and associated emotions. In describing the functions of the triune brain metaphorically, one might imagine that the reptilian brain provides the basic plots and actions; that the limbic brain influences emotionally the developments of the plots; while the neomammalian brain has the capacity to expound the plots and emotions in as many ways as there are authors.

A major problem is to discover how the three evolutionary formations, so radically different in anatomy and chemistry, communicate with one another. Whatever the biochemical and biological signalling devices, it must be inferred that they involve nonverbal coding. Stated otherwise, there are indications that with the evolution of the forebrain structures underlying the three mentalities in question, no provision is made for intercommunication by the use of words. And this, we suppose, must be a source of many human dilemmas and conflicts.

It is commonly asserted that people are governed by their emotions. In writing about Pinel, *Graham* (1961) described how he appealed to Aristotle's theory of balancing the passions as a means of treating what we would today call psychosomatic disease and other conditions commonly ascribed to the emotions. There is a long tradition for speaking of the instincts and the emotions in the same breath, as though they could be equated. *Freud* (1949) was high on the list of those who thought so, and at the age of 77 in his new introductory lectures said: 'In popular language we may think that the id stands for the untamed passions.'

It would seem, however, that developing insights call for a clearer separation of protomentation associated with 'instincts' (prototypical behavior) and emotional mentation identified with our affects. I would like to raise the question that because of their subjective obtrusiveness, perhaps a disproportionate emphasis has been given to the importance of emotions and that we should keep in mind the possibility that the emotions may oftentimes be passive reflectors of psychic states rather than determinants of actions.

It seems likely that another reason that we give more emphasis to the emotions than to protomentation underlying prototypical behavior is that no one, not even our most gifted poets, dramatists and novelists are able to articulate the subjective states that accompany our proclivities and those conditions in which we are driven by impulses and compulsions. Here we have a real 'alexithymia'[1]. In closing, I would suggest that one should keep in mind that protomentation may be more basically involved in human actions than emotional mentation, recalling symbolically that 'the reptile does what it has to do' (*MacLean*, 1975a).

References

Bridgman, P.W.: The way things are, 333 pp. (Harvard University Press, Cambridge 1959).

Broca, P.: Anatomie comparée des circonvolutions cérébrales. Le grand lobe limbique et la scissure limbique dans la série des mammifères. Revue Anthrop. *1:* 385–498 (1878).

Falck, B. and Hillarp, N.A.: On the cellular localization of catecholamines in the brain. Acta Anat. *38:* 277–279 (1959).

Freud, S.: New introductory lectures on psychoanalysis, 239 pp. (The Hogarth Press and The Institute of Psychoanalysis, 1949).

Grange, K.M.: Pinel and eighteenth-century psychiatry. Bull. Hist. Med. *35:* 442–453 (1961).

Greenberg, N.; Ferguson, J.L., and MacLean, P.D.: A neuroethological study of display behavior in lizards. Abstract Soc. Neurosci. *2:* 689 (1976).

Hallowitz, R.A. and MacLean, P.D.: Effects of vagal volleys on units of intralaminar and juxtalaminar thalamic nuclei in monkeys. Brain Res. *124* (in press, 1977).

Juorio, A.V. and Vogt, M.: Monoamines and their metabolites in the avian brain. J. Physiol. *189:* 489–518 (1967).

MacLean, P.D.: Some psychiatric implications of physiological studies on frontotemporal portion of limbic system (visceral brain). Electroenceph. clin. Neurophysiol. *4:* 407–418 (1952).

MacLean, P.D.: The limbic system and its hippocampal formation. Studies in animals and their possible application to man. J. Neurosurg. *11:* 29–44 (1954).

MacLean, P.D.: Contrasting functions of limbic and neocortical systems of the brain and their relevance to psychophysiological aspects of medicine. Am. J. Med. *25:* 611–626 (1958).

---

[1] See elsewhere in this volume discussion of alexithymia by Sifneos, Nemiah, Heiberg, Borens, Taylor, Stierlin, and Freyberger.

MacLean, P.D.: Mirror display in the squirrel monkey, *Saimiri sciureus.* Science *146:* 950–952 (1964).

MacLean, P.D.: The brain in relation to empathy and medical education. J. Nerv. ment. Dis. *144:* 374–382 (1967).

MacLean, P.D.: The triune brain, emotion and scientific bias; in *Schmitt* The neurosciences second study program, pp. 336–349 (The Rockefeller University Press, New York 1970).

MacLean, P.D.: Cerebral evolution and emotional processes. New findings on the striatal complex. Ann. N.Y. Acad. Sci. *193:* 137–149 (1972).

MacLean, P.D.: Effects of pallidal lesions on species-typical display behavior of squirrel monkey. Fed. Proc., Fed. Am. Socs exp. Biol. *32:* 384 (1973a).

MacLean, P.D.: The brain's generation gap. Some human implications. Zygon J. Relig. Sci. *8:* 113–127 (1973b).

MacLean, P.D.: A triune concept of the brain and behaviour. Lecture I: Man's reptilian and limbic inheritance. Lecture II: Man's limbic brain and the psychoses. Lecture III: New trends in man's evolution; in *Boag and Campbell* The Hincks memorial lectures, pp. 6–66 (University of Toronto Press, Toronto 1973c).

MacLean, P.D.: On the evolution of three mentalities. Man-Envir. Syst. *5:* 213–222 (1975a).

MacLean, P.D.: Role of pallidal projections in species-typical behavior of squirrel monkey. Trans. Am. neurol. Ass. *100:* 110–113 (1975b).

MacLean, P.D.: The imitative-creative interplay of our three mentalities; in *Harris* Astride the two cultures, Arthur Koestler at 70, pp. 187–213 (Random House, New York 1975c).

Nietzsche, F.: Thus spoke Zarathustra; in *Kaufmann* The portable Nietzsche (Viking, New York 1954).

Parent, A. and Olivier, A.: Comparative histochemical study of the corpus striatum. J. Hirnforsch. *12:* 75–81 (1970).

Ploog, D.W. and MacLean, P.D.: Display of penile erection in the squirrel monkey *(Saimiri sciureus).* Anim. Behav. *11:* 32–39 (1963).

Paul D. MacLean, MD, Laboratory of Brain Evolution and Behavior, National Institute of Mental Health, *Bethesda, MD 20014* (USA)

Proc. 11th Eur. Conf. Psychosom. Res., Heidelberg 1976
Psychother. Psychosom. *28:* 221–225 (1977)

Alexithymia – an Inherited Trait?

A Study of Twins

Astrid Heiberg and Arvid Heiberg

Psychiatric Institute, and Institute of Medical Genetics, University of Oslo, Oslo

A fundamental question in considerations about etiology is whether a condition is inborn or acquired. The twin method, although with several minor disadvantages, is commonly considered the most efficient research method in this respect.

The difference between monozygous and dizygous twins is commonly considered to be due to the genetic component. The difference between the twins in a monozygous pair is considered to be due to environmental differences or interactions between environment and the genetic component, and the same is assumed to be true for dizygous twins.

The varying ways of measuring whether a trait is genetically determined or not all take into consideration the size of the difference between monozygous twins and between dizygous twins, and if the difference in monozygous twins is smaller than in dizygous twins, the condition is commonly considered to be inherited. A great many statistical methods have been proposed for the estimation of the heritability, but no general agreement has been reached which is the better method.

The twins we investigated were not collected for the purpose of studying alexithymia at all. They were sought out and invited to come to an investigation of blood lipids, and some anthropometric studies.

Because of the burden of work to contact so many twins and because of their value as a scientific material in many respects, we decided to ask for their cooperation in two other studies. One being the alexithymic one, and the other being a study of personality traits. The twins had a positive attitude towards scientific investigations, and were willing to cooperate even though some feelings of exploitation were voiced.

They were all obtained from the twin registry at the Institute of Medical

Genetics at the University of Oslo. All lived in the greater Oslo area. Their zygosity was determined by more than 20 genetic marker systems, so that a chance for a dizygotic pair to be labelled as monozygotic was less than 0.5%. All dizygotic pairs differed in one or more genetic marker systems. Altogether 15 monozygous and 18 dizygous like-sexed pairs were collected. The twins were generally living together or had separated within a few years. There was no difference between the monozygous and the dizygous twins as to sex, education and age. The mean age at the time of the investigation was 24.6 years in the monozygous twins and 25.3 years in the dizygous twins.

To measure alexithymic traits we used a questionnaire, constructed by Prof. *Peter E. Sifneos* and then translated into Norwegian. It is an interviewer's questionnaire, a forced choice yes or no, and the questions designed to elicit the alexithymic traits, are as shown in table I.

These questions, however, are scattered among 15 other questions like 'Is he above average intelligence?', 'Has he a high socioeconomic status?' etc.

The interviewing of the twins and the handing out of the questionnaires was performed by a psychologist who studied personality traits. He was, and still is, uninterested in the concept of alexithymia, filling in our forms and questionnaires was something he did to get access to the twins. He had about 1 h interview with each twin and filled in his form after the interview.

Our findings were as shown in table II. There is very little difference between monozygous pairs, the so-called intrapair difference was zero in 11 out of 15 pairs, while the intrapair difference in dizygous twin pairs was quite large. This is shown mathematically in table III where the intrapair variances are found to be 0.5 in monozygous and 3.9 in dizygous twins. If one com-

Table I. Questions for alexithymic traits

	Alexithymic
Tendency to endless description of details instead of feelings	yes
Ability to find appropriate words to describe feelings	no
Rich fantasy life	no
Use of action to avoid feelings	yes
Use of action to avoid conflicts	yes
Inappropriate feelings	yes
Description of circumstances instead of feelings connected to an event	yes
Preoccupation with external events rather than with feelings and fantasies	yes

Table II. Intrapair differences

Interviewer's rating scoring difference (range 0–8)	monozygous	dizygous
0	11	3
1	2	5
2	1	3
3	1	2
4	0	2
5	0	3

Table III. Variances of alexithymic trait scores

	Monozygous	Dizygous
Intrapair	0.5	3.9
Interpair	3.1	1.2
Common interpair	2.0	

pares the variance in dizygous twins with the one in monozygous twins, this ratio, the F ratio is highly significant. It is also common to calculate the difference between pairs, and, mainly because of the small sample, this interpair variance is different in monozygous and dizygous twins. The common interpair variance is also calculated and the advantage of this parameter is the smaller confidence interval.

Table IV shows different comparison of variances: the interpair and the intrapair variance in monozygous twins are comparad and are highly significant as is the difference between the common interpair variance and intrapair variance. The differences between the interpair variances in dizygous twins are smaller than expected, and the interpair variance is not as large as the difference within a twin pair.

Table V shows the so-called intraclass correlation coefficients which can be calculated from these data. Depending on which of the variances is used, the numerical value differs slightly. The intraclass correlation coefficient is larger in monozygous than in dizygous twins, and this also points to a genetical influence and is in fact quite high for such a type of study. Identical answers within a twin pair would give a correlation coefficient of 1. Complete

Table IV. Comparison of variances

Comparisons	d.f.	F ratio
Interpair MZ/intrapair MZ	15/15	7.9[1]
Common interpair/intrapair MZ	33/15	4.0[1]
Interpair DZ/intrapair DZ	18/18	0.4
Common intrapair DZ/intrapair DZ	33/18	0.6

[1] $p < 0.01$; MZ = monozygous; DZ = dizygous.

Table V. Alexithymic traits: intraclass correlation coefficients

	Twin group	
Interpair variance	MZ	DZ
Specific	0.7[1]	−0.5
Common	0.6[1]	−0.3

[1] $p < 0.01$.

Table VI. Different estimates of heritability of alexithymic traits

	Interpair variance	
Parameter	specific	common
H value	0.87	
r_{mz}	0.72	0.60
r_{dz}	−0.53	−0.33
$\dfrac{r_{mz}-r_{dz}}{1-r_{dz}}$	0.82	0.70
$2(r_{mz}-r_{dz})$	1.0	1.0

lack of similarity would give a coefficient of 0. Our results, a coefficient of 0.7, are significant at the $p < 0.01$ level.

In table VI different estimates of the heritability of alexithymia are summarized under different assumptions. The so-called H value is very high and all these estimates point to a high degree of heritability of alexithymia, although we have to remember that the confidence intervals are large.

Generally though, these data point strongly to a hereditary component as an important factor in alexithymic traits.

As this was a somewhat unexpected finding, we scrutinized our data to discover whether any obvious bias was present.

The twins were selected from a twin registry for completely different purposes. They were, at the initial presentation, considered healthy. They were young adults so that the environmental factor was mostly common. They were generally well educated so that those who had a capacity for fantasy should have a chance to develop and express it. The male/female ratio in the two groups were about the same. All these seem to be rather ideal conditions.

Then, what about our tool, the questionnaire, is it fit, that is, valid, to elicit the alexithymic properties? Our study cannot answer to that, but, by what you have heard of these questions, it seems difficult to think of a more valid way of measuring.

The scoring was not easily biased, as the scorer was not informed about the zygosity of the twins until after the scoring was finished.

The greatest difficulty, as in so many studies, is the question of the number of the patients. Our sample is small, consisting of altogether 66 persons, and the confidence intervals are necessarily large. It is, however, probably very hard to find enough numbers of concordant or discordant monozygous or dizygous twin pairs to answer this question more fully, but efforts should be made.

In conclusio, therefore, we maintain that alexithymic traits as judged from this twin study seem to be largely inherited.

As a clinician, I am not too happy about this conclusion. It is nicer in a way to regard a condition as acquired or learned because then we have a chance to treat it by relearning, etc. But again, I want to attract your attention to the fact that alexithymic traits seem to be evenly distributed in our material. It was not a question of being alexithymic or not, but of the degree and extent of an alexithymic tendency. There is, therefore, good reason to compare alexithymic problems to other inborn impairments like dyslexia, impaired hearing, etc., and our attitude should not be fatalistic. On the contrary, we should try to diagnose this condition as early as possible to provide the alexithymic with the appropriate training. Fantasy life is a prominent factor in a child's daily life, and a study on alexithymic traits in children should therefore be easier than in grown-ups. I seriously hope that the child therapists will take up this challenge.

Discussion

Dr. König: Like Dr. *Nemiah* I cannot help being impressed by the twins study Dr. *Heiberg* presented and as a clinician would join her in not feeling too good about the results seeming to establish alexithymia as an inherited trait. However, a different inter-pretation of her results is possible. Dr. *Heiberg,* you told us that the twins with whom you worked were selected for a different purpose. There were no psychosomatic patients, so your study is apt to bring out hereditary components of alexithymia in a normal population. But it is possible that an acquired component of alexithymia is present in psychosomatic patients and I would think it is necessary to do the same study with psychosomatic patients who are also twins which is very difficult. But I think it may be possible to get an answer by comparing the amount of alexithymia you found in your twins with the amount found in a control group of psychosomatic patients. I wonder if you have done anything like this or thought about it and I would be interested in your results.

Dr. Heiberg: These are complex questions. It certainly would be interesting to make a later follow-up study on the twins we have because they are still so young that they have not yet run through their risk period for different diseases.

Dr. Gottschalk: There are three questions I have for Dr. *Heiberg,* somewhat similar to what Dr. *König* has asked. Number *one* is, would you not, still at this stage of your re-search, ask the twins which ones have any type of somatic disorders. Even if they have none at the age of 20, one would have to wait until towards the end of their life, since many psychosomatic disorders start then. *Secondly* you did not tell us how many of the fraternal twins were of a different sex. And *thirdly,* how many of these twins were reared in the same families or were reared in different families; that fact would be somewhat relative to any conclusions regarding an environmental versus a genetic effect in your studies. If they were reared in the same families, environmental influences cannot be ruled out.

Dr. Heiberg: We did ask whether they had any somatic complaints but these were so few that they could not give us any statistical evidence. Half of the twins were male and half of them female. It was the same sex ratio in the monozygous and the dizygous groups. All the dizygous pairs were same-sexed. All the twins were raised within their own families.

Dr. Shands: It is possible to comment on the genetic question indirectly through the notion of development in the technological sense. The people gathered here are among the most 'developed' persons from the most developed nations in the world; evidence I have collected in a random way suggests that psychosomatic diseases occur in undeveloped people in developed countries.

Inkeles and Smith, in a book called *Becoming Modern* discuss the ethnic correlation with modernity, noting that certain groups, East Indian Parsis, Nigerian Ibos, Swiss Prot-estants and Eastern European Jews have the capacity for learning the techniques of development differentially, thus suggesting some kind of genetic predisposition to develop-ment that is the other side of a resistance to psychosomatic disease.

Dr. Zador: I would like to ask Dr. *MacLean* two questions. He referred to the pheno-mena of limbic epilepsy and I would like to ask him if he refers to the same clinical entity that we referred to as the temporary lobe epilepsy; if it is the same? Secondly, I would like to ask him if he would comment on the system for the internal organs, cardiovascular, alimentary system and so on, and if it is so, what is the connection between the visceral brain and the vegetative representation of the cerebral cortex?

Dr. MacLean: Briefly (since my talk encroached upon the time left for discussion), I'll answer the first question by saying: yes, I do equate limbic epilepsy with temporal lobe epilepsy and more generally with what was originally described as psychomotor epilepsy. As for the second question, I do not think I would go so far as to say that the limbic system serves as a kind of biological computer *solely* with respect to internal functions. But I will say that the limbic system is beginning to look more like a 'visceral brain' than I intended to imply when I so referred to it in 1949, with the intention of circumventing the narrow implications of the term rhinencephalon that has commonly been applied to the same constellation of structures. I used the word 'visceral' in its original 16th century sense, meaning strong, inward feelings. I found, however, that physiologists objected to this term because they interpreted 'visceral' in the narrow sense as applying only to the glands and hollow organs, including the blood vessels. Consequently, I reverted to *Broca*'s descriptive term 'limbic' when referring to the cortex of the limbic lobe and structures of the brain stem with which it has primary connections – hoping that the neutral, descriptive word 'limbic' would not give people, especially my colleagues, unpleasant 'visceral' feelings! This is how the term 'limbic system' crept into the literature in 1952.

Dr. Hoppe: What we heard this morning from Prof. *MacLean* and *Nemiah* was a very interesting presentation focusing on the vertical connections of brain structures, especially between the limbic system and the neocortex. I suggest that in addition to these very important vertical connections, the horizontal cerebral connections and the different cognitive styles of the two cerebral hemispheres should also be considered. I dope we will have time to discuss this topic this afternoon when I will present my paper about com-missurotomized patients. It seems to me that in any discussion of psychosomatic phe-nomena, the difference of cognitive styles of the two hemispheres should not be overlooked.

Dr. Groen: To give a full discussion of Dr. *MacLean's* paper one would have to be Charles Darwin himself, because, as you realise, Dr. *MacLean* continues in the great tra-dition of this great man. Today he not only gave us a description of the biological develop-ment of the brain in the course of the evolution of man, but also of the parallel role which behavior and especially emotional expression played in this evolution. This is exactly in the spirit of what Darwin did: after having elucidated the *Origin of Species,* he wrote another pioneer book (the first psychobiological study I would say) on 'The expression of the emotions in animals and man.' Dr. *MacLean* has similarly given us a synthesis of the development of brain structure, brain function and behavior in the course of the evolution. I would like to ask two questions: If we compare the human brain with that of other mammals, is not the development of the prefrontal and temporal cortex, where speech and verbal thinking are localized a new, fundamental and typical human addition to the triune brain of the other mammals? It is through the capacity of verbal communications, by means of a word language, which the human brain can learn to speak and to understand that the human species has developed a culture which no animal has achieved to that degree. I would like to ask you therefore whether when we consider the *human* brain, instead of classifying it also as a 'triune' brain, we had better call it a 'quadrune' brain because of this new development of word-language localised in the prefrontal and in temporal areas superimposed on the triune brain of the other mammals.

My second question pertains to the interpretation of Dr. *Heiberg*'s findings, which we have heard earlier today. She found on comparing a form of behavior (this is what alexithymia is) in monozygous and heterozygous twins that there was more concordance among the monozygous than among the heterozygous, and, as usual in twin research, she concluded that this demonstrates that alexithymia is hereditary. On the other hand, as illustrated by her figures, there were definitely also a number of nonconcordant twins among the homozygous, as far as alexithymia is concerned. One must therefore consider that there is also a nonhereditary factor underlying this form of behavior; otherwise alexithymia would have been completely concordant in 100% of the monozygous twins. As this example shows once more, most forms of human behavior are partly hereditary and partly acquired. Now, Dr. *MacLean*, isn't that just what one would expect for almost any form of behavior in a mammal (and certainly in man), because the development of the neocortex which you described has enormously increased the capacity to learn? This is what distinguishes the mammalian from the reptilian brain and thereby mammalian from reptilian behavior. The reptilian brain, like the fish brain, can do very little more than it is born with. But the mammalian brain can learn much more. The ethologists in Leiden University have been able to teach sticklebacks to modify their behavior somewhat. These fishes can indeed learn a few new behavior patterns when rewarded, like food seeking and sex behavior, but most of their behavior patterns are inborn. But in mammals and in man, although some behavior patterns are still predominantly hereditary, the capacity of developing learned behavior is much larger. Therefore, the conclusion that alexithymia is partly hereditary, but also partly acquired, seems to be in harmony with the structure and functions of the human brain in general. Would you agree to this generalization from your brain and behavior studies?

Dr. MacLean: Again, briefly, there is no doubt about the importance of the extensive, horizontal connections of the neocortex both as they relate cortical areas in one hemisphere and between the two hemispheres. Years ago in using strychnine neuronography, the disappointing thing to us was to find how few *direct* horizontal connections exist between limbic cortical and neocortical structures. It seemed that the organization for getting messages back and forth between the limbic and neocortex must be somewhat like that in government, with the emphasis being on vertical lines of communication! Prof. *Groen*, thank you for those nice comments. I will simply say that it was primarily my purpose to emphasize the importance of the large 'reptolimbic' formations of the brain. In this respect it is significant to point out that in rats and other rodents one can destroy by a drug or X-ray the matrix cells that form the neocortex, provided that treatment is applied just at the time of their migration. The remaining forebrain of such animals consists essentially of the reptolimbic formations. Except for somewhat poor performance in spatial learning, it is impossible to distinguish these animals from normal animals. For example, they are entirely capable of mating and rearing their young. But to say this in no way depreciates the role of that giant computer that you referred to, Dr. *Groen* (the neomammalian formation), that sits above the other two formations; and emphatically yes, I had no intention at all to deny its importance in my presentation! Finally, I think that you gave a very nice answer to the two last questions!

Dr. von Rad: I have a short question that I would like to put to Dr. *Heiberg,* that is to say to Dr. *Sifneos.* Everybody is referring and relying on the Beth Israel questionnaire and I would just like to know if it has in the meantime been standardized. Has it ever been used on a normal population? If this has not yet been done, do you think anyone can do so?

Dr. Sifneos: The answer to the first question is 'no' and to the second 'we are planning to'.

Dr. Weiner: I would like to congratulate my friend, *John Nemiah,* for his comments and scholarly review. Nonetheless, I would like to ask him two questions: Alexithymia is a widespread characteristic not only of 'psychosomatic' patients. In his view, does it play an etiological pathogenic or a sustaining role in psychosomatic disease? First, if it is common to all psychosomatic patients, why does one patient develop one disease and not another? Second, there is a strong body of evidence that the factors that are etiologic are not the same as the factors that are pathogenetic or that sustain a disease. In short, the question that I have for him is: If alexithymic patients develop psychosomatic disease, why does one patient develop an ulcer, another hypertension and a third arthritis?

Dr. Nemiah: You know quite well, Herbert, that I am not going to be trapped by your question on specificity! That, as we are all aware, is a central conundrum in our field. What I was in essence trying to do was something perhaps more modest – to suggest the kinds of models that might explain psychosomatic symptom formation, and to indicate the role of alexithymic characteristics in this process. In the terms you suggest, we should consider them etiologic but at the same time should emphasize that they are not alone a sufficient condition.

Dr. Weiner: John, as you well know, Alexander tried by his specificity hypothesis to come to grips with the question of the 'choice' of a disease. Today, we can partly answer his question. But it cannot be answered if we go back to an emphasis on the commonalities that characterize these patients, or any one single factor that determines the 'choice'.

Dr. Nemiah: In other words, we must beware of the single-factor etiological model.

Dr. Weiner: Right. Patients with these diseases share certain common characteristics but they also differ as Alexander was wont to emphasize.

Dr. Nemiah: I would agree completely with you there, Herb. In linking alexithymia with psychosomatic disorders, we are not suggesting that it is 'the cause'. We are merely saying that it appears to be a feature common to many patients with such illnesses and that it must have some relationship to their production as one of a number of factors that in combination lead to a clinical disorder.

Proc. 11th Eur. Conf. Psychosom. Res., Heidelberg 1976
Psychother. Psychosom. *28:* 230–235 (1977)

A Social-Psychological Approach to the Specificity of Psychosomatic Diseases

Karola Brede

I think, many of you will agree when I start my paper with the claim that physiology, the psychology of neuroses and social psychology were all united to give their share to the development of a homogeneous psychosomatic (PSS) theory. Keeping this frame of reference in mind, I shall confine myself to present some thoughts on the possible function of social psychology. As to the claim of a *unified* PSS theory I understand my statement to be part of this venture, as modest as it may be.

No matter which methodological approach PSS research was obliged to, its students had to consider that the social sciences were to be given their share in the discussion of strategies that are able to explain PSS disturbances. As for myself, I would like to introduce you to a hypothesis which has received positive proof, though it may appear to you a bit daring. This hypothesis is as follows: When one assumes that PSS disturbances can be understood adequately only by means of the psychoanalytic theory of neuroses, then I would suggest that their *specificity,* as compared to that of neurotic disturbances, has to be localized in sociocultural factors. These factors are related to the genesis of PSS disorders, and ought to be considered when the genesis of PSS disorders is drafted. Today it is no longer adequate to explain PSS disorders through the relationship of 'psyche' to 'physis' only. The explanation of PSS disorders has to be extended to include the influence of society, if the quality of explanation is ever to be satisfactory. That is to say, the intimate involvement of the individual with society will have to be examined closely.

Putting the question in this way, two problems already well known to PSS medicine, become a focus of concern: (1) PSS disorders are measurable pathological deviations within a physiological context or lesions of the organic substratum, in both cases in the sense of the valid conception of pathology, the natural sciences have developed. A methodological difficulty, therefore, arises – namely, that of extending the explanatory approach of the social sciences into processes of which evidence can be given only in physiological terms. (2) If the specifity of PSS disorders is to be localized in sociocultural factors, the psychopathological and the social-psychological analyses have to be carried out from the point of view of a theoretically unified concept. This becomes important, because of the supposed inner connection between the production of symptoms and the sociocultural mediation of action, in general.

Though the first mentioned problem of an adequate concept of the organism in the social sciences is indispensable[1], I shall only go into the second problem of the connection between psychoanalysis and 'socioanalysis' in the case of neurotic symptom formation.

If I assume that PSS disorders can be understood on the grounds of the psychology of neuroses, then this means: PSS disturbances are based on an inner (psychodynamic) conflict which occupies and consumes, so-to-speak, the psychic functions of perception and memory. The emotional-motivational mobility, therefore, will be reduced when the individual is interacting with others. Such a conflict, no doubt, has a deep bearing on the personality organization and on the biography of this individual. He can only generate incomplete conflict resolutions. If a conflict of this kind leads to self-regulation (Eigengesetzlichkeit) of psychic functions and if these functions, therefore, are governed by dynamics hardly to be changed – these conditions given, the PSS patient finds himself practicing an autoplastic resolution, his symptoms being situated in his body and within this area of conflict resolution in somatic processes. As *Mitscherlich* (1954) assumes, these processes take place within the body as a somatic field of expression. In general, we do not associate with this field the capacity to generate meaningful actions or to participate in them. The somatic field of expression contributes to the factual situation in the respect that the PSS patient is not perceptibly conspicuous as far as his social behavior is concerned (sozial unauffällig). While

---

[1] As far as I can see there is at present hardly a chance for a concept of the organism that is apt to the requirements of the social sciences, and at the same time would allow deduction of the genesis of *specific* psychosomatic disorders from the postulated unified psychosomatic theory. When I suggest a sociocultural specificity of psychosomatic disorders on the following pages, I shall, therefore, relate to differences in comparison to neurotic disturbances only.

hysteria and compulsive neurosis consist of symptoms, by which the patient deviates from social expectations, the PSS patient complies with the normative requirements of the very social situations, he is acting in. He is, in a psychologically complex sense of the word 'adapted' (angepasst), that means that adaptation and disorder are perfectly married.

The PSS patient appears socially integrated, also when his personality is evaluated according to criteria derived from the functionalist theory of socialization. This includes criteria which are supposed to tell, whether the integration into systems of action, like the family, the generation, work, etc., has been accomplished by the individual or not. If students of PSS medicine investigate the 'socializatory' context of PSS patients, i.e., familial relationships and relationships within other reference groups that are emotionally relevant, they have, sometimes scarcely mentioned, the explicit intention,to discover and identify conditions within the interactional field of the PSS patient that might specify the etiology of PSS disorders. Further, I believe it is important to investigate, whether the interaction within a family testifies the habitual dealing of the family with sickness or whether the style of handling one member in the family *makes* the sickness (I assume, that Mr. *Stierlin* will discuss these questions more in detail); neither shall I enter into questions, resulting when the emotional-motivational processes under the surface of familial interaction are taken to draw conclusions about the personality of the patient. I will confine myself to considerations about the socializatory approach which, as I hope, will lead a little further to solving the problems that emerge when the *genetic specificity* of sociocultural factors in illness is discussed.

It is assumed, in the theory of the socialization process as a *sociological* appraoch to personality development, that the individual acquires his competence to interact in social situations by societal influences. The family as an institution that transmits sociocultural values and norms to the growing child, even under conditions of constraint, is in the center of these considerations. It is usually *so,* that this approach to the socialization process is reduced to an understanding of growth according to which development is an adaptational process to social standards, norms and values. It defines the socialization process positively (*Parsons and Bales, 1956*) and yet at the same time inadmissibly as successful social integration of the individual. In general, this approach can only differentiate socially integrated and 'deviant' behavior. A behavior is deviant if the individual does not comply to normative expectations, when, therefore, his behavior is situationally inadequate, and when socially approved room for action is transgressed by the individual.

PSS disorders cannot be localized within this frame of reference, for a violation of social norms or of the approved room of interaction, allowing to speak of a deviance, is not at hand. The PSS patient carries out his psychodynamic conflicts within the limits of socially approved behavior.

One could surmise, on the one hand, that theoretical incapacity of this approach is the reason why it does not apply to PSS disorders. This fact might, on the other hand, also be instructive as far as the PSS syndrome is concerned. The inconspicuous social behavior which characterizes the PSS patient, gives rise to the conjecture that the patient by his psychodynamic situation has a share in the symptom formation, and that this share consists of a highly integrational achievement through which the generated PSS symptom is resorbing the social deviance (*de M'Uzan,* 1974). The PSS patient, at the same time, complies to the expectations that belong to the exceptional rules governing the role of the sick, in general; like every patient with an organic disease, the PSS patient's actions are appropriate to the rules of the sick. By that I mean, the patient may withdraw, in part or entirely, from the obligations the healthy fulfills; he cannot be held responsible because of his condition, etc. If, however, the generating of PSS symptoms and at least the major traits of the sick role (*Parsons,* 1958) – the need to be cared for and the readiness and will to recover – are inseparably tied to each other, then this would be the proof for a relationship between the psychoanalytic approach to neuroses and social-psychological conditions, specifying the symptom choice as the PSS expression of a conflict. This relationship is described a bit more precisely below.

According to the PSS assumptions I am referring to, the compliance to interactional rules the PSS patient demonstrates can only be produced via the mechanisms that govern the formation of neuroses. In general, the individual is capable to consciously or preconsciously conform with the normative expectations of others. This will be the case if the individual enacts fundamental qualifications such as tolerance toward ambivalent feelings and if he can evade one role obligation in favor of another, if necessary. In regard to the PSS patient, on the contrary, one has to assume (1) that the very compliance with normative expectations and his actions as a sick person have been produced *unconsciously*; (2) that the PSS patient in comparison to his *competence* to interact, is overstrained; the range of *motivation* which should be at the disposal of the patient if he is to bear conflicts is a victim to the dynamics of the pathogenic psychosomatic process, and (3) if one, however, assumes that the patient is acting with an unconscious intention, there is at least one indispensable condition to be mentioned: a social pattern that is related to the patient's behavior, especially to the PSS symptoms, must contain elements that correspond to his regression. This holds exactly true for the normative aspects of the sick role. It is affirmed by the sick role that the symptom formation is not consciously intended by the individual, and the unconscious libidinal gain in disease is socially licenced as (acceptable) regression. The individual's share in his sickness merely consists of a mode of experience that is determined by unconscious guilt feelings[2]. This is the function of interactional rules the individual is following when he accepts the sick role.

I assume that the PSS symptom is related to the *rules* of social inter-action in a *meaningful* way. The capability to refer to rules makes up the *generative* nature of the *ego achievement*. That is, the patient is bridging the gap between the symptom and the role enactment as a sick person not consciously by far. By 'bridging the gap' I do not mean the often referred to conception of secondary gain. Since the unconscious conflict is dealt with in the somatic field of expression, the individual through this expression is following the rules imbedded in the sick role, a role, therefore, the normative structure of which corresponds to elements of the neurosis. The ego achieve-ment the individual is accomplishing thereby, I call generative.

The PSS symptom, however, is to be looked upon as a symptom in the sense of the psychology of neuroses. The symptomatic PSS manifestation, therefore, is meaningful at the psychopathological price of *regression* and *compulsion to repeat*. The ego achievement of the PSS patient which is related to the symptom formation remains limited by these psychodynamic processes. An additional point of view, specific to PSS disorders shows up if the function of the ego is not investigated in the perspective of social inter-

---

[2] Many clinical details from the interview and therapy reports to be found in *de M'Uzan* (1974) and in *Nemiah and Sifneos* (1970), for example, seem to support these consi-derations. Regarding the 'pensée opératoire' and fantasy activity, *de M'Uzan,* however, leaves it to descriptive information. It is, therefore, difficult to conclude from these obser-vations on genetic aspects of the PSS process. *Nemiah and Sifneos,* on the other hand, tend to a psychological-physiological pluralism of theoretical approaches. It is, therefore, rather impossible to assess the theoretical place of their observations and also their correspondence to the observations their French colleagues had made. Hence, even if one would clear up methodological objections against the investigations of *Marty et al.* (1963), *Nemiah and Sifneos* (1970), and *Sifneos* (1973), there would remain the prior task in psychosomatic medicine to develop a unified psychosomatic theory that is sufficient to the current demands of theory building. This is necessary if all the results from empirical research are to be examined regarding their definite meaning.

action, but in the perspective of the unconscious, that is, if one stresses the defensive function of the ego. In this perspective, the following is to be said: By the production of PSS symptoms, the defensive activity of the ego is alleviated. The PSS symptom is *not* the debarred unconscious content, but the functional *equivalent* of defense, because the conflict conforms in all cases to the sick role. That is, through its interactional rules the socio-cultural system has a discharging effect on the burden of individual neurosis. The price to be paid by the PSS patient, however, demonstrates that these processes are imbedded in a complex relationship of control between society and its individual members.

References

Marty, P.; M'Uzan, M. de et David, C.: L'investigation psychosomatique (Presses Univ., Paris 1963).

Mitscherlich, A.: Psychosomatik vom Standpunkt der Psychoanalyse. Med. Klin. *49:* 1789–1793 (1954).

M'Uzan, M. de: The psychodynamic mechanisms in psychosomatic symptom formation. Psychother. Psychosom. *23:* 103–110 (1974).

Nemiah, J.C. and Sifneos, P.E.: Affect and fantasy in patients with psychosomatic disorders; in *Hill* Modern trends in psychosomatic medicine, vol. 2, pp. 26–34 (Butterworths, London 1970).

Parsons, T. and Bales, R.F.: Family. Socialization and interaction process (Routledge & Kegan, London 1956).

Parsons, T.: Definitions of health and illness in the light of American values and social structure; in *Parsons* Social structure and personality, pp. 257–291 (Free Press, London 1958).

Sifneos, P.E.: The prevalence of 'alexithymic' characteristics in psychosomatic patients. Psychother. Psychosom. *22:* 255–262 (1973).

Dr. phil. *Karola Brede,* Sigmund-Freud-Institut, Myliusstrasse 20, *D-6000 Frankfurt/Main* (FRG)

Proc. 11th Eur. Conf. Psychosom. Res., Heidelberg 1976
Psychother. Psychosom. *28:* 236–242 (1977)

Some Reflections about the Conception of 'Psychosomatic Patients' in the French School

Johannes Cremerius

After *Ruesch* (1948) and *MacLean* (1949) had, at the peak of the American specification research, already drawn attention to the fact that certain personality traits independent of the type of disease are common to all patients who suffer from psychosomatic diseases, since 1960 some French psychosomatists – *David, Fain, Marty, de M'Uzan* – have again taken up this field of research. They describe a 'psychosomatic structure' which they compare with the neurotic, genital, perverse and psychotic structure and differentiate it from these. As characteristics of the 'psychosomatic structure' they mention: *operational thinking* with mental deficiency of contact towards the object, incapability of imagination, sterility of verbal expression, somatization instead of verbalization, incapability of admitting drive impulses to consciousness – in a direct or in a defensive way; *disorders of the ego* in the sense of partial mental immaturity and rigid, fragile defence organisation, lack of capacity to symbolize, emptiness of relations in the object relation and being cut off from the own unconscious. These patients lead an automatistic, mechanistic life; *psychosomatic regression* to a primitive system of defence and to the earliest stages of somatic development – even to the interaction between fetus and mother (*Marty,* 1951), and finally *projective duplication.*

From the *diagnostic aspect* you can find migraine, allergy, urticaria, essential hypertonia and gastroduodenal ulcus, as well as functional and conversion hysterical syndromes. Besides that, the authors mention glaucoma and phthisis. Most of the serious psychosomatic diseases are lacking, such as anorexia nervosa, colitis ulcerosa, diabetes, bronchial asthma, malign types of obesity caused by voracity and those hypochondriac organ sensations which are an expression of the earliest narcissistic disturbances of bodily feelings.

From the *sociologic aspect* the group consists of patients from the lower education and income class.

Furthermore, two methodical particularities should be mentioned: the system of selection and the method of the acquiring of data. The *selection* takes place in such a way that 3rd class patients of the Parisian clinics for internal medicine, surgery, etc., are chosen for an interview.

The *acquiring of data* takes place within the scope of a public exploration, in the presence of students and younger doctors. Everyone of us knows patients who more or less distinctly show the mentioned structure. Doubtlessly, it is more frequently and more distinctly found in psychosomatic patients than in patients with other neurotic disorders. But we can also find it there – and not as a rarity. Now, I put forth the thesis that the 'psychosomatic structure' described by the French authors is not disease-specific. As proof, I will show you two groups for comparison. One group of psychoneurotic patients *without* bodily symptoms from the same education and income class, a second group of psychosomatic patients from a middle income and education class from my private practice. The group of psychoneurotic patients coincides with the French group not only in the social composition, but also in the system of selection. Concerning the method of acquiring data, however, we differ from our French colleagues inasmuch as we make the exploration without the presence of other persons. The group of psychosomatic patients from my private practice are either sent to me directly by doctors or they come spontaneously.

The result of the *comparison between the group of the French authors and the group of my psychoneurotic patients* shows a far-reaching accordance: the psychoneurotic patients also talk about themselves, their body and closely related persons as if they were things; fantasies are hardly ever expressed; the verbal expressions are sterile and banal; their ego is weak, shows a fragile defence structure and a defective capacity of symbolizing; the patients hardly seem to have any access to their unconscious; in critical situations of their life they get serious forms of regression like drunkenness, depersonalization, affected actions and somatization; they have nothing to say, especially nothing about their conflicts; they talk about happenings, not about experiences.

In contrast to the French authors I could not notice the 'emptiness of relations', the lack of affective contact with the researcher and the 'projective duplication'. I want to explain the difference between these two collectives by the method of the acquiring of data, that means by an artefact. *Schneider* supposes that the situation in which the exploration takes place can only be felt to be hostile, and that it must bring forth primitive defence mechanisms which hinder any possibilities of producing fantasies.

I'll now come to the *comparison of the French group with the group of psychosomatic patients* from my private practice, to a kind of check-test in comparison with the first group. Firstly, we have to notice here that this group is less homogeneous to analyze than the first one. Whilst an analytic treatment was possible only in a few cases there, here it takes place with many patients. These are generally those patients who come to the consultation hour already with the wish for treatment or who soon get the wish in the initial conversations. Many of these patients complain of difficulties in life and interior conflicts besides their bodily troubles. With them neither in the first conversation nor during the treatment which lasted up to 5 years were signs of a 'psychosomatic structure' to be found.

The other part of the patients from the private practice distinctly differs from that formerly described. These patients come to the consultation hours without any clear ideas about psychoanalysis, and expect that something will be done with them or they hope to get rid of their troubles without their neurotic problems being touched. With this group of the patients who rarely agree to psychoanalytic therapy, many characteristics of the so-called 'psychosomatic structure' are to be found. Especially the deficiency of contact, the incapability of imagination, the lacking of access to their own unconscious, and the difficulty to admit drive impulses, rigid defence organization and somatization instead of verbalization and communication. However, I never saw the completely matured state of the so-called 'psychosomatic structure', which means a picture of the pregenital patient.

My experiences in my private practice coincide with those of the analysts who treat psychosomatic patients who come to them spontaneously and who belong to the middle education and income class. These analysts – *Alexander, Garma, Monsour, Orgel, Oston, Sperling,* to name only a few – classify these patients like I do as neurotics, carry out the analysis in the standard method and report about good success.

The result of my research is that the so-called psychosomatic structure is not disease – specific. It is also to be found in patients with psychoneurotic disorders *without* bodily symptoms, and in the rule it is missing in all psychosomatic patients from the middle class, who come to the private practice of an analyst for treatment. Where the patients who show the so-called psychosomatic structure coincide, however, is that they belong to the same social class. Therefore, I have come to the conclusion that it is a characteristic of a certain social class. The check-test with the group of the psychosomatic private patients confirms my thesis.

My expression 'specific of a class' is only an abbreviation for a complex summoning-up of facts. But I do not mean that it is a given characteristic of a social class in the sense as one talks of characteristics of animal species. On the contrary I take it to be on the one hand based on historical and social conditions, and on the other to be caused by the examination – situation, in which the peculiarity of one class shall be defined with the standard of another, which, in addition, is the ruling class. This procedure was found to be incorrect by the ethno-psychologists as much as 50 years ago. Furthermore, I do not mean difficulties of understanding in the sense of speech barriers as Bernstein for example described them. The difficulties of understanding are easier to understand and comprehend if one takes note of the world of fantasy of the researching analysts. This world is, even for psychoanalysts who do not belong to this school, unfamiliar, astonishing and sometimes totally incomprehensible. What must it then be like for other people, particularly for those who belong to the lower education class?

The other result of my research is that there is a correlation between the so-called psychosomatic structure and the system of selection. It is to be found in all those whom we ask, perhaps I had better say urge to the examination because we need them for research and for teaching, in those who are sent to us, and in those who come to us with the hope that we will cure their bodily troubles without touching their neurotic background. This group is not bound to a certain education or income class. The characteristic described here of a lacking or disturbed relation to the doctor, the nonunderstanding of the therapeutic offer, his refusal to the offer or the incapability of accepting it, is found in every social class. The factor of readiness, of 'maturity' I consider to be especially important. For the analytical work, especially for transference, it is of decisive importance whether someone wishes a psychoanalytic treatment of his own accord, or whether he does not feel the necessity for it. The lacking or missing maturity normally frustrates the treatment – independent from the fact whether the patient has a psychosomatic or a psychoneurotic disturbance. And from this we conclude that there are two contrasting experiences: (1) those of the analysts who in their private practice treat psychosomatic patients who come to them with the wish for a therapy and whom they treat like psychoneurotics successfully with psychoanalytic treatment, and (2) those of the analysts who for their research work have to 'fish for' patients in clinics and institutions, who neither have any insight into the nature of their bodily disorder nor feel the necessity of a therapy, and with whom they diagnose special personality traits and the in-capability of being therapeutically treated.

Therefore, it is not astonishing that all of us who have done such a research were able to state more or less similar traits with the psychosomatic patients as the French authors.

If the so-called psychosomatic structure is not disease-specific, but a characteristic on the one hand of the lower social class, on the other hand of those patients who, independent of their class, cannot see or accept the connection between the pathological disorder and their biography, that means who are lacking the readiness for a therapeutic contact, we must ask our-selves what the nature of this structure is? First of all I must emphasize once more that here we are dealing partly with an artefact, which originated from the method of selection and exploration by the authors. Thereby, personality traits of the patient were caricatured. What is described as psychosomatic structure seems far more likely to originate in the pathology of pregenital disorders and in that of schizophrenic diseases. Besides that, we must state that this is a very complex structure in which material from the observation level is mixed with material from the interpretation level without marking the limits. The things we have for observation can be classified conceptually in two ways. First of all with the help of ego psychological terms. From this opinion the traits named by the French authors appear as defence movements of the ego, as reaction formation and repression with the aim to prevent emotions and fantasies to reach consciousness. Secondly, the objects for observation can be classified with the help of terms of the psychology of development. From this opinion the traits appear as disorders of socialization. These people did not develop the usual connection between emotions and words, and therefore suffer from the incapability of expressing inner processes in words or fantasies.

For both factors it is true that they play a role in the etiology of all types of neuroses, although to a different extent. Based upon my comparing researches of the two named collectives I can state, however, that a disorder of socialization as a cause of the so-called psychosomatic structure is more frequent with patients of the lower social class than with patients of the middle class. Already the social psychiatrists *Hollingshead and Redlich* (1958), *Pflanz* (1962) and *Häfner* (1969) have detected that a correlation exists between social class and type of disease.

They have shown that there is a correlation on the one hand between lower class and psychosomatic disease, and on the other between upper class and mental disease.

At the end of my reflections, I have come to the conclusion that the so-called psychosomatic structure of the French authors is not disease-specific. What they have observed would be better if it were described in terms of the defence theory and the psychology of socialization. A fundamental factor for the construction of the so-called psychosomatic structure doubt-lessly is due to the fact that the authors examined patients who were frighten-ed by the situation in which they were examined, who did not understand what was wanted of them and who did not feel any necessity for a therapeutic conversation.

I am sorry that I cannot go into detail with a further argument against the thesis of the psychosomatic structure. It originates in the exploration of the course of a disease, which has shown us that neurotic aspects of a case can on principle change the field of manifestation. Thereby psychosomatic diseases change for example into psychoneuroses or psychosocial disorders (*Cremerius*, 1968). What happens then with the psychosomatic structure? Where is the wind when it doesn't blow?

At the end I would like to state that the psychosomatic structure also doesn't coincide with the general experiences in life. Are for instance the poets and artists, are our friends and acquaintencies our psychoanalytic col-leagues, all those whom we know to suffer from psychosomatic diseases marked by psychosomatic structure without fantasy, by emptiness of relation and by projective duplication? Marcel Proust suffered from asthma and Sigmund Freud from migraine and functional heart and circulatory disturbances. I think that there are still a lot of open questions in the 'chose psychosomatique'. It is this that I wanted to draw attention to.

References

Cremerius, J.: Die Prognose funktioneller Syndrome (Enke, Stuttgart 1968).
Cremerius, J.: Schichtspezifische Schwierigkeiten bei der Anwendung der Psychoanalyse. Münch. med. Wschr. *117:* 1229–1232 (1975).
Fain, M. et Marty, P.: Perspectives psychosomatiques sur la fonction des fantasmes. Revue fr. Psychanal. *28:* 609–622 (1964).
Häfner, H.: Inzidenz seelischer Erkrankungen in Mannheim 1965; in Sozialpsychiatrie (Hogrefe, Göttingen 1969).
Hollingshead, A.-G. and Redlich, F.-C.: Social class and mental illness (Wiley, New York 1958).
MacLean, P.D.: Psychosomatic disease and the 'visceral brain'. Psychosom. Med. *11:* 338–345 (1949).

Marty, P.: Aspect psychodynamique de l'étude clinique de quelques cas de céphalgies. Revue fr. Psychanal. *22:* 5–35 (1951).

Marty, P. et M'Uzan, M. de: La 'pensée opératoire'. Revue fr. Psychanal. *22:* 5–35 (1963).

Marty, P.; M'Uzan, M. de et David, C.: L'investigation psychosomatique (Presses Universitaires de France, Paris 1963).

M'Uzan, M. de et David, C.: Préliminaires critiques à la recherche psychosomatique. Revue Psychanal. *24:* 19–39 (1960).

Overbeck, G.: Objektivierende Untersuchungen zur Ich-Struktur und Objektbeziehung von Patienten mit psychosomatischen Störungen; Habil.-Schrift, Universität Giessen (1975).

Pflanz, M.: Sozialer Wandel und Krankheit (Enke, Stuttgart 1962).

Ruesch, J.: The infantile personality. The core problem of psychosomatic medicine. Psychosom. Med. *10:* 134–139 (1948).

Prof. Dr. med. *J. Cremerius,* Lehrstuhl für Psychotherapie der Universität Freiburg i. Br., Habsburger Strasse 62, *D-7800 Freiburg i. Br.* (FRG)

Proc. 11th Eur. Conf. Psychosom. Res., Heidelberg 1976
Psychother. Psychosom. *28:* 243–251 (1977)

Family Dynamics and Psychosomatic Disorders in Adolescence [1]

Helm Stierlin, M. Wirsching and W. Knauss

Man, an animal endowed with awareness (and even awareness of awareness) faces complex tasks of reconciliation. In particular, he needs to differentiate self from nonself, inside from outside, one's own thoughts, wishes, expectations, hopes, etc., from those held by others. We may speak of a self-other differentiation which must include self-other integration: increasingly, the differentiated psycho-social organism must fit in with larger systems, with a 'community of otherness' (*Friedmann,* 1976), as represented by his parents, siblings, spouse, children, friends, and society at large.

Success in such self-other differentiation and -integration hinges on intrapsychic and interpersonal channels and tools of communication – channels and tools which must safeguard individuation even under stressful conditions, especially those requiring empathy and closeness. We must communicate with, and tune ourselves into, our inner world, and our emotional undercurrents. And we must communicate with others, to whom we need to convey, as clearly and effectively as possible, our needs, wishes, and expectations. A breakdown of such intra- and interpersonal communication may result in opposite types of deadlocks: individuation may overreach itself, as it were; here boundaries become too strong and rigid, and independence turns into isolation. Or boundaries stay too soft, permeable or brittle and individuation gives way to fusion with, or intrusion by, others.

Such failures in individuation derive from, as well as reflect, alienation from self, or alienation from others, or both (*Stierlin,* 1970).

To emphasize the relational dimension in individuation, we prefer to speak of '*related individuation*' (bezogene Individuation) rather than 'individuation'. Related individuation implies that higher levels of individuation

[1] Supported by the Robert-Bosch-Stiftung, Stuttgart.

require ever higher levels of relatedness. At the same time, the term counteracts the bourgeois 'illusion of a personal individuality' which already Sullivan (1950) decried.

Psychosomatic disorders, we submit, imply the just-mentioned kinds of alienation, and thus signal a derailment of that intrapsychic as well as interpersonal dialectic which the term 'related individuation' evokes.

We believe that the concept of alexithymia, staking out this conference's main theme, brings into view important features of such derailment, features we found in many, albeit not all the psychosomatic patients we came to know.

From an Individual to a Family Perspective

To explore related individuation in psychosomatic disorders we need to focus not only on intrapsychic dynamics but must take into account *all* members of the relational system. This then involves us in a family perspective which charts these members' individual contributions (wishes, expectations, actions, etc.) as well as relevant (overt and covert) systems forces. For relationship systems reflect more than the sum of individual contributions, just as water is more than the sum of hydrogen and oxygen.

The concepts of the transactional modes (or scenarios) of binding and expelling, and of the delegating process, as developed by *Stierlin* (1972, 1974, 1975) try to provide a framework within which we may assess impaired related individuation in families with psychosomatic patients.

Binding in Psychosomatic Disorders

Where a binding scenario prevails, a child's age-appropriate differentiation-integration and hence related individuation vis-à-vis, as well as separation from, his parents is delayed, if not forestalled.

Binding can operate on three major levels: a mainly affective level, on which the child's dependency needs are exploited and manipulated; a mainly cognitive level on which the binding parent (or parents) substitute his or her own distortive ego for the child's discriminative ego, and a third level, on which loyalty needs are fostered as well as exploited.

Id-level binding frequently implies massive regressive gratification which fosters a passive dependent, if not symbiotic disposition, as we find it frequently in psychosomatic disorders, particularly those involving the digestive tract (i.e. ulcus, ulcerative colitis, etc.).

Ego level binding implies mystification by means of bewildering and double-messages: a dependent, mystified child often becomes confused as to how he should read his inner signals.

Finally, massive binding may occur on a superego level primarily. Here the child is in the grips of an intense, albeit invisible, loyalty and develops a strong sense of obligation. There results, therefore, an intense breakaway guilt whenever he attempts separation in thought or action. Such ever-present breakaway guilt, too, locks a child into the family ghetto and, in addition, may contribute to overexertive and self-destructive life styles as we observe these frequently in certain types of psychosomatic disorders (e.g., patients suffering from thyrotoxicosis).

Expelling in Psychosomatic Disorders

However, while features of the binding mode have thus far stood out in psychosomatic family research, those of the expelling mode also appear important.

The expelling mode contrasts with the binding mode. Here the child is rejected and neglected; i.e. expelled rather than bound. Such expulsion may bear upon a child's disposition to psychosomatic disorders in a number of ways: first, at critical developmental phases, the child lacks vital care and stimulation. This then may result in extreme oral rage and frustration as well as in lifelong repair needs and needs for contact. Second, there is a centrifugal rush out of the family into premature pseudoindependence. This may then result in an uneven biopsychological differentiation-integration. Third, expelled children are likely to lack a sense of importance, as well as a capacity for concern, loyalty and guilt. Such lack may cause a person either to surrender to self-destructive drift, or to resort to an overcompensating (narcissistic) seeking of importance.

Delegating in Psychosomatic Disorders

In addition to, and interweaving with, the above dynamics, those of the delegating process frequently interfere with 'related individuation'. In this process there recur elements of the binding *and* expelling mode, reflecting centripetal *and* centrifugal forces. The push and pull of these forces shines forth in the original meaning of the Latin word 'delegare': to send out and to entrust with a mission (or missions). Central to delegation is the loyalty bond which binds together delegator and delegate.

Within limits we consider delegation to be a necessary and legitimate relational process: in being delegated, our lives receive direction and meaning, they become anchored in a chain of obligations across generations. In serving as delegates we have a chance to prove our loyalty and fidelity, to show our integrity by faithfully fulfilling missions which answer not only a personal but also transpersonal calling. But this relational process may derail and this may happen in three major ways. First, difficult missions may over-tax an individual, as they are incompatible with his talents, resources, and age-appropriate needs. This leads to his psychological exploitation and, at the same time, induces in him an uneven development. Typically, this happens when a child of only mediocre gifts is delegated to become the shining aca-demic star that his parent (or parents) failed to become.

Second, there may be a conflict of missions as when missions that originate in one or more delegators conflict with each other, pulling the delegate in different directions. Thus, one parent or parents may delegate a son to be-come a dissolute playboy, and to thus serve as excitement provider, while he has also to become a well-behaved theology student. Third, there may be a conflict of loyalties which subjects the delegate to massive guilt should he betray one delegator for the sake of another.

Psychosomatic disorders, according to our clinical experience, frequently reveal characteristic conflicts of delegation. For example, we again and again find psychosomatic patients to have been commissioned to take the place of a deceased and unmourned sibling. Inevitably, such a child becomes for his parents a focus of constant worried agitation and of an overprotective re-gressive gratification. At the same time, he remains tightly locked into the family orbit. As a consequence, all this child's efforts to achieve higher levels of related individuation remain seriously curtailed. In many other cases a regressively gratified child may have to fulfill a repair mission for parents which grows out of these parents' deprivation by their own parents: they now 'give' to their child as they once needed to be given to by their parents. Also, we found many psychosomatic patients entrusted with the mission of be-coming noncomplaining conformist achievers in the service of their parents' restrictive, bourgeois ego ideals.

Related Individuation in Adolescence

Mahler et al., (1975), above other psychoanalytic authors, explored individuation in early childhood. Yet *Blos* (1962), *Jacobson* (1964), and others reminded us that a second period of life, i.e. adolescence, is equally important to successful individuation: the adolescent drives toward autonomy and identity by internationalizing and tolerating conflicts and by actively seeking partners and values outside his or her family of origin. This drive is fueled and shaped by societal expectations as well as by psychophysiological developments that affect the adolescent's total being. His aggressive and libidinal drives intensify, his defensive organization realigns, and his relational vicissitudes increase. *Freud* (1958), *Blos* (1962), *Erikson* (1950), and others have amply described these processes.

Disturbances of the Individuation Process in Psychosomatically Disturbed Adolescents

We submit that adolescents with psychosomatic disorders allow us to explore in 'statu nascendi' those disturbances of the individuation process which befall large numbers of psychosomatic patients. Also, therapeutic interventions appear more promising in this age group.

We emphasize the work with all members of an adolescent's family. Currently, we are engaged in a research project with psychosomatically ill adolescents and families. The adolescents suffered from either asthma, neurodermitis, duodenal ulcer, colitis or ileitis. In our research we employed questionnaires, conducted home visits and clinical interviews, and engaged the whole family in a consensus Rorschach procedure. From this project we would now like to present a characteristic example of a failure of related individuation. It concerns an 18-year-old girl suffering from duodenal ulcer. In describing her case we shall stress the following aspects bearing on the individuation process: (1) The nature of the forces binding the family together. (2) The central expectations or missions (*Stierlin,* 1974) the adolescent has to fulfill in her family. (3) The conflicts over guilt, merits, and loyalty *Boszormenyi-Nagy and Spark,* 1974) which arise in the separation process.

Brief Overview of Family A

The family lives in a modern suburban bungalow. The father, an engineer aged 50, invites us into the house. His wife, aged 51, has a slight Spanish accent. She finally calls her 18-year-old daughter, Eva, a tall, pale, nervous girl with dark curly hair – the psychosomatic patient. Eva's symptoms first occurred when she was 8. She had surgery for a stomach perforation 3 years ago and a two-thirds resection plus vagotomy last year. Her periods stopped a year ago.

The family at once connected the onset of her symptoms with two events: (1) the girl's younger sister's death from a malignant tumor, and (2) serious quarrels between the two mothers-in-law which entailed quarrels between the two parents.

Since the girl's stomach symptoms appeared after the last operation disagreements between parents and daughter came more to the fore. The main problems concerned pocket money, helping at home, school and time spent out of the house. Both parents complained about the daughter being out of the house too much of the time. When Eva moved into a room of her own, her mother viewed this as an act of desertion. Both parents have chronic physical complaints. Mrs. A. suffers from a circulatory disorder, her husband from gastritis and cystitis.

Sketch of the Family History

Mrs. A. was born in Spain. Her father was German and died of cirrhosis of the liver before her birth. When she was 11 she was sent to a boarding school in Germany. Two years later her older brother died in the Spanish Civil War and her one older sister also settled in Germany. The rest of the family moved to the town where they still live.

Mr. A. grew up as a single child in a relatively poor family. His ambition was to rise socially, yet he never moved away from his family's place of birth.

In the first years of their marriage the young couple lived under one roof with Mr. A.'s parents. After their first daughter Eva was born, the little girl became strongly attached to her grandparents, yet lost her grandfather when she was only 3½ years old. Mrs. A. worked until her second child, Betty, was born 5 years after Eva. Little Betty developed a malignant tumor of the salivary glands and died at the age of 3.

With that event the family's whole life changed. Mrs. A. has since alternated between apathy and rage. Till today she 'cannot forget' and must talk compulsively to everybody her about lost child. In contrast to her, Eva said at the funeral: 'We do not want to come to the cemetry every day from now on.' She has since stayed in the car when her parents visited her sister's grave. She wants to forget and cannot bear it when her mother talks incessantly about the dead Betty.

Interpretation

Interpretating this family's dynamics we shall chiefly focus on the impaired process of related individuation. This impairment came across in the family's inability to solve their problems by dialogue. Pathological mourning determined centrally the members' communications. Feelings of despair and resignation were almost tangible but could not be verbalized. Instead, all members clung to an illusion of total harmony. Yet the more they became locked into a clinging dependence, the stronger became explosive forces aiming at expulsion and division with a resulting retrait into resignation. In such prevalence of binding forces the parents were unable to accept the individuality of their daughter and came to see her age-appropriate moves out of the family as desertion. But also Eva could not act independently as she remained bound-up in stubborn opposition to her demanding parents. On the 'id level' she became bound by her parents' overprotectiveness, and her mother's regressive gratification of her. On the superego level there arose massive 'breakaway guilt'. To some extent, these binding forces originated with Betty's death 10 years ago. But the family was already strongly bound-up before the pathological mourning set in. Even today both parents remain strongly bound to their own mothers.

An important factor impairing Eva's individuation was her mission to serve as replacement for the lost Betty. This turned Eva into a 'bound delegate' of her parents, i.e. one whose missions interfered with an age-appropriate adolescent separation. So far, her symptoms bespoke a compromise: she took the role of the dependent little girl and became to her parents a source of renewed concern and (pathological) mourning.

In living up to her parents' expectations, Eva was victimized but also became strategically placed to operate the guilt lever on her parents. Thus, she permanently blamed them for her desolate physical condition. The parents, on their part, tried to cope with *their* guilt by *blaming* Eva. In this way, complex problems of guilt and of mutual accounting came into play.

To sum up, we see Eva's attempts at related individuation fail because of the prevalence of strong binding forces. These forces originated with parents who had been frustrated and isolated from one another for a long time and with a child who, in taking her dead sister's place, tried to act as her parent's loyal delegate. At the time being, Eva is bound by regressive gratification. The family's style of relating alternates between clinging dependence and harsh, disillusioned distancing. Potentials for a genuine dialogue have almost totally disappeared.

Therapeutic Implications

Our therapeutic endeavors must take into account the above relational or systems forces. But these endeavors must frequently differ depending on whether we deal with acute or chronic psychosomatic disorders. Whenever a presenting patient has a chronic psychosomatic (or, for that matter, psychiatric) condition we must expect not only a costly and uneven, but also *stable* state of restrictively related individuation. At the same time, we can expect a stably integrated relational and family system in which the patient's chronic symptoms and complaints have become functional to other members of the system. For example, a young woman's rheumatoid arthritis and consequently restricted sex life may, among other things, serve not only the function of muting her concerns over her own frigidity, but also of 'protecting' her husband's impotence. In addition, her rheumatoid arthritis may help her to remain bound-up with an overprotective mother, thereby providing this mother with meaning and a purpose in life while alleviating her own breakaway guilt. Therefore, a therapist must be wary not to interfere too abruptly with a precarious relational homeostasis. At the same time, he must take into account, and dare to employ, the positive resources which may inhere in the very binding and delegating processes that are here at issue. What to do or not to do, may then become for him or her, no less than for his patient(s), a matter of conflict and reconciliation.

In the light of the above, our therapeutic interventions with the aforementioned family are guided by the following main goals: (a) To set in motion a mourning process that frees Eva from the burden of replacing the dead Betty and allows her parents to accept Eva as Eva. (b) To 'unbind' the family and to thereby facilitate Eva's age-appropriate separation. As a result, each member should be able to recognize the other as an individual with his or her own wishes, hopes, feelings and goals. (c) To bring together the parents, i.e. anull their 'emotional divorce'. At the moment, the only thing they share is their concern for Eva. To make a go of their marriage, they would have to develop new common interests.

Individual Psychotherapy versus Family Therapy

Any attempt at mere individual treatment would very likely leave unaffected or unwittingly aggravate elements of dynamic importance, such as the members' shared pathological mourning and the parents' schismatic marriage.

Moreover, a forced separation of Eva from her family would probably cause a conflict of loyalty with a resulting family crisis. The worsening conditions of father and/or mother would then possibly entail a premature termination of the therapy. Therefore, we would suggest here and in similar cases a therapeutic approach which not only includes the identified patient, but the family members as well.

Family Dynamics and Psychosomatic Disorders in Adolescence   251

References

Blos, P.: On adolescence. A psychoanalytic interpretation (Free Press, New York 1962).
Boszormenyi-Nagy, I. and Spark, G.: Invisible loyalties (Harper & Row, New York 1973).
Erikson, E.H.: Childhood and society (Norton, New York 1950).
Freud, A.: Adolescence. The psychoanalytic study of the child, vol. 13 (1958).
Friedmann, M.: Healing through meeting. A dialogical approach to psychotherapy and family therapy; in Smith Psychiatry and the humanities (Yale University Press, New Haven 1976).
Jacobson, E.: The self and the object world. (International Universities Press, New York 1964).
Mahler, M.S.; Pine, F., and Bergmann, A.: The psychological birth of the human infant. Symbiosis and individuation (Basic Books, New York 1975).
Stierlin, H.: The functions of inner objects. Int. J. Psychoanal. 51: 321–329.
Stierlin, H.: Family dynamics and separation patterns of potential schizophrenics; in Alanen and Rubinstein Proc. 4th Int. Symp. Psychother. of Schizophrenia (Excerpta Medica, Amsterdam 1972).
Stierlin, H.: Separating parents and adolescents. (Quadrangle, New York 1974).
Stierlin, H.: Von der Psychoanalyse zur Familientherapie. (Klett, Stuttgart 1975).
Sullivan, H.S.: The Illusion of personal individuality. Psychiatry 13: 317–332 (1950).

Prof. Dr. Helm Stierlin, Psychosomatische Klinik, Abt. für Psychoanalytische Grundlagenforschung, Mönchhofstr. 15a, D-6900 Heidelberg 1 (FRG)

Discussion

Dr. König: I think I can be brief. I want to address myself to Mrs. *Brede* but what I have to say also applies to the presentation of Dr. *Cremerius* and the link is motivation for treatment. What Mrs. *Brede* has presented sounds very theoretical but her ideas have helped me in understanding what is happening in the hospital in which I am working – one of the largest German psychoanalytic hospitals.

Mrs. *Brede* told us that psychosomatic patients have a great tendency to comply to social norms, they want to belong by complying to social norms and they often live in social groups where having conflicts is not 'in', where you do not belong if you have conflicts but where you do belong if you have some symptom of organic sickness. We have many patients in the hospital who have come from such social groups. They comply at first to the therapy norms of the hospital which are introduced by the staff *but are also supported by the patients who have already begun treatment* and this motivation by compliance changes in the course of treatment into what we call genuine motivation. So I think that what Mrs. *Brede* has presented helps us to understand why for so many psychosomatic patients an inpatient treatment is indicated; these patients could not be motivated in an outpatient setting.

Dr. Zador: I would just like to ask Prof. *Stierlin* how would he elaborate between the parallel of the process of identification and invisible loyalties; another question, what is the therapeutical process to being the invisible loyalties, which I assume are unconscious up to the conscious level and to deal with the complex.

Dr. Stierlin: This question is difficult to answer. But let me say this: when you look at a family rather than at an individual patient, you observe quite different phenomena. The observational setting is different, the focus is different and therefore the phenomena one sees are different. But there is a further problem: our observations are guided by our observation and we are still lacking those sophisticated concepts which are needed to guide our observations on families. This applies also to the concept of invisible loyalties which *Ivan Boszormenyi-Nagy* elaborated and which I integrated into my delegation concept. As I see it today, the concept of delegation refers to enduring and multigenerational relational structures within which also identifactory processes play a central role. I am presently engaged in further analyzing how the concepts of identification and delegation relate to each other.

Proc. 11th Eur. Conf. Psychosom. Res., Heidelberg 1976
Psychother. Psychosom. *28:* 253–259 (1977)

The Role of the Family in Symptom Selection and Perpetuation in Psychosomatic Illness

E. M. Waring

Introduction

Morton Reiser has cogently discussed how different physical, psychological, and social etiological factors may play a more or less significant role at different points in the course of a psychosomatic illness. It is surprising that the role of family dynamics has had such little impact either as predisposing, precipitating, or perpetuating variables in most psychosomatic theories. For example reviews of family process in psychosomatic illness by *Reissner and Grolnick* have appeared only recently, but have raised important theoretical issues. It is only in the last several years that the pioneering work of *Lieberman and Minuchin* in describing family therapy in the treatment of psychosomatic illness, specifically asthma, ulcerative colitis, and anorexia nervosa, have appeared in the literature. Despite the above which has focused on psychosomatic illness in children, practically no literature exists on family process in psychosomatic illness in adults.

This paper arises out of our clinical research and experience using family therapy with chronic, frequently treatment-resistant, adult psychosomatic patients. The majority of these patients are chronic pain problems and cardiovascular patients demonstrating the 'giving up – given up complex'. The discussion which follows is based on newer concepts of family process exemplified by the work of *Bowen, Framo, Minuchin,* etc., and hopefully will shed some light on some perplexing theoretical issues in the study of psychosomatic problems.

Significant other Specificity

The perplexing theoretical problem of psychosomatic symptom specificity has eluded precise definition. Earlier research attempting to define specific personality traits or unconscious psychological conflicts in specific psychosomatic illnesses has gradually been displaced by the current 'non-specificity' model. But the question of why this specific symptom and why this specific member of the family remains fascinating. The area most ignored in the psychological and environmental factors has been the family. The concept of 'significant other specificity' steps away from individual psychodynamics or interpersonal issues and utilizes family systems concepts such as the 'transgenerational hypothesis' of *Murray Bowen,* family projective identification *(Framo),* and the concept of operant rewarding for matching random physical symptomatology to the specific unconscious system of the significant other.

Let me elaborate. First, within the nuclear family, the family's 'affective system' tends to effect one child or one spouse and not the other family members. The reasons why the specific patients become involved are complex and must include the parental dynamics as well as the prevailing multi-generational family system. For example, *Bowen*'s multi-generational family system suggests that often the child who becomes sick with the physical symptom is the child who is viewed by the family as most behaviourally similar to a member of the parent's nuclear family.

For example, in one family the son through the course of his first 12 years had many physical symptoms including partial deafness, headaches, a skin disorder, etc. These symptoms were accepted and managed within the family context, but when he developed symptoms of abdominal pains suggesting ulcer symptoms and because he was identified with the grandfather who had also suffered from ulcers, these symptoms motivated the family system to seek outside help.

Framo's application of the concept of projective identification applied to family systems to the transference of the family as a whole is also useful here. Who is selected as the identified psychosomatic patient represents a projective identification of 'the significant others introject of the parent who was ill or was wished ill'.

Thus, object-related needs, both conscious and unconscious, form a diadic unit in which the partners use scapegoating or projection to fit or split off internal objects. Thus, a partial explanation of the 'who' may be found in the family's affective system, both through the multigeneration hypothesis of *Bowen* and also through the function of family projective identification introduced by *Framo*.

Once the 'who' develops the symptom is selected, the why this particular symptom is a more perplexing theoretical issue, but our clinical observation suggests that the operant rewarding of a symptom which matches the unconscious 'wishing ill' of the significant other may be as important a variable in symptom selection as the identified patient's individual constitutional predisposition and his individual psychodynamics. For example, a patient we have seen had had many psychological symptoms and physical symptoms over the course of his marriage. However, he was injured in an industrial accident in which he burnt his hands. There resulted a chronic dermatitis which was refractory to standard dermatological treatment. The chronicity of this problem when examined in the context of this man's family related to a long-standing sexual incapability. His wife was frigid and 'hated the thoughts of him touching me' to the point that when he attempted to have intercourse she actually vomited. A fantasy he had that if his hands did not improve he would chop them off was in keeping with the unconscious wish of his wife in this particular clinical situation. In summary, the concept of 'significant other specificity' needs further study, but may prove relevant to the question of why a particular family member becomes ill, why he becomes ill with physical symptoms as opposed to psychological symptoms, and why he develops the specific physical symptoms.

Sick Role Homeostasis

Although introducing this theoretical concept as a perpetuating factor in adult psychosomatic illness, it may play an even greater etiological role in predisposition particularly in childhood psychosomatic disorders. This concept as it applies to psychosomatic illness is derived from the works of *Ackerman* and his focus on family 'roles', *Bowen* and his concept of family 'triangles', the structural-family therapeutic model of *Minuchin* and co-workers, and our own work with adult chronic pain problems. This formulation is focused not only on the impingement of the family on the effected members as in previous interpersonal dynamic research, but also directs our attention to the patterns of involvement and interaction of the family itself.

Ackerman conceptualized the breakdown of the healthy process within the family as a breakdown of 'role complementarity'. In a family where parental roles and marital roles are dysfunctional and non-complementary, the 'sick role' may provide this family system with homeostasis.

Clinically, the families rigidly maintain the 'sick role' to prevent the eruption and disruption if the failure of role complementarity is acknowledged and recognized. Put simply if the symptom persists, the family may need it.

The 'sick role' also allows the family to interact differently with the extrafamilial social system. The sick role allows an interaction with physicians as opposed to mental health workers or the court system in the case of a crazy or bad family member. This frequently enmeshes the physician in a family affective system in which he seldom if ever perceives the function he is providing to the homeostasis of the family. The important point here is ably demonstrated by the expression 'I am in pain' which relieves the family of responsibility and a physician assumes responsibility for the patient as opposed to the expression 'You are a pain' which would lead the family interactional system in a different direction.

The theoretical concepts of *Murray Bowen* are even more illuminating with reference to symptom perpetuation in adult psychosomatic problems. He suggests that there is a great tension in all families and particularly between the marital diad, between ego fusion or dependency, and differentiation of the self or autonomy.

The marital couple uses three major ways of controlling the intensity of this conflict within the family. The first is marital conflict. The second is the dysfunction of one of the spouses, either psychologically or physically. This is the usual pattern in adults with chronic psychosomatic pain problems. The third way is transmission of the problem to one of the children. The child becomes the focus of the problem and breaks down with psychosomatic illness under the burden of carrying the family disorder. The above raises an important question as to why some families select to go outside of the family system in the direction of physicians as opposed to the direction of mental health counsellors or the judicial system. In other words why do some families initiate help seeking around 'the physically sick role' as opposed to the crazy role or the bad role.

Two important clinical observations we have made suggest that further studies of sick role homeostasis are indicated. First, the parental psychosomatic breakdown in one of the spouses frequently occurs when a child who has been 'triangulated' and suffered from psychosomatic symptoms abandons the family system. Second, the symptom itself or the physician who has been asked to treat the symptom, particularly in chronic pain problems, is invited to play the part of the departed child by reacting to the system rather than responding to it. This concept confirmed through the work of *Minuchin* will be discussed further.

The 'Better Sick than Dead' Family Myth

The final theoretical construct in understanding the role of the family in perpetuating psychosomatic illness attempts to answer the question of why certain families opt for the 'sick role' in the form of psychosomatic illness.

The 'better sick than dead' family myth is commonly seen in psychosomatic families and is theoretically derived from several sources including the concept of 'alexithymia' introduced by *Sifneos,* communication theory as seen in the work of *Haley* and particularly our own clinical research with cardiac patients who have manifested the phenomenon of 'giving up – given up complex'.

One of the characteristics of individual psychotherapy with psychosomatic patients is their difficulty in verbalizing affect and tolerating unconscious impulses and fantasies. This resistance to a lessening of control of primary process and affect has been referred to as 'alexithymia' in individual patients by *Sifneos*. In fact, the literature on individual therapy has suggested that the exploration of unconscious conflict with psychosomatic patients can and frequently does worsen their physical symptom and most therapists are now suggesting a more supportive and non-insightful approach.

The families of psychosomatic patients mirror this individual phenomenon and are characterized by a kind of cohesion that mitigates against any form of expression of hatred or dysphoria. These feelings are strongly repressed within the family as a whole. Clinically, we have found with patients with the giving up-given up complex that bringing the wife and patient together and encouraging verbalization of the anger and sadness about the impending death has remarkable effect in terms of improving the patient who has 'turned to the wall'. As the patient improves, he frequently verbalizes that he was aware that significant others felt this anger and sadness, but could not verbalize it.

A particularly poignant example of this is the marital disharmony and arguing manifested by a couple in which the husband continued to work hard as a carpenter and they fought about how hard he worked. Through family intervention they became aware that the husband was working hard so that he could leave his wife something to remember him by when he died, whereas his wife wished that he would stop working so that they could enjoy what time they had left to them. The fraying up and verbalizing of the anger and sadness that they both felt about impending death led to symptomatic and psychological improvement in his cardiac condition.

This leads to communication theory concepts of family myths as expressed through *Haley and Satir*. Our experience with patients with the giving up-given up complex and also in chronic pain problems is that the family myth is 'better sick than dead' expressed both through the individual member and the family itself. Our concept that one of the perpetuating factors is the fear of the expression of unconscious death wishes has been supported by the work of *Finch and Hess* in children with ulcerative colitis.

Finally, Minuchin has demonstrated in his work with asthmatics that there may be some specific interactional family dynamics in the psychosomatic family. These include the concept of 'infantilization of the patient' introduced by *Meissner* and a characteristic finding of many researchers that these families have a type of cohesion which is reminiscent of *Wynne's* concept of 'pseudo-mutuality' in schizophrenic families. These families harbour magical dependency wishes towards physicians. They characteristically have few outside contacts with society outside of the family and their major one is through the physician. Thus, the 'sick role' is conferred with enormous power within the family and the physician frequently is invited to be triangled as being responsible for not only the symptom but also the functioning of the family. Clinically this occurs when the physician feels helpless and enraged and is not sure in the treatment of these chronic physical disabilities what he is reacting to. In fact, he frequently is reacting to the dysfunctional set of the diadic marriage in which role complementarity has never been present.

Implications

First, the above theory suggests that to ignore the family (both nuclear and current) in chronic psychosomatic illness is to invite therapeutic failure. We have found family assessment to be an integral part of the assessment of adult chronic psychosomatic patients and frequently specific family therapy is also recommended.

Where in specific cases family therapy has been an integral part of our treatment program, particularly in the field of the 'giving up – given up' complex and the chronic pain problems, we have found the following points to be useful in management:

(1) A systems approach to the family dynamics and family interaction allows the physician to enter the system without introducing guilt in individual members thus overcoming one of the greatest resistances to individual therapy with psychosomatic patients.

(2) The presenting physical symptom must be diffused. Like the individual patient who focuses some much of his attention on physical symptoms, the family does likewise. Unless some symptomatic relief can be offered the family will generally refuse to entertain the possibility that family dynamics are contributing. Thus, we use whatever method necessary to remove the presenting symptom including operant conditioning, biofeedback, sodium amytal interviews, narcotics, etc.

(3) The involved physician who has been triangulated into the family system must be diffused. This physician must participate in at least the first few family sessions and give the responsibility for illness back to the family.

(4) We have found that the ventilation of anger and sadness in the family system is frequently curative in both chronic pain problems and the giving up-given up complex in very few sessions and with no worsening of the individual's psychosomatic illness.

Second, I have introduced three concepts: 'significant others specificity', 'sick role homeostasis', and the 'better sick than dead' myth which I believe can provide the basis for further empirical research into a beginning insight into the role of family dynamics and symptom selection and symptom perpetuation.

E.M. Waring, MD, Department of Psychiatry, Victoria Hospital, *London, Ont.* (Canada)

Proc. 11th Eur. Conf. Psychosom. Res., Heidelberg 1976
Psychother. Psychosom. *28:* 260–271 (1977)

The Pathology of the Self as a Basis of Psychosomatic Disorders

Renata Gaddini

Mental Hygiene Unit, Department of Pediatrics, University of Rome, Rome

The concept of 'self' has been used in psychoanalysis for a long time with different meanings. In my presentation, the word 'self' is used within a maturational context based on a developmental theory. In this context, the 'self' is the outcome of the infant's total bodily experience of the first months of life. These are sensations which, in the course of growing, are gradually elaborated in a process of mentalization.

In January 1971, in a letter to his French translator, who had questioned him about the word 'self', *Winnicott* (13) wrote:

'For me the self, which is not the ego, is the person who is me, who is only me, who has a totality based on the operation of the maturational process. At the same time the self has parts, and in fact is constituted by these parts. These parts agglutinate from a direction interior-exterior in the course of the operation of the maturational process, aided as it must be (maximally at the beginning) by the human environment which holds and handles and in a live way facilitates. The self finds itself naturally placed in the body, but may in certain circumstances become dissociated from the body or the body from it. The self essentially recognizes itself in the eyes and facial expression of the mother and in the mirror which can come to represent the mother's face. Eventually the self arrives at a significant relationship between the child and the sum of the identifications which (after enough of incorporation and introjection of mental representations) become organized in the shape of an internal psychic living reality. The relationship between the boy or girl with his or her own internal psychic organization becomes reinforced or modified according to the expectations that are displayed by the father and mother and those who have become significant in the external life of the individual. It is the self and the life of the self that alone makes sense of action or of living from the point of view of the individual who has grown so far and who is continuing to grow from dependence and immaturity towards independence and the capacity to identify with mature love objects without loss of individual identity. "And, further on:" I feel that your use of the word *le moi corporel* may be necessary but one would like to leave it that the self is not always putting emphasis on the body to the exclusion of a more abstract self that certainly does, however, belong to the concept of a healthy functioning brain.' In this drawing (fig. 1) *Winnicott* (13) meant to represent the formation of the self, as he describes it.

The personality structure, in this view, is something which forms itself around the self. Psychoanalysis has given the greatest attention to the structure, but it has failed to consider the self, which is the central nucleus underlying it. The growth of the mind implies the growth of structures, which allow the elaboration of elementary experiences. Leibnitz' famous statement that

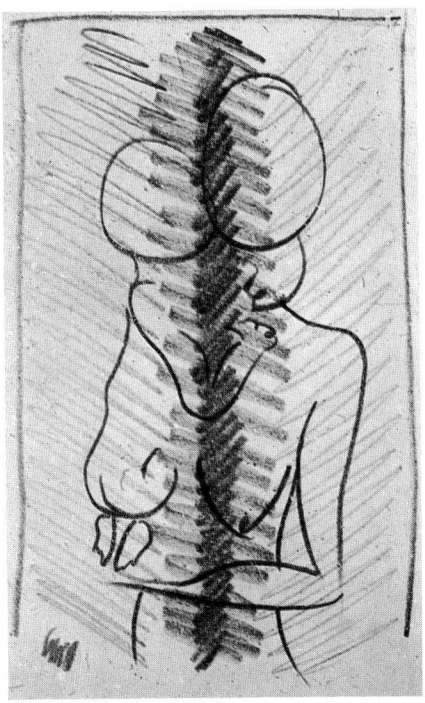

Fig. 1. Formation of the self (*Winnicott*, 12).

'Nihil est in intellectu quid non fuerit in sensibus' may have been in *Bion*'s mind when he found out for himself that 'Feelings and thinking are based on sense data' (1). The longitudinal studies of growing up children have taught us that this is the rule, i.e., that in the process of growing the child goes from sensations to perceptions and feelings and symbols, and finally, to thoughts (table I). The schemata which we have developed (6) indicate *early symbolization,* such as we find in the transitional object, as the first *observable* step in the development of secondary process thinking. But the substrate of the transitional object (TO), the matter on which the TO is *created* by the infant at times of anaclitic depression (mother's absence), these are early sensations experienced by the child at the beginning of life, at times of fusion at the breast (in arms). My figures (fig. 2) indicating that babies born in the autumn and winter more often become attached to woolen objects, while spring and summer babies tend to hold objects made of linen or nylon, show how early these sensations are experienced (7). The going-to-sleep situation implies separation (from reality, outside world, mother); this is a regularly recurring, anxiety-determining situation. In the face of such stress, the baby tries to relive the reassuring reunion with the mother. He recaptures the feeding situation, when he was fused with the breast, the nipple was in his mouth, and the wrapping blanket with which his mother was holding him was caressing his cheeks or other uncovered parts of his body. He may then use the thumb or the pacifier instead of the nipple, and the crib's blanket instead of the wrapping blanket: but the underlying fantasy is the original one, that of being fused with his mother (4, 5).

Table I. Schema of the growing child

Developmental moment	Dominant mode	Process
Perinatal and neonatal period	sensations	autistic world
Early months	infant enters own body conception and outside world perception, i.e., world of relationships	in relating to object infant is stimulated and kept alive
Later	sensations and perceptions elaborated in feelings and thoughts	psychic development as a process of differentiation; capacity for mentalization (mental metabolism)

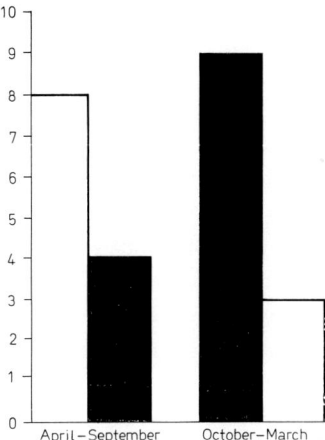

Fig. 2. Type of transitional object adopted. Open = Nylon, silk, linen, cotton; hatched = wool, plush.

It is on the basis of these longitudinal studies that I have been able to individuate the quality of the mother-infant interaction which pertains best to the particular infant's specific developmental stage, to allow his growth out of physical self. The energy freed from narcissistic investment, originally maintained and fostered by mother's attitudes towards the child, can now be directed towards the external environment. In those cases in which there has been a poor quality of mother-child interactions we find that growth and the whole process of individuation are held back, so that the child remains incarcerated in his own physical self. In stressful situations different psycho-somatic symptoms will then shape themselves, in the precarious yet pervasive organic apparatus.

Seen from this angle, the psychosomatic symptom takes place when the mother has failed her interactional task during the child's infancy, a time when the child has not yet developed the necessary mental apparatus to endow an object, once associated with the mother, as a symbol for the mother (8).

The self, in fact, is the first organization of the individual just born, while he tries to adapt to the new homeostasis. He works at its formation in the very first few months. In the organization of the self there is the contri-bution of the mother touching her baby, and, in so doing, delimiting, defining and demarcating her infant's body limits, and the innate contribution of the baby. It is through the converging of these two contributions that the baby's self originates.

Winnicott's (13) representation inspires an almost plastic view, with a central nucleus based on the innate contribution of the child (of his id), and a periphery determined by the infinite points of mother-newborn mutual contacts, and mother-infant in his first months. It is a skin-to-skin contact, the moment mother lifts her baby, or holds him, or put him back in his crib, or when he is moved in space to be put to the breast, or for his daily care (washing, dressing, etc.). The wholeness of these peripheral sensations of skin-to-skin contact and of his body impact in space are what matters for the child to build his sense of Self.

On the basis of this primordial entity, which is bodily, but implies a relationship, will later develop the ego, in the course of growing, in the complex interplaying of the symbiotic fusion of the 'to and fro' which is typical of this phase of child development. Mother's ego will be the supporting element for the child's ego construction, as it is expressed in her daily maternal functions. Her ways of meeting his complete dependence, and of gradually allowing independence (autonomy) will be fundamental in determining the quality of the child's ego. It is on the basis of these ways, which represent mother's potentials towards that particular child, that we talk of a 'facilitating' or, on the contrary, of a 'pathogenic' environment (table II).

The functioning of the body (the various organs' function) is the language of the body; this body language, on its way to becoming mental (somehow), is the language of the self (9, 12). Everytime we refer to the self we find ourselves immediately dealing with a mental activity which in some way is related to (has to do with) the body (II). We see, among the functions of the self, the control of organic reactions of the body.

Sanders and Condon's (10) recorded data show us that from the first days on, the neonates move in precise and sustained organisation, which is in synchrony with the articulated structure of adult language. *Mutuality* and *specificity* of cues between mother and neonates are clearly shown in these studies (table III). Keeping these data in mind we can easily see that at this early level of maturation an altered development of the child's self may easily occur, on the basis of a poor interaction and of early environmental difficulties. If the interaction between mother and infant is pathogenic (6), and the early child's environment has failed in the first months, early psychosomatic responses may arise. A less specific vulnerability to all sort of illnesses and physical injury may be found in other cases (10), the undergoing

Table II. Pathogenic, borderline, and facilitating environments: their effects at 2 stages of development

Environment	Mother	Infant	Early somatic response	Later response
Pathogenic	not available	let down	vomiting	no transitional object
	not predictable	apathic	screaming, crying	nonrelating child
	feeding not recipro-	nonprotected transitions	constant sleep	self-rocking
	cating event	between sleep and waking,		annihilated
	protective function	hunger and satiation		psychotic
	lost	does not get to know mother		
	does not get to know			no capacity for creative playing
	her infant			no abstract symbolisation
	separated from infant			
	in nursery			
Borderline	spoils with untimely	let down at times	regurgitate	language difficulties
	frustrations	resents nonavailability	3-months colic	masters meaning of symbols
	resents dependence	untimely experience of	sleeping difficulties	principally on somatic level
		frustration	dermatosis	psychosomatic symptoms
Facilitating	knows her infant	knows mother	extending world	intermediate area between
				psychic reality and external
				reality
	adapts to needs	transitions clear between	development of transitional	symbolic functioning
	frustrates when	sleeping and waking,	object of phenomena	cultural experiences
	necessary	hunger and satiation		creative

Table III. Correspondence of infant movements with recorded speech and nonspeech sounds

Study	Sound	Baby	Total occurrences	Total discrepancies	Agreement, %
4	speech (word boundaries)	A	146	19	87
5	disconnected vowels	E	167	97	42
		C-	124	51	59
6	tapping sounds	E	27	15	44
		C	34	16	53

of somatic illnesses being itself one of the early signs of the failure of the interaction between the soma (the internal world) and the psyche.

We have seen that the child first lives his experiences on a physiological basis. It is at a further step of his development that he organizes himself on a mental basis, in order to master them. Nevertheless, I would not call the mind a functional organizer, in Spitz' sense. The word *organizer* is a biological concept, and, in my view, it should not be used for the mental function. It is true that mental functions originate on the basis of biological functions: there is no mind without brain. But soon the mental function enters its own functional differentiation, which is the highest level of differentiation of all biological functions. From now on the mind has its own growth, and has nothing biological except its origins. This is to say that the original models of mental experiences are biological, in so far as they are bodily experiences. But soon they become mental experiences, a long way differentiated from biological.

The young child lives his physical experiences, while growing, with disintegration anxieties and fears. Mental activity comes just at a point when the child can use it (he is in need of it) to master them. In the child's mind fantasy takes place, to save him from disintegration. Reality belongs to the body, in early life. It is *all* in the self when a child is a few months old, there is no external reality. But fantasy is lived through the body, it is materialized through the body, it turns to reality only through bodily experiences. This is the puzzling leap from the mental to the physical that Freud referred to. We can solve it only by studying carefully the process of development. Let's take the example of rumination. In rumination the infant *makes the fantasy of being the nursing mother* (i.e. he lives again the experience which once he has lived in omnipotent fusion with his mother). This fantasy is lived in a way which is inextricably connected with his own previous bodily experiences and gets materialized through his own body. The vomiting, with which nearly all ruminators initiate the syndrome in the first months of their life, is an organic automatic response, which can be self-destructive. In those cases where there is no vomiting preceding rumination, we find, with no exception, a sudden interruption of breast feeding, and/or a separation from mother, with loss of comforting habits, like a pacifier, or thumb-sucking. In other words, the infant has gone through a sudden and severe bodily frustration. As soon as he biologically can – never before the 3rd month – what does he organize for himself, with the act of ruminating? An entirely satisfying bodily experience, which is a defense against frustration and against being let down. In rumination the infant undergoes a number of bodily modifications which repeat (or imitate) as blueprints, the previous bodily experiences with mother, which are now lost. The food, or milk, is repeatedly brought back into the mouth, and the mouth is full of milk, and then in part it flows into his mouth corners, and in part is again swallowed. It is typically the tongue which initiates the process of rumination, in function of the lost nipple (or thumb, or pacifier). But this time the child can recreate the experience of self-feeding indefinitely, reproducing those sensations which were connected with his mother' feeding him. With this imitative fantasy he masters his self-loss, and controls his fears of disintegration (2, 3).

What is the difference between the *imitative fantasy* of ruminators and the maturative illusion of the normal 3-month-old infant, who 'creates' for himself the breast? The 'created' breast, for the normal infant, is a fantasy which has a bodily correspondence. The child wishes for his mother's breast, and his mother's breast, in fact, is there. It is his omnipotent illusion which makes him think he has created it. Soon frustrations will come, and he will have to learn that omnipotence does not last forever. But his illusion has been the basic element of his maturational process, and has derived from it a powerful incentive for developing mentalization. Illusion, in the first months of life, belongs to normal development of mental activities and of thinking. There is no maturational value in the fantasy of the ruminator (2). The fantasy which underlies rumination is a pathological fantasy on the part of the infant; just as the self-rocking babies have the fantasy of being the rocking mother (or, as *Winnicott* (13) would say, enact the pathological representation of the reunion with the mother), in the same way the ruminating babies make the fantasies of being the feeding mother, and they recuperate in the autistic self-feeding the omnipotent control. No evaluation

Table IV. Incidence of perinatal complications, and distribution according to sex in asthmatic children and controls

	n	Perinatal complications, %	Sex distribution, %	
			males	females
Asthmatics	100	36	74	26
Controls	100	16	49	51

takes place in the process: it is an end to itself, and the child does not mature. This psychosomatic syndrome is a time-marking condition, insofar as it indicates a pathology which can only take place at a particular level of development, and which is dependent on maternal and infant factors.

I would like to point out correlations which I came across while studying 'developmentally' some asthma cases (table IV). Though limited in number, I see them as indicative. Speculating on these randomly selected children, I found myself wondering which is the element through which perinatal adversities from pure propensity to illnesses, acquires inclination towards specific illnesses. Is it the mother's preoccupation about her child's fragility reflected back to her infant in the beginning of life at the basis of child's vulnerability, acting as an adverse factor in the early formation of the child's self? In which relationship fear of breakdown (as spelled for us from *Winnicott* (14) in his posthumous paper), in the way we see it manifested in some asthmatic patients, stands in respect of fear of separation? What does the latter have to do with the scarcity of symbolization (which implies fantasy life) as expressed by the noncoexistence of a transitional object in the case of severe psychosomatic patients (6)? In our longitudinal study it appears in a statistically significant way that those children who had a TO are the children who, at the age of 4 years, have more capacity for creative play.

Behaviorally, the child capable of creative play is, for me, the child who can put on scenes, pretending that objects and persons are there who are not, in fact, there, and who can give value and dramatic life to his scenes, to master anxiety and thus getting relief. The child capable of creative play has been studied in contrast to the child whose play consists of pure physical activity implying excitement, provocations, and testing out of the mother and/or outside world. What I find *dynamically* in the child who can play dramatically at the basis of his behavior, are the capacity for *concern*, and the capacity for *contributing* to the outside world with his own fantasy life, which belongs to his inner world. These dynamic characteristics are not found in the child whose playing consists of physical excitement and provocation. On the contrary, we see in such a child a high degree of dependence on the mother, and a continuous need of the other, in order to exist. Separation implies for him fear of disintegration and of breakdown, in *Winnicott*'s terms.

Both the capacities which we find in the dramatically creative child – the capacity for concern, and the capacity for looking at the outside world from his own point of view, investing the latter with the child's own inner world, are characteristics basic to the nature of TO. Looking at play from the TO point of view, we can recognize in it the original consolatory ambit in which the earlier TO had come to life. We see, in playing, the continuation of the bridge function between self and outside world, which is typical of TO. Playing, too, implies an external reality – a place and time where the play takes place and an inner reality which the child contributes to it.

The significant difference between TO and playing is, in our view, the entirely private character that the former has, in contrast to the latter. I find myself speculating whether and how much incapacity for playing has to do with the 'pensée opératoire' of some psychosomatic patients, and whether creative play could be considered a predecessor to imaginative thinking.

We intend to explore further the area of self-creativity while the children of our longitudinal studies grow up. What is basic to self-creativity, seen as the capacity for contributing to the outside world with one's inner world, is the existence in the individual of a total separate self, as I have described it as the optimal developmental outcome of the process of integration. On clinical grounds, we can say that we rarely find self-creativity in the young psychosomatic patient. Behaviorally, as we know, he or she tends to depend on mother for breathing and eating, and basic physiological functions; namely, for existing. But how are things at the beginning? The mother of Mauro, a 4-year-old boy with severe asthma, who tells us about *her own* breakdown at the time her 4-month-old baby was first weaned, may give us some clues: 'It was awful. He (the baby) had taken no more than two drops of cow's milk when he started to choke and became all swollen. He was allergic to cow's milk, how could I know. He had a spasm in his throat, and was going to die. Luckily, I was quick in making him vomit and in taking him to the hospital, right away. He went on with cortison for a long time, because of his allergy'.

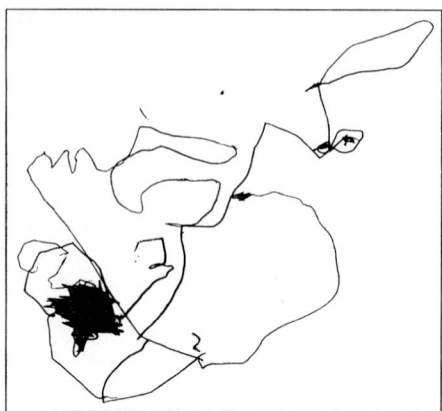

Fig. 3. Non-integration of the self in an asthmatic 4½-year-old child. 'A little mountain'. Note the composition in pieces of his 'ensemble' and the lack of fusion and integration with the presence of the 'black hole' in one part (constant characteristic). Where extension of the main figure is represented, this is typically an isolated image of self, with a bond to the main piece, lest 'he' is lost in the space. This is true even when the tie to the mother is closer: the missed sense of fusion and integration, with its relative fear of 'falling for ever', are evident in these drawings.

Let us now, for a moment, try to see how this mother's 'fear of breakdown' may have been experienced by the baby. Obviously, this infant was not felt by the mother as separate from her own self, and the problem of weaning, implying separation, was crucial to her. She *saw* her child dying in the separation, and the child *felt* this dying element (disintegrating) which was implicit in his separation from the mother. He is now one of those children who *need* the mother in order to breath. It is striking the element of non-integration which can be seen in this child's drawings, and greatly contrasting with his high intelligence and performance capacities at non-creative levels (fig. 3).

In *Winnicott*'s terms, 'breakdown' equates with 'a failure of a defense organization, related to the individual past experiences and to the environmental vagaries'. He suggests that in the area of psychoneurosis it is the castration anxiety that lies behind the defenses, whereas in the more psychotic phenomena 'is the establishment of the unit self that is indicated'. The loss of psychosomatic collusion, with depersonalization as a defense, and the loss of the sense of reality (of the more psychotic states), with primary narcissism as a defense, are found close in his enumeration of the primitive agonies, nonintegration and disintegration being the elements of closeness.

The conclusion of my presentation implies that it is the defenses of the self which have to be strengthened, if we want to contribute within the psychosomatic approach to individual susceptibility to disease. This can be best done in terms of prevention, which is, for me, support without interference in the natural processes that characterize a young child's relationship with his mother.

References

1   *Bion, W.:* Learning from experience. Chapt. XII, XIX (Heineman, London 1962).
2   *Gaddini, E.:* On imitation. Int. J. Psychoanal. *50:* 475–484 (1969).
3   *Gaddini, E. and Gaddini, R.:* Rumination in infancy; in Dynamic psychopathology in childhood (Grune & Stratton, New York 1959).
4   *Gaddini, R.:* Transitional objects and the process of individuation. J. Am. Acad. Child Psychiat. *9:* 347–365 (1970).
5   *Gaddini, R.:* Re-union symbolizazion in infancy. Proc. 13th Int. Congr. Pediatries, Vienna 1971.
6   *Gaddini, R.:* Early psychosomatic symptom and the tendency towards integration. Psychother. Psychosom. *23:* 26–34 (1974).
7   *Gaddini, R.:* The concept of transitional object. J. Am. Acad. Child Psychiat. *14:* 731–736 (1975).
8   *Gaddini, R.:* Transitional object and the psychosomatic symptom; in *Grolnick and Barkin* Transitional Phenomena (in press, 1976).
9   *Gaddini, R.:* Psychosomatic disorders in children; in *Wittkower and Warnes* Psychosomatic approach to medicine (in press, 1976).
10 *Sanders, L.W. and Condon, W.:* An investigation of change of infant caretaker interaction over the first two weeks of life; in *Rexford, Sander and Shapiro* Infant psychiatry (Yale University Press, New Haven 1974).
11 *Winnicott, D.W.:* Through pediatrics to psychoanalysis (Tavistock, London 1958).
12 *Winnicott, D.W.:* Somatic illness in its positive and negative aspects. Int. J. Psychoanal. *7:* 510–516 (1966).
13 *Winnicott, D.W.:* Letter to J. Kalmanovitch in Paris, Jan. 19, 1971; published in part in Introduction to fragment d'une analyse (Payot, Paris 1975).
14 *Winnicott, D.W.:* Fear of breakdown. Int. Rev. Psychoanal. *1:* (1974).

Prof. Dr. med. *Renata Gaddini,* 13, Via Sebastiano Conca, *I-00197 Roma* (Italy)

Proc. 11th Eur. Conf. Psychosom. Res., Heidelberg 1976
Psychother. Psychosom. *28:* 272–277 (1977)

The Significance of the Transitional Object for Psychosomatic Thinking

M. Mitscherlich

In 1953, *Winnicott,* in his work entitled 'Transitional objects and transitional phenomena' was concerned with objects of importance to children from the age of 6 months onward, such as the corners of bed linen, little pieces of cloth, or teddy bears, and which become essential for the child, especially when he feels lonely and left by his mother. The transitional object may change in the course of time and eventually may be disregarded.

According to *Winnicott,* the transitional object is the first possession independent of the self. He emphasizes that it has a real existence and that it is independent of the individual self. Originally the maternal breast belongs to this self; by means of his fantasy of omnipotence the infant exercises a magic power over it. At this point there is a unity in the representation of the self and the object. If the transitional object interferes, this unity is disrupted and a reality-oriented development sets in. Domination over the transitional object is not exercised by means of magic fantasies of omnipotence, but by muscular manipulation.

The transitional object is a creative achievement of the child and also an illusion, like the ideas that are the basis of religion and art. Illusions reconcile the inner and outside world. They are modes of conflict solution. In this case the solution of the conflict consists in the fact that for the infant the transitional object means the maternal breast. The baby symbolizes it for the time being and later on symbolizes the maternal personality.

Winnicott associates the transitional object with the origin of symbolizing, but he does not develop that idea any further. This is the starting point of the author's own deliberations.

The term 'symbol' is not used here as defined by psychoanalysis, but in accordance with *Ernst Simmel* and *Susanne Lange*. It implies the ability to give things a meaning, that means, to symbolize them. On the highest cognitive level this ability is realized in language. The given meaning is binding for all those who speak that language. The transitional object is the manifestation of this human potential.

These explanations suggest that the transitional object may be regarded as a valuable means of diagnosing psychic development in early childhood. It helps to explain the relation of the subject to the object and shows the first reality-based division between the representation of the self and the object; furthermore, it suggests that the phase of the magic fantasy of omnipotence begins to be overcome; it indicates a development that is oriented towards real being and clears the field for active, individual efforts. In short, it means a first separation from the mother and the incipient autonomy of the child.

Moreover, the transitional object constitutes the successful attempt at a conflict solution. The conflict originates when the urges of the child are not fulfilled and the mother is not always at the child's disposal. This deprivation makes it possible to distinguish between hallucinated magic omnipotence and objective reality, i.e., to differentiate between the real and the hallucinated object.

The above mentioned deprivation is on the one hand the *conditio sine qua non* for the coming to terms with reality, but on the other hand it is a reason for a state of tension which can be differentiated as mourning, narcissistic mortification, irritation, anger, and aggression. The more frustrating the interaction between mother and child is, the more strongly the destructive aggression will be directed against the mother. Since the mother, however, is vital for the child, these aggressions cause fear. The transitional object succeeds in averting threatening fear and anarchical aggressions. In doing so it acquires decisive significance for the solution of conflicts in the child. *Winnicott* supposes that the transitional object is a normal, ubiquitous phenomenon in the life of a baby. If the transitional object is lacking or if it persists, it is to be assumed that the development in question has not taken place. A reality-based separation between the subjective and the objective has not come about – a separation being the premise for coming to terms with reality.

The therapeutic relevance of the transitional object will be discussed in the light of a case history. A 30-year-old married student, the mother of two children, came to see a young colleague *(Dr. Grüttner)* after having tried to commit suicide three times and complained that she was not able to take her final exams, because she was not in a position to organize her written work. This young colleague supervised the case under my guidance. He had enormous difficulties to overcome in order to work with the patient. She rejected each of his interventions with the argument that she did not understand anything, that she was stupid and passive, and that she did not know whether the sky was outside of her or within her. It was not until a 1-hour talk about her transitional object, in connection with the discussion about the relationship with her mother and her grandmother, that a new, fertile phase of treatment commenced.

She said that she had never had a pain in the neck, but when she cried plaintively, her mother came running to her and gave her a little blanket. This she slobbered on and threw down. Consequently, by nightfall, there were up to six or seven baby towels around her bed. She gave them the name 'Ladl'. After the patient had talked about her Ladl, the therapist was able to understand her better. He understood her oral craving and the boundless nature of her wishes and the lack of an object permanence. He understood her statement that she made when quoting Pavese, to the effect that it would only be meaningful to communicate with those people who are willing to be together with one day and night. Quite obviously it was now possible for him to communicate with the patient in terms that were intelligible to her. This became apparent when in the next session the patient brought with her a list of first names, such as Fridolin (that might be translated as 'Freddy') and Nestmann (that might be translated as 'nest-man'), and submitted it to him; she had copied the names out of the telephone directory. It seemed that she no more used the analyst as a function, but was trying instead to comprehend him as an individual. It was very revealing that she was not yet capable of calling him by name. The character of the Ladl made itself felt here, too. The behaviour of the patient in the analytic process could be newly understood by the therapist in connection with the transitional object and his interventions could be arranged in accordance with it. A new situation of transference and counter-transference came into being. The analysis could be continued in a satisfactory fashion.

A 31-year-old patient suffering from juvenile diabetes that was difficult to regulate and who was also suffering from severe vomiting came in for treatment. Within 2 years she succeeded in overcoming the vomiting as a result of taking part in psychoanalytic group therapy. After the lapse of 2 more years, she began an individual psychoanalytic treatment. In the fifth session she brought a little towel with her that she kept with her all the time and tried to make a groove in the middle of it in order to then roll it up with great pressure. At the same time she told me that as a child she had to lie in the groove of the bed between her father and her mother. When an aunt wanted to adopt her, her mother refused categorically, saying that she had to remain home in order to prevent the old goat – meaning the husband – from jumping on her. For the first time she described the painful relationship with her mother; she was an illegitimate child and daily had to experience that her younger brother, who was born in lawful wedlock and was suffering from diabetes, enjoyed a treatment by the mother that was absolutely different from hers. While she was reporting this, she was extraordinarily agitated and was hardly able to speak; she was gasping for breath, wheezing, shouting, and weeping. Finally she said that she believed she was going mad. Her body was not her own body, but that of her mother, the phallus, with which she penetrated into her mother's body in order to destroy her; at the same time she was extremely disgusted.

She experienced her own body as a part of her mother's body. A separation between her own body and that of her mother had not come about. The patient identified with the function her mother had given to her. She identified with the aggressor. In the same session she expressed deep-rooted hatred she had never shown before, a hatred which was directed towards destroying the mother and which by means of transference was directed towards the therapist.

Could it not be possible that this destructive aggression is an expression of the fact that the patient was not regarded as an autonomous self, but as a function? (And that it is furthermore very difficult for the therapist to endure that hatred for a longer period of time?)

Finally, I want to talk about a patient who was taken ill with *myasthenia gravis (pseudoparalytica)* and who had no transitional object, but according to what he said, in the second year of his life already had an imagined object that he called 'Buck'. This imagined object was diametrically opposed to the transitional object.

Whereas the transitional object is a materially visible thing, that can be handled and has a real existence, the imagined object was a psychic phenomenon created by the patient himself and exercised a predominantly controlling function.

Buck sat on chimneys, in the corners of rooms, was not visible and was not allowed to be seen. But its controlling power could be constantly felt by the patient and aroused feelings of fear in him like those his mother used to arouse in him. Buck symbolized the magic and omnipotent control, i.e. the mother. But at the same time Buck was his own creation and by means of it he also controlled his own dangerous mother, that means that there was a unity between the subjective and the objective. Buck belonged to the realm of the magic, controlling omnipotence which controls the child at the beginning of his life. I have already referred to that phenomenon. The patient was fixated in a phase of his development that already in its early stages failed to demonstrate a grasp of reality.

My speech on 'The interaction approach of psychosomatic thinking as illustrated by a case of *myasthenia gravis pseudoparalytica*' will give a detailed report on that problem.

Mrs. *Gaddini* in her work entitled 'early psychosomatic symptom and the tendency towards integration' has furnished evidence of the fact that children suffering from psychosomatic illnesses in early childhood have no transitional object and *Hoppe* found out, though in a fewer number of cases, that the psychosomatically ill also have no transitional object or one that comes into existence only much later.

If this statement can be verified on the basis of a larger number of patients, the following hypothesis would be possible.

The transitional object gives us information on the cognitive and emotional development and on the unfolding of the subject-object relationship of the baby and the relationship with his own body that in analogy with the transitional object is experienced as a body independent of the maternal body and that exactly like the transitional object is manipulated by its own actions produced by muscular movement. If the transitional object is lacking, the separation between the self's body and the body of the object, the mother, is lacking too. The body itself is not integrated into the self and is not subject to it. It belongs to the outside world and is controlled by magic fantasies of omnipotence, such as are normal at the beginning of life before the first separation takes place. The transitional object obviously constitutes a beneficial counter-regulation against repression on this first symbiotic level. If, moreover, it becomes apparent that the psychosomatically ill lack transitional objects or if they persist, it is to be assumed that these persons have not completed a certain step in their development, namely, that of symbolizing, of the separation from and reunification with the mother, the first object. It means that separation and reunification do not take place on the level of the symbol, in the way that this is brought into being with regard to the transitional object, but on the level of being, in the somatic field. Up to now it has become obvious that psychosomatic illness is regarded as an incorporation of the object which is associated with deep-rooted hatred, the object implying both, the destruction of the self's body and the injury to the self's body.

References

Cassirer, E.: Wesen und Wirkung des Symbolbegriffes (Wissenschaftliche Buchgesell-
  schaft, Darmstadt 1956).
Cassirer, E.: Philosophie der symbolischen Formen, vol. 1, 2 (Wissenschaftliche Buchge-
  sellschaft, Darmstadt 1973).
Langer, S.: Philosophy in a new key (Harvard Univ. Press, Cambridge 1942).
Winnicott, D.W.: Transitional objects and transitional phenomena. Int. J. Psychoanalyt.
  34 (1953); Collected papers (Tavistock, London 1958).

Prof. Dr. med. *M. Mitscherlich*, Weezer Strasse 2, *D-4000 Düsseldorf 11* (BRD)

Proc. 11th Eur. Conf. Psychosom. Res., Heidelberg 1976
Psychother. Psychosom. *28:* 278–284 (1977)

Primary Socialisation and Alexithymic Defects in Symbol and Concept Formation

S. Zepf

The title of my lecture states explicitly that symbol and concept formation are to be its general subject, and no doubt some of you may be expecting a systematic discussion of the manifold problems connected with this field of research. However, I am afraid I must disappoint you on this score: simply to skim over these problems would by far overtax the 15 min allowed. This limit obliges me to narrow my subject down to the language of the psychosomatic patient which is striking for its lack of subjective connotations. The perspective in which I shall be looking at this phenomenon is, I must point out, one opened up recently by *Lorenzer* (4, 5) in his studies on language, symbol formation, and interaction. In Hannover we have chosen this angle for the following reason: from a genetic point of view 'alexithymia' can, like its clinical manifestation, also be described as a deficiency. Such problematical constructions such as 'irreversible denial' thus become superfluous.

Before we get down to the discussion I have to acquaint you with *Lorenzer*'s conception of language acquisition in childhood. *Lorenzer*'s main interest lies in the development of a 'non-subjective theory of the subject'. Herein he is indebted to a language theory for which *Lorenz* (3) in particular, is a major exponent and which sees the acquisition of language inextricably bound up with the individual's real life experience. In this theory parts of reality are shown to a 'languageless' listener and predicated for him by a speaker. In the following step of regulation the listener can differentiate these predicated parts from one another. Predication refers to the act of associating a sound complex with an object or a series of movements in a learning dialogue. Regulation denotes the following faculty: once several objects or series of movements are predicated, the assignment of one predicator can be followed by the rejection of other predicators for the same. To take an example: the series of movements – bowing – and – going for a walk – must first be differently predicated before the predicator 'going for a walk' can be rejected for – bowing – and vice versa.

Lorenzer takes up these two notions and applies them within his own conception. He likewise considers language acquisition to be a process of conveying language which sets in in primary socialisation when the first objects speak to the child. However, unlike the above-mentioned learning dialogue, the first dyadic relationship of mother and child in the primary unit does not involve a confrontation of two separate partners, nor is there such a thing as an object distinct from the child to which certain sound complexes could be assigned. What we have here is the predication of a relationship, to be more precise, of an interaction actually being performed at the time of predication. In other words, the subject of predication is a realisation of one of the forms of interaction mutually agreed on by mother and child in the course of establishing a reciprocally gratifying relationship during the prelanguage stage, and which have been stored up as engrams in the child's memory. For instance, when the mother-figure speaks a word, let us say 'mummy' and in so doing implicitly points to the interaction being currently performed, this form of interaction is named for the child. It goes without saying that this act of predication must be performed repeatedly if the sound complex 'mummy' is to be absorbed engrammatically and be fused with the engram of the interactions to which it belongs. At this stage, however, although the word 'mummy' is now internalized, it is still a long way from becoming a symbol. *Lorenzer* rightly points out that this fusion of the sound complex 'mummy' is for the time being just one more element in a circle of interaction, an element with the quality of a signal and thus a means of activating the interaction engram but not of reflecting on it. The decisive step is still lacking, a step which, when constantly repeated, enables the individual to overcome the compulsive rigidity of signal-bound and unconscious behaviour and to reflect on his life practice, stored up in engrams at his conscious disposal. *Lorenzer* demonstrates how this qualitative step is to be envisaged by means of the concepts 'differentiation' and 'identity' formation. I have modified these in a diagram for my own purposes (fig. 1).

This diagram is to be read as follows:

(I) A form of interaction, for example a warm-gratifying one, actually being performed is named. 'Mummy' is the initial predication. The same process is repeated, occasionally interrupted by a second form of interaction, in this case a cold-frustrating one.

I. Introduction of the initial predication 'Mummy' in a first form of interaction (IF$_1$), e.g., warm-gratifying (w-g). The mother then displays cold- frustrating (c-f) behaviour in a second form of interaction (IF$_2$).

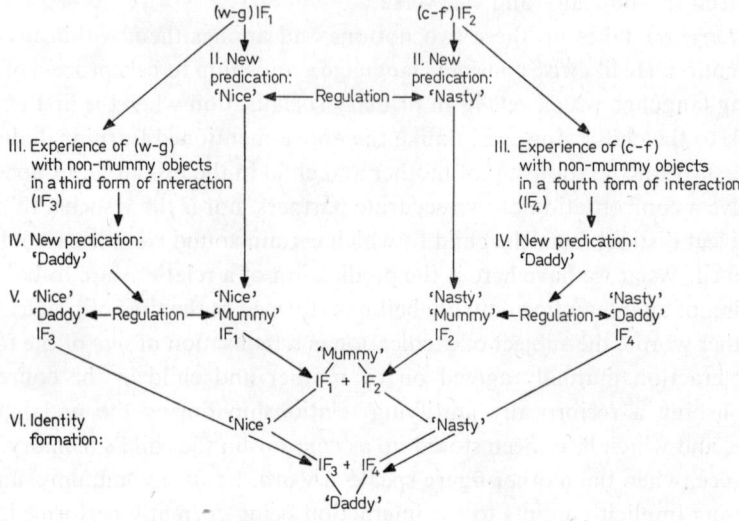

Fig. 1. Symbol formation.

(II) New predicators are introduced which are assigned to certain interactions and rejected for others: 'nice' is assigned to the first form of interaction and rejected for the second, 'nasty' is assigned to the second and rejected for the first.

(III) The child then experiences these warm-gratifying and cold-frustrating qualities again in interaction with non-mummy objects,

(IV) Both these new interactions are assigned the same predicator, for example, 'daddy'.

(V) A further regulatory step takes place: the warm-gratifying form of interaction is split up into 'nice mummy' and 'nice daddy' and the cold-frustrating one into 'nasty mummy' and 'nasty daddy'.

(VI) Integration and formation of the following identities: (a) 'mummy' as 'nice and nasty'; (b) 'daddy' as 'nice and nasty'; (c) 'nice' as 'mummy and daddy', and (d) 'nasty' as 'mummy and daddy'.

Lorenzer localizes symbol formation in the following step: in the course of assigning sound complexes and rejecting them, sound and interaction engrams are brought into mutual relationships to one another. A sound engram becomes related to various interaction engrams and vice versa. At the central nervous level structures crystallize which, as symbols, can be evoked independent of actual interaction. Words gradually become substitutes for their respective interaction engrams. A language system is set up which renders the individual's life history available for him as his repertoire of conscious plans for action.

To sum up, if we examine our scheme carefully, there are three things to note: (1) at the very beginning, words do not designate sharply delineated and already distinguishable objects, but rather forms of interaction; (2) When centered onto the symbolic object representation, the different forms of interaction constitute the different meanings of the object for the subject, and (3) it becomes obvious that in this process of language acquisition drive activities are woven up into the existing semantics of language.

However, a critical glance will show us that the conceptions of predication and regulation alone do not suffice to comprehend adequately how individual structures of consciousness take shape. For if we conceive symbols as those instruments with which secondary-process, abstract-logical and reality-orientated thinking operates, that is to say as the instruments with which the individual can anticipate interaction on the basis of his previous experience in the form of a 'trial run', then we must think of symbols as being concepts. And this presents us with a problem, for then we are obliged to show how content and realm of a symbol are formed. Let us just call to mind the studies of *Rapaport et al.* (6) on concept formation: it is precisely because concepts have a content and a realm that they permit us to categorize our experiences according to logical principles, to judge what they 'belong to' and thus to plan our activities in advance and in accordance with reality. Now, if we ask how the content of a symbol is formed, then we recognize immediately how insufficient our diagram is. Predication and regulation do of course constitute a necessary prerequisite for symbol formation. What they do not do is to permit us to explain satisfactorily how the content of a symbol is formed. We have contended that in regulation, predicated interaction is broken up by means of the assigning and rejecting of names. Yet were the different forms of interaction merely distinguishable by their names, then the realm of the future symbol would have been formed, but not the content, and with that I mean the invariant identical quality common to all those objects and relationships reflected in the scope of a certain symbol.

In order to legitimate the following considerations I would normally have to demonstrate each step of my argumentation very carefully. In this first attempt to pinpoint the emotionless language of the psychosomatic patient I nevertheless must confine myself to a rather simplified presentation. It will cause us no problem to postulate that the content of a symbol as the content of a concept must be regarded as a product of abstraction. Where does it come from? This analytic product must result out of a comparison of differing forms of interaction, out of a process in which their abstract identical qualities are conceptualized in sound engrams. The contrary process can then take place in which the concretion of particular forms of interaction as differing cases of an identical quality is possible. However, what we must remember here is that the identical is only definable in contrast to the non-identical. Not only must the identical qualities be perceptible in the non-identical, but also the non-identical qualities in the identical. Thus, the synthetic act of concretion must not only be regarded as the product of the analytic act of abstraction, but also as its necessary precondition.

Perhaps I can illustrate this complex matter by taking the content formation of 'mummy' and 'nice'. Our diagram showed that the mummy object does not exist for the child 'as such', isolated from the child's experience. 'Mummy' is always mummy-in-a-specific-type-of-interaction which constitutes one of the concrete forms in which 'mummy' is experienced, for instance as warm-and-gratifying or as cold-and-frustrating. Now, if 'mummy' is to be abstracted from these two differing forms of interaction as their identical nature, then a number of abstractions must already have taken place, for example, 'nice' and 'nasty'. The different nature of the two manifestations of 'mummy', the non-identity of warm-gratifying and cold-frustrating could otherwise not be understood. Supposing we turn our attention to the process in which 'nice' is to be abstracted as the identical quality: we have no choice but to presume not only that 'nice' must have been interacted in differing forms of interaction but also that this 'differentness' must be conceivable, for example, as nice-in-relation-to-mummy and as nice-in-relation-to-daddy. In this case likewise, abstractions are necessary and these again preclude other abstractions.

There can now be no doubt that the symbolic level can hardly be attained on the basis of four forms of interaction and four predicators, as one might suppose looking at our diagram. If we roll our two postulates into one we can make the following formulation: The development of symbols must be regarded as a process of mutually dependent abstractions requiring a wide range of interaction and the introduction of innumerable predicators. These factors alone can guarantee that the abstract identities, those qualities remaining invariant in spite of the changing forms of interaction, can be conceptualized in sound engrams. This is the way the individual's subjective life experience is bound up into the objective semantics of his language.

This brings me to the central point of my discussion, the language of the psychosomatic patient. Going through the literature it strikes one that the primary socialisation of the psychosomatic patient has one outstanding common feature. In a vast proportion of cases the mother figure is described as narcissistic, as overprotective or as engulfing. The following quotation from the painstaking study carried out by *Garner and Wenar* (1) may stand for a whole host of similar findings and may serve to illustrate the empirical correlation of the termini just mentioned: 'With no exception, all these mothers were (...) uninterested in the child except as a self-enhancing asset. (...) Caretaking and training are done either in a wooden manner or with distaste and the infant is clearly regarded as (...) a source of (...) anxiety and frustration (...). Maternal (...) frustration may have been relieved occasionally by moments of impersonal, objective contact, but the spontaneous gestures of affection, the unanticipated gift, the "extras" that delight child and mother, were (...) missing.'

If, as we may certainly deduce from the quotation, primary socialisation suffers from a deficit in forms of interaction, a restricted practice so to speak, it follows that the individual's consciousness cannot take shape out of his life experience. The practice of primary socialisation does not get beyond the level of the 'protosymbol', and that means that it does not attain consciousness.

Needless to say, this postulate confronts us with a serious problem. If we do not want to find ourselves at variance with basic tenets of modern language theory we must identify the formation of consciousness with the development of language. Are we not then forced to conclude that the psychosomatic patient remains without language and without consciousness, a conclusion which is totally at odds with the facts? To contend this would be short-sighted and would overlook the fact that the meanings of language, the contents of concepts are not just acquired in the process of symbol formation but equally through metalanguage definitions as well as through demonstrated practice in which the individual is not allowed to participate. Language must necessarily be acquired: a different accentuation of the basis of content formation in a semantic system in the making, the tendency towards an 'exemplary' type of practice in which others do the interaction and the subject, to use *Holzkamp*'s (2) distinction, has little 'direct' practice of his own, all this has dire effects on the individual's language.

Let me summarize these effects briefly: a meagre system of forms of interaction is unfolded which, however, does not necessarily mean that the system of predicators need be similarly reduced. On the contrary, a great number and variety of predicators can have been introduced. But, and this is the crux of the matter, because in this type of language acquisition the relationships to predicated objects are either completely blocked or kept at a rudimentary level, the predicators have simply a denotative reference and are not anchored in an ensemble of connotative references to the individual's life history. For these individuals, objects are merely 'used' in an instrumental fashion. Their predicators can appropriately be termed as 'signs'.

Lorenzer himself considers the sign to be the result of defence mechanisms, yet there can be no doubt that in terms of his theory restricted practice in primary socialisation must produce a similar effect. Admittedly, the aetiological processes differ, but the result is in both cases lacunal language. As long as the individual's life experience is not absorbed into the content formation of concepts, the individual is bound to manifest that very same emotional emptiness described in the literature under the heading of 'alexithymia'.

I must confess that I have had to simplify my arguments in a way that does not really do the subject matter justice, but perhaps I have nevertheless managed to give you some insight into the basic points of our reasoning. Although it was not possible to outline the connections to basic tenets of psychoanalysis at every point, I hope it became obvious that an epistemological investigation into symbol and concept formation can throw fresh light on the concept of 'alexithymia'.

References

1   *Garner, A.M. and Wenar, C.:* The mother-child interaction in psychosomatic disorders (Urbana 1959).
2   *Holzkamp, K.:* Wissenschaftstheoretische Voraussetzungen kritisch-emanzipatorischer Psychologie; in *Holzkamp* Kritische Psychologie, p. 75 ff. (Frankfurt 1972).
3   *Lorenz, K.:* Elemente der Sprachkritik (Frankfurt 1970).
4   *Lorenzer, A.:* Sprachzerstörung und Rekonstruktion (Frankfurt 1971).
5   *Lorenzer, A.:* Zur Begründung einer materialistischen Sozialisationstheorie (Frankfurt 1972).
6   *Rapaport, D.; Gill, M., and Schafer, R.:* in *Holt* Diagnostic psychological testing, p. 191 (New York 1968).

Dr. med. habil. *S. Zepf,* Medizinische Hochschule Hannover, Abteilung für Psychosomatik, Postfach 610180, *D-3000 Hannover* (FRG)

Proc. 11th Eur. Conf. Psychosom. Res., Heidelberg 1976
Psychother. Psychosom. *28:* 285–293 (1977)

The Implications of the Specificity Concept for the Treatment of Psychosomatic Patients

Jan Bastiaans

Introduction

With regard to the concept of psychosomatic specificity *Groen* (1971) recently has asked 'Where do we stand now'?

In fact, this question has been a most burning one during all the years of development of modern psychosomatic medicine. The psychosomatic specificity concept is part of the more general concept of reaction specificity. It is related to the concept of 'choice of neurosis' (Neurosenwahl) and to a certain extent it deals with specific manifestations of neurosis.

The starting point for a discussion on reaction specificity is given in the well known S-O-R model, which implies that certain situational stimuli or stresses may evoke in a certain organism or personality a certain reaction or chain of reactions. Psychosomatic specificity implies that specific situational stresses may lead to specific conflict situations. The elaboration of the conflict results in specific psychosomatic conditions. *Groen* and co-workers have described how psychosomatic patients cannot act out their frustrations in violence, depression, weeping or complaining to the key figures in their environment. These authors elaborated two schemes to illustrate their view (table I, fig. 1).

This scheme implies that in case of development of psychosomatic disease a certain type of personality, as determined by both genetic and acquired factors, is supposed to be sensitive to certain environmental stresses. How the behaviour of one individual may become a stimulus or stress for another individual is diagrammatically expressed in figure 1.

This scheme has been extensively described by *Groen and Bastiaans* (1974) in their paper on 'Psychosocial Stress, Interhuman Communication

Table I

P (personality)	+S (Stress) $\longrightarrow$ B (Behaviour, c.q. Disease)	
Genetic	Physico-chemical	externally directed:
Developmental	biological	motoric
Experience	interhuman	mimic
		vocal (verbal)
(conditioning, learning)		internally directed:
		endocrine
		vascular
		visceral
		secretory

A Model of Human Interaction

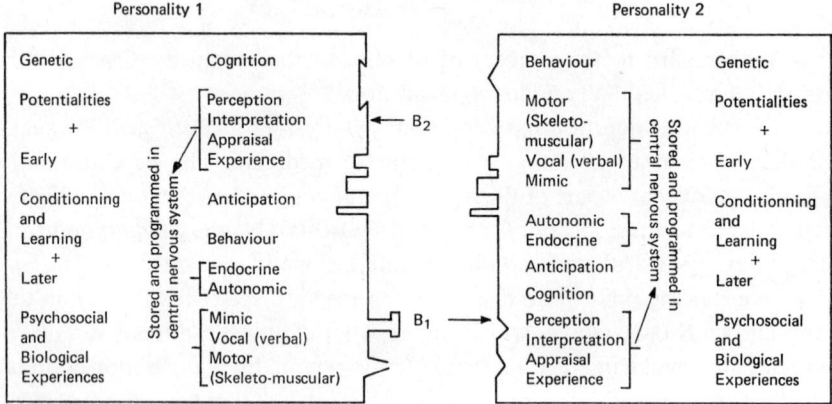

Fig. 1. The behaviour of personality 2 is the stimulus (or stress) for personality 1 and vice versa $B_1 = S_2$ and $B_2 = S_1$.

and psychosomatic Disease'. It implies an elaboration of the S-OR- model. Still, it has also its restrictions because it does not depict the continuous dynamic development that takes place in the behaviour of individuals toward each other in the course of their childhood, adulthood and senescence. Nor does it illustrate the continuous evolution and change in the subgroups in which people live and that influence and modify the ways of their communication. In the frame of this congress it may be clear that 'alexithymia' is implied in the scheme as an inefficient manner of communication which in itself may be determined by the other factors included in the scheme.

In the related paper *Groen* and *Bastiaans* have answered the question 'where do we stand now'. Their concept is: Man is a social animal living in a human culture. In this culture he has to maintain his social and internal homeostasis (i.e. his health) in continuous communication with his fellow men and, especially, with the key figures in the social subgroups to which he belongs.

Every society and every social subgroup has its own psychosocial stressors that consist of the behaviour patterns of its members, which require more than the usual cognitive appraisal, anticipation and adaptive behaviour. Successful coping with these stressors leads to gratification; failure to cope leads to frustration.

A Clinical Example

Some years ago the author has introduced a technique called 'microanalysis of the first interview'. This technique is known in Germany under the title 'the translation of the complaint' (die Übersetzung der Klage). A case used for the illustration of this technique, is the following. A 26-year-old unmarried female typist is referred by a departmental dermatologist to a psychoanalytic institute. She suffers from atopic dermatitis. Some symptoms of nervousness have given rise for a psychiatric examination. At the start of the first interview the psychiatrist asks the patient what trouble she has. The striking first answer is: 'Tenseness and fears and the constant necessity to scratch, mostly at the end of the day and in bed before going to sleep I scratch my whole skin till it is open.'

In reaction to the second question of the psychiatrist 'does it itch you', the response behaviour of the patient is marked by: (1) a rather aggressive and active response including denial, protest, rationalization of the cause of the complaint; (2) a rather depressive continuation of the response when the therapist does not react in an understandable way, and (3) a continuation of the response behaviour marked by anxiety at the moment the therapist also reacts in an inadequate way to the symptoms of depression: possibly this occurs also at the moment the patient more or less consciously perceives that she is inclined to attack the psychiatrist in an indirect way.

Thus, within the frame of the first minutes of the interview it becomes clear that the patient at least disposes of three adaptation strategies activated by expectations and stresses induced by the therapist. The psychiatrist primarily is interested in the psychological aspects of atopic dermatitis. The psychological examination leads to the conclusion that the patient is marked by a personality profile as often found in cases of this disease. Further analysis of the situational factors reveals that the three main response strategies are evoked by different situational stimuli.

In situations in which the patient felt threathened by the possibility that a dear friend could leave her she predominantly reacted with overt anxiety (fears). In situations, in which she really was left alone and felt rejected, she tended to react with depressive behaviour. Finally, in situations in which she tried to prevent threatening rejection by a controlled fight-behaviour, she reacted with scratching and eczema. Thus, the three specific reaction patterns were not used alternating or simultaneously independent of the environment, but highly dependent on the specificity of the constellation.

This example may be used to illustrate how one-sided it is to relate the specificity of the response to a certain personality core only or to the situational constellation only.

Safety and Specificity

Bastiaans (1975), following the ideas of *Sandler* (1960) has added that the best indicator for a successful coping with the environment, which results in homeostasis and health, is given in the feeling state of safety. He is of the opinion that in psychosomatic medicine the safety concept has been neglected all too long. Its meaning can be described best with the help of the scheme shown in figure 2.

Under normal circumstances an optimal feeling state of safety is reached in positive and pleasurable communication and interaction. But frequently this optimal pathway is blocked. The only way to reach safety which remains open after such a blockade, is the pathway of power and the related manifestations of aggression.

But the power-way to reach security and safety implies isolation of the personality or group in the form of 'armours', 'forts' or 'castles'. On the

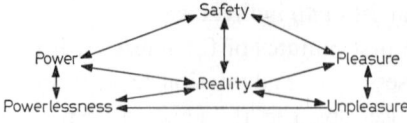

Fig. 2. Realization of safety.

personality level this implies nearly always intrapsychic isles or jails of self-centeredness, narcissism, autism or comparable defence structures. One of the manifestations of a certain isolation strategy or isolation development may lead to the symptom or syndrome of alexithymia. The author is of the opinion that psychosomatic disease and psychosomatic syndromes can be understood best as the result of a deficient coping strategy to reach safety and security along the pathway of optimal communication. At the same time they are the result of a strategy to reach the highly wanted feeling state of safety along the pathway of power, defence against powerlessness, including specific manifestations of emotional isolation.

Some Remarks about Alexithymia

It has been stated sufficiently that alexithymia may have different origins. The author is not convinced that every psychosomatic patient has a constitutional deficiency of the capacity to verbalize special and dangerous emotions. At the moment the wall of psychosomatic rigidity has been broken in the course of the therapeutic process, it usually becomes clear that psychosomatic patients are not different from psychoneurotic ones with regard to their constitutional and acquired capacities for verbalization of inner experiences. The author has been able to clarify this with the help of an LSD-technique in which psychoanalytic-oriented psychotherapy and some LSD sessions are combined. Sometimes, even after a quarter of an hour after the beginning of an LSD session, a so-called alexithymic patient may change into a personality who is very well able to verbalize strong repressed emotions. There is a wide range between the autistic and/or mutistic child that is unable to establish verbal communication with its environment, the so-called normal psychosomatic patient and the more or less mutistic victim of the stresses of the severe traumatic man-made disasters. The most striking complaint of the representatives of the last group is: I cannot tell you what I went through. You cannot understand me because you have not gone through it yourself. On this level these patients are really alexithymic as long as, in the therapeutic situation, the climate of human understanding and safety has not pervaded their autistic defence.

The essence is that activated emotions may turn from friends or allies into enemies at the moment that their intensity becomes a threat of a danger to the patient.

Such emotions have to be repressed for survival purposes. With enemies it is difficult to speak. Hence, the advice: Let the therapist try to turn these enemies into friends. Let the patients accept their emotions. Try to realise this in a therapeutic process in which training in verbalization can be realized in a climate of safety and human understanding. Emotions have feedback function but this function cannot be used if emotions cannot be associated with images, symbols, words.

The Specific Interrelation of Psychiatric and Psychosomatic Syndromes

For educational purposes the author constructed the model shown in figure 3.

When homeostasis is threathened by stressors from the outside or the inside, the human organism primarily reacts with the well-known sympto-matology of shock and alarm, usually given in the syndromes of general nervousness, anxiety and other manifestations of arousal. The author has described this as the symptomatology of traumatisation. All the arousal reactions may stimulate the use of the right strategies for coping and adaptation. Failure of such an intrapsychic process leads to the development of the clinical syndromes.

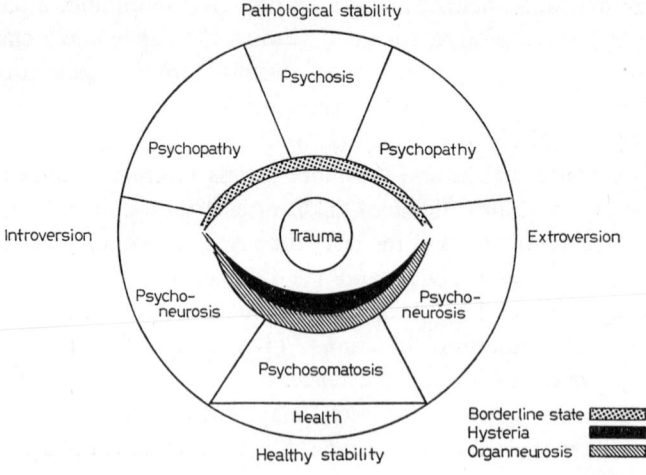

Fig. 3. The interrelation of the different psychiatric and psychosomatic syndromes.

Since many years, *Groen, Bastiaans* and their coworkers have advocated that the psychosomatic and the organ-neurotic modes of adaptation have to be regarded as the result of a constant intrapsychic struggle of the individual not to behave towards the environment in an overt hysterical way.

Hysteria in this view is regarded as a very general and ubiquitous phenomenon which implies an exaggerated but inefficient strategy to obtain help, support, love and attention. In some cultures the hysterical way of coping is more accepted than in other cultures. The main finding of the author is that once, in the psychotherapeutic sessions, the psychosomatic wall of defence has been broken the underlying nucleus of hysteria may become overt. The related conclusion has been that many West-European and American societies are both hysterogenic and anti-hysterogenic. This has to be kept in mind by every therapist who is engaged in the treatment of psychosomatic patients.

Consequences of the Specificity Theory for the Treatment of Psychosomatic Patients

Though the specificity theory and all its modifications (complete specificity, relative response specificity, multidimensional and unidimensional specificity) has been criticized and rejected by many workers in the field, the most striking finding is that only few colleagues really have had the opportunity to observe the psychological differences between psychiatric and psychosomatic patients and those between different groups of psychosomatic patients in a clinical setting which allows observation and examination of large series of special groups. Based on this experience the author is still of the opinion that the specificity concept cannot be rejected. The personality profiles of psychosomatic patients, as described by the pioneers and especially by the Amsterdam group, are still valuable. Guidelines for the first approach of the psychosomatic patient have been formulated by the author in his paper for the Rome congress in 1975. These are described under the headings of: (1) Introductory phase of psychotherapy. (2) Exploration of psychosomatic rigidity. (3) First approach to specific superego components. (4) Evaluation of the expected or wanted role of the therapist. (5) Focusing on repressed feelings, emotions and affects which ask for immediate expression. (6) Focusing on the expression of phantasies and dreams. (7) Focusing on deeper repressed feelings, affects and emotions. (8) Focusing on the optimal balance of passivity and activity.

In fact these guidelines are based on the analysis of the more or less specific manifestations of more or less normal mental or emotional isolation. The author has described these manifestations with the help of the above-mentioned concepts of psychosomatic rigidity, psychosomatic narcissism, psychosomatic self-centeredness. Basic in the therapy is that even a relative decrease of the intensity of these specific modes of self-defence against stress and anxiety may give rise to the disappearance of the specific behaviour.

Therefore, it may be repeated: because psychosomatic patients are marked by a forced adaptation to reality, the therapy has to be directed on a behavioural change which results in a shift from forced adaptation into flexible and smooth adaptation. It is well known that such a shift may be promoted by the use of different techniques: (1) relaxation therapies; (2) techniques which alleviate the pressure of an all too strict superego; (3) techniques which strengthen the ego capacities for adaptation; (4) techniques which focus on the decrease of more or less specific situational or environmental stresses and demands, and (5) techniques which focus on improvement of adaptation by the use of psychopharmacology.

To What Extent Does the Knowledge of Psychosomatic Specificity Facilitate the Treatment of Different Psychosomatic Disorders?

Since 1952, *Groen* and his coworkers have repeatedly stressed the necessity of special guidelines for the approach to different psychosomatic groups. Patients suffering from ulcerative colitis predominately need a supportive and assertive fatherly or motherly understanding and approach. The asthmatic patient, oversensitive for dominance, needs very flexible and above all non-dominant understanding, sometimes even submissive therapeutic behaviour. The ulcer patient, usually involved in repressed problems of rivalry and competition, asks from his doctor that he behaves as an understanding comrade, certainly not as an authoritarian boss or rival. In the same way some key formulations have been given for the approach of patients suffering from essential hypertension, rheumatoid arthritis, psychosomatic skin diseases, etc.

Today, it may be repeated that unfortunately many of these important clinical findings have not irradiated sufficiently in teaching and international literature. But even the best generalization of this kind of experience into the literature would not be sufficient to induce at least, the idea that something of value and of truth might be in it. A remarkable fact in working with psychosomatic patients is that nearly every therapist can approve the psychosomatic hypothesis only after a period of personal experience in the domain of psychosomatic therapy. The psychosomatic patient has also been defined as a personality marked by a certain hidden delusion of 'autonomy in isolation'. The intrapsychic formula is: 'do it yourself', because being dependent on the environment is interpreted as a threat or a danger. This attitude, which is frequently so characteristic for representatives of the medical profession and the social sciences, is also an infectious one.

In being engaged in the psychosomatic area, one is sometimes subconsciously inclined to identify oneself too much with the dominant adaptational strategies of the object of examination, i.e., the patient. The only remedy in this situation is the advice to the therapist: If you cannot accept even the slightest defence or presentation of the psychosomatic specificity hypothesis, try to analyze the problem yourself. The truth is not in the essence of a transferred theory, but in the careful description of what you can observe with all the instruments which are at your disposal.

References

Bastiaans, J. and Groen, J.J.: Psychotherapy of internal diseases; in The affective contact, p. 368 (Strengholt, Leiden 1951).

Bastiaans, J.: The place of personality traits in specific syndromes: cause or effect? in *Wisdom and Wolff* The role of psychosomatic disorder in adult life (Pergamon Press, Oxford 1965).

Bastiaans, J.: Die Übersetzung der Klage. Z. Psychother. med. Psychol. *21:* 5, 167 (1971).

Bastiaans, J.: Neue psychodynamische und psychobiologische Aspekte der Hysterie. Praxis Psychother. *50:* 159 (1974).

Bastiaans, J.: Das erste Gespräch mit psychosomatischen Patienten; in *Jores* Praktische Psychosomatik (Huber, Bern 1976).

Bastiaans, J.: Der Beitrag der Psychoanalyse zur Psychosomatischen Medizin; in Die Psychologie des 20. Jahrhunderts, Band II (Kindler, Zürich 1976).

Bastiaans, J.: Psychotherapy in psychosomatic medicine; in *Antonelli* Psychosomatic medicine (Pozzi, Rome 1977).

Groen, J.J.: The challenge of the future: the prevention of psychosomatic disorders. Psychother. Psychosom. *23:* 283–303 (1974).

Groen, J.J. and Bastiaans, J.: Psychosocial stress, interhuman communication and psychosomatic disease; in *Spielberger and Sarason* Stress and anxiety, vol. I. (Wiley, New York 1975).

Sandler, J.: The background of safety. Int. J. Psychol. *41:* 352 (1960).

Prof. Dr. *Jan Bastiaans,* Psychiatrische Kliniek, Jelgersma-Kliniek, Rhijngeesterstraatweg 13, *Oegstgeest* (The Netherlands)

Proc. 11th Eur. Conf. Psychosom. Res., Heidelberg 1976
Psychother. Psychosom. *28:* 294–304 (1977)

Group Psychotherapy of Somatizing Patients

Charles V. Ford and Kahlila D. Long[1]

Introduction

Any busy private practice or hospital clinic has a number of patients for whom some type of psychological assistance is indicated (1, 2). However, many of these patients complain primarily of physical symptoms and do not recognize the underlying emotional problems. These patients may have 'classical psychosomatic' diseases such as ulcerative colitis or peptic ulcer disease. Others with little objective evidence of organic disease are often perjoratively labeled 'crocks', 'hypochondriacs', or 'hysterics'. Both types of patients, too often, receive increasingly superficial treatment as they are referred from physician to physician or clinic to clinic. They not only do not recognize their emotional distress but often are resentful of any implication that there is a possibility of a psychological problem. These patients usually do not follow through with referrals to a psychiatric clinic and when they do they are poorly motivated, irregular in keeping appointments, and fail to engender therapeutic zeal in their therapists. Group therapy is one means of treatment which has been proposed for these difficult patients.

Literature Review

Group therapy of 'psychosomatic patients' has been described in the literature since shortly after the turn of the century (3). The techniques of

[1] Dr. *Ford* is Adjunct Associate Professor of Psychiatry, University of California, Los Angeles, Calif., and formerly was Head Physician, Psychiatric Liaison Service, Harbor General Hospital. Mrs. *Long* is the psychiatric social worker for the Psychiatric Liaison Service, Harbor General Hospital, Torrance, Calif.

group treatment have varied considerably, one extreme being essentially inspirational and educational lectures (4) and at the other end of the continuum, psychoanalytic insight oriented methods (3, 5, 6). Interpretation of therapeutic results has also varied. One author found that group therapy was contraindicated for hypertensive patients because it increased their blood pressure (7). Other authors report differing degrees of improvement. *Milberg* (5) found that patients with different types of dermatitis almost invariably had had improvement of their skin lesions and the majority of patients continued treatment to modify personality change by insight into their conflicts. *Stein* (3), whose orientation is that of psychoanalytic technique, has stated that over 50% of patients improved with group psychotherapy and that this occurred through 'their ability to become aware of emotions psychologically and to express them by more purely affective means such as anger, shouting and weeping'. Specific somatic changes were not detailed.

In another communication, *Stein et al.* (6) reported upon their experiences with psychoanalytically oriented group psychotherapy of peptic ulcer patients. They found commonly expressed feelings of deprivation, resentment, rivalry and greed. The authors also detected strong passive-dependent longings and deep seated sexual conflicts. Over an 18-month period there was a diminution of ulcer symptoms coinciding with some decrease of emotional tensions and loosening of their previous rigid patterns of interacting. Therapy, however, did not eradicate the basic personality problems which they thought to be generally severe. *Fortin* and *Abse* (8) have also reported on their experiences with peptic ulcer disease patients. These patients were male college students who were seen in intensive (3 h/week) analytic group therapy. Members of this group showed improvement in the academic and psychosexual functioning and after some time had diminution of ulcer symptoms. However, such symptoms were apt to reappear when the patient experienced unusual stress.

Sclare and Crocket (9) treating asthmatics in Scotland found that group therapy failed to favorably influence the respiratory manifestations of bronchial asthma. However, there were favorable well-defined personality changes in these patients including increased tolerance and acceptance, reduced anxiety and tension, less rigidity and improved socialization. They found these changes to be consistent with those usually found in neurotic patients treated by group psychotherapy. Group discussion themes of anger and hostility were very common and the therapist was able to relate repressed anger to asthmatic attacks.

Groen and Pelser (10) in a detailed controlled study of Dutch patients with bronchial asthma found symptomatic improvement and decreased mortality in those patients treated with group psychotherapy and ACTH or other indicated symptomatic drugs compared to control groups where only symptomatic therapy and/or ACTH were utilized. Anger dependency conflicts and repressed sexuality were prominent in these patients. Over the course of treatment some patients were noted to have improved the manner in whichthey handled interpersonal conflicts. 'Blind' evaluation via Rorschach testing indicated a significant decrease in the number of 'oppressive' responses from those asthmatics who received group therapy compared to those who did not (11).

An important distinction in the treatment techniques of Drs. *Groen* and *Pelser* was that their groups were led by internists who utilized the group sessions for concurrent symptomatic treatment and patients were actively questioned about their health. *Groen* and *Pelser* hypothesized that having the entire treatment in the hands of one physician may both have facilitated transference and improved the somatic results of therapy as well as having a positive influence on group attendance.

They also noted that a number of factors were indicative of a poorer prognosis including advanced age, history of hospital admission for testing, unfavorable home situations, unemployment or unfavorable relationships with the employer, group behavior which included lies or concealed information, and lack of introspection.

A group method was used by *Mally* and *Ogston* (12) to treat women with numerous somatic complaints. These patients were generally middle-aged and all were supported by public assistance or relatives. They seemed to be the least successful members of their families educationally, economically, socially and maritally. Their energies were directed toward the goal of being cared for and they magically expected medical clinics, etc., to meet these needs. Group sessions (1½ h weekly) involved competitiveness for the interest and concern of the leaders but there was a gradual increase of social cohesiveness and mutual support. Dependent longings, resentment and hostility were common features in these women who also reported sexually unsatisfying marriages. After several years of treatment there was a significant reduction of visits that group members made to the medical clinics.

Despite the fact that reports concerning group psychotherapy of psychosomatic patients come from widely dispersed geographical locations there is a remarkable similarity in the descriptions of patient characteristics. Prominently mentioned are features of resentment, underlying hostility, dependent longings and repressed sexuality.

Rational and Details of Group Psychotherapy for Psychosomatic Patients

A plan for group treatment of somatizing patients was developed by the Psychiatric Liaison Service at Harbor General for both theoretical and practical reasons. From a theoretical stance it was believed that 'psychosomatic' patients have difficulty expressing and communicating affect and a group experience might facilitate the patient's affective responses and thereby be therapeutic. An additional hypothesis was that these patients use physical symptoms as a means of establishing and maintaining interpersonal relationships. It was hoped that a group setting might offer an alternative method of relating to others.

From a more practical standpoint, the authors' experience with these patients indicated poor compliance with scheduled appointments and thereby ineffective use of the therapists available time. Group treatment allowed more flexibility in patient attendance. Another important issue was the personal discomfort of the therapists in treating many of these patients individually. These nonverbal, nonpsychologically minded and frequently clinging dependent patients made therapy emotionally draining. It was hoped that a group approach could effectively reduce the therapist's discomfort by diluting the dependency and by reducing the need for continuous activity by the therapist.

It was specifically planned that the therapeutic interventions would primarily focus upon affect and secondarily on group process and/or psychodynamic material.

Patients comprising the groups came from a variety of sources. Some patients had been in individual psychotherapy with either one of the group therapists or were referred by another therapist who felt that group experience would be useful. Over one-half of the patients were referred from the hospital's psychiatric consultation clinic. These patients saw one of the group therapists in 1–4 individual sessions and would then be started in a group. It was explained to them that they were being referred to a group consisting of people who had both physical and emotional problems. No promise of improvement of the physical complaint was made and patients continued their medical care in the appropriate medical or surgical clinic. Although it was the original intent to restrict the group to patients having 'classical psychosomatic' illnesses we soon found that patients could not be categorized so easily and soon any patient who appeared to 'somatize' his or her psychological discomfort was considered a possible candidate for one of the groups.

The patients were representative of the population served by our publicly supported hospital. They were of various racial origins and few were employed at time of referral. Age has ranged from 20 to 70 years, the majority being in the range 40–55 years. Women outnumbered men by approximately 2:1. Typical medical diagnoses included rheumatoid arthritis, ulcerative colitis, essential hypertension, pain syndromes of various organ systems and hypochondriacal neuroses.

The groups meet weekly for approximately 75 min. They are open-ended in that there is no prescribed number of sessions and patients join and terminate the group at various times. Average attendance at a meeting is 4–6 patients although total membership in each of the groups is 8–12 persons.

The original group is now in its 7th year. Subsequently two other groups have been established, one is now starting its 6th year and the other is in its 2nd year. Some patients have been in one of the groups for as long as 5 years.

The primary therapist of the first group was originally the psychiatrist in charge of the Psychiatric Consultation Service and the co-therapist a psychiatric social worker. At the present time the primary therapist for all three groups is the psychiatric social worker who uses social work graduate students as co-therapists (see below).

Clinical Experience with the Groups

Rather than recount details of the three groups and the specific interactions of each, comments will be limited to generalities transcending the three groups.

Group members with few exceptions were rejecting of any association of physical symptoms to emotional life. They were resentful that they had been referred by their physician and viewed the referral as either a real or potential rejection. If they acknowledged any difficulties in their lives it was because of their maltreatment by their marital partners, children, parents, physicians, etc. They saw themselves as victims rather than perpetrators of conflictual situations and would question, 'Why do these things keep happening to me?' Group discussion was preoccupied with these issues and/or details of physical illnesses, medical treatments or complaints concerning the hospital clinics. For example, there were many complaints about the length of waiting time at the pharmacy. Complaints about physicians were common and there was resentment that the doctors 'can't find a cure'. The patients often looked for 'magical' answers as if only the right doctor or drug could cure their illness. Not infrequently religion would be interjected in a similar fashion with the hope that a higher authority might intervene and relieve their distress.

Efforts of the therapists to redirect the above conversation topics were only minimally successful as group members tended to reinforce each other's resistances rather than to confront each other.

The therapists, in keeping with the planned goals of therapy, made little in the way of interpretations concerning childhood experiences but rather tried to facilitate expression and recognition of affects. It became readily apparent that this was no easy task and one that had to be handled with consumate skill. The primary affect involved was that of anger. Group members related considerable 'resentment' and told tales of mistreatment with varying degrees of expressed or latent anger. However, when questioned or confronted with this anger it was denied. If any significant amount of anger was mobilized in a therapy session the patient generally missed the group the following week. In fact, any session in which the therapist felt some success in getting the group to discuss or deal with affectual issues would be followed by poor attendance at the next meeting by all members. Patients particularly avoided terms such as anger, hostility, rage, etc. They instead used words such as irritation, annoyance, resentment. The therapists learned that it was more therapeutically advantageous to use the patients terminology. For example, an obviously angry patient when asked why he was 'angry' would deny his anger but if asked why he was annoyed might then respond to the question.

The therapists' early experience with the groups was to be too active in fostering affective issues and some patients never returned to the group. Paradoxically, the therapists had had the feeling that they (the therapists) were being too passive and not sufficiently active in therapeutic interventions.

With the most successful group of patients it has taken over 4 years before they could examine issues related to anger at more than a superficial level without adversely affecting attendance. In this group there has gradually developed the capability to verbalize their pattern of avoidance of affectual responses toward each other rather than avoiding the group itself.

In terms of behavior observed in the group setting we were unable to distinguish differences between the various diagnostic categories. Although specific diagnoses were established there appeared to be more similarities than differences, for example, in comparing patients with rheumatoid arthritis with those having back pain considered to be of hysterical or hypochondriacal origin.

Sexual issues were also skirted by group members on the whole. However, sexuality did not seem to have the same degree of importance to these patients as did anger and the group members appeared relatively uninterested in the sexual aspects of their lives. However, sexual problems have been brought up for discussion in instances where a patient felt secure in the group after a lengthy attendance or if a specific meeting was attended by members of only one sex.

Relationships with the marital partners were viewed as being more conflicted in the area of dependence rather than sex. Patients complained that in a variety of ways they were being deprived by the significant others in their lives without any self-realization that their demands were excessive or not realistic.

A major difficulty in these groups was the problem of attendance. Not only was absenteeism common but often patients would start the group, attend once or twice and then fail to return. This, of course, was destructive to the attempts to maintain group cohesiveness and continuity of therapy. With increasing experience, some patterns of introducing new patients to the groups emerged. Those patients who had had the opportunity to see one of the therapists individually for approximately ten sessions, starting with the goal of eventual referral to a group, seemed to do the best. They appeared to develop sufficient attachment to the therapist to continue through the anxiety of attending the initial group meetings. Patients seen only once or twice often failed to follow through with a referral to the group or were early dropouts. Patients seen extensively before referral to the group appeared to have significant difficulty in 'sharing' the therapist with the group and often failed to make the transition from individual to group therapy.

A somewhat fortuitous event changed our view as to what type of therapist is more ideal for the group. Initially, the primary therapist was the physician and this extended over the first several years. However, other commitments necessitated a leave of absence with the psychiatric social worker assuming the role as primary therapist. With the physician out of the group patients were less preoccupied with details of illness and medications and the therapist found it easier to redirect the conversation. There was also an increase in the expressions of resentment toward physicians and feelings of being 'passed on' for their medical care. Because of this reduction in preoccupation with somatic topics the physician is no longer considered the primary therapist and does not attend the group. He remains, however, as the consultant and discusses the week to week meetings with the psychiatric social worker who, as the primary therapist, is assisted by student co-therapists.

Therapeutic gains in these somatizing patients have been modest. Two patients have had complete relief of presenting symptoms. Both had developed pain syndromes fairly acutely in response to situation difficulties. However, for most patients the use of somatic symptoms appeared lifelong and characterological in nature. Some of these patients appeared to make fewer medical clinic visits after starting the group but this observation must be viewed cautiously as patients tended to be referred at times that they were making frequent visits. Some patients appear to have made gains in the quality of their interpersonal relationships or marital situations. Others have made little overt movement but we are encouraged in that those who have improved did so after lengthy therapy with little evidence of progress initially.

A few patients have used the groups in an antitherapeutic fashion. These patients were those who felt under some pressure to seek therapy from the referring physician, attended sessions in a negativistic manner and then proclaimed that because they were no better physically they had proved that they had no psychological problems.

Discussion

As previously mentioned, group psychotherapy of psychosomatic patients is not a new technique. However, evaluation of the efficacy of the method of treatment is fraught with methodological difficulties because of numerous interacting variables. Even an attempt to define 'psychosomatic disease' leads into controversy. What constitutes improvement is also a difficult question. Most chronic diseases that are considered 'psychosomatic' do not have easily measured indices of severity. Psychological parameters such as 'happiness' or 'human relatedness' are even more intangible and less measurable.

This report of clinical experience must be considered anecdotal and reflecting the subjective biases of the authors. However, despite the scientific shortcomings of our experience some observations and comparison with the experience of others will, hopefully, be useful. We personally feel that we have learned from our experience and are now more skilled in working with 'psychosomatic' patients.

The various diagnostic categories of patients with physical complaints did not demonstrate specific differences in our treatment situation. Patients with 'classical psychosomatic' illnesses, hypochondriacal neurosis, hysterical personalities, etc., tended to have more similarities than differences. For practical purposes these patients could be grouped together and considered to be somatizing patients.

The concept of 'emotional illiteracy' (13) or 'alexithymia' (14, 15) was repetitively demonstrated. These somatizing patients had considerable difficulty with the expression, recognition, and description of affect. In fact, we were surprised with the degree to which these patients, who were for all appearances resentful and angry, could not consciously recognize their anger and demonstrated behavior to avoid any potential confrontation with their own, or others', expression of anger. This intensive discomfort with affect and lack of introspection means that the therapist must proceed more cautiously than with the typical neurotic patient and must be accepting of what appears to be little therapeutic work for prolonged periods of time.

It must be questioned, however, whether these findings of alexithymia are specific for patients with 'psychosomatic illness' or whether this is more reflective of the patients' lower socioeconomic status. Of note, *Schwab et al.* (16) have found some correlation between psychosomatic illness and lower socioeconomic status. We are planning a controlled study comparing alexithymic features between those patients applying to the adult outpatient psychiatric clinic versus those referred to the psychosomatic clinic.

In comparing other authors' experience with group therapy of psychosomatic patients we find similarity in the preoccupation with themes of anger, dependency, and repressed sexuality (6, 9, 10, 12). Our treatment results, however, appear more modest than those reported by some (3, 5, 6, 8, 10). This may be related to the fact that our lower socioeconomic status patient population reflected those characteristics related to a less favorable prognosis as reported by *Groen and Pelser* (10). Our patients were certainly different than descriptions of those who had been treated in some of the insight-oriented groups (3, 5, 8).

Another major consideration is the effect of difference in technique. The Dutch group solicited comments about health and responded to them. In contrast we attempted to minimize any concern with physical complaints and deliberately would redirect conversation topics. Admittedly, it is difficult to argue with someone else's success but we continue to have some reservations about encouraging the patients to utilize the defense that we are attempting to modify. However, anxiety provoking methods of treatment for alexithymic patients have been regarded as contraindicated by *Sifneos* (17) and our experience confirms that these patients do have a minimum capacity for tolerating either anxiety or anger. If too aggressively challenged they will not remain in treatment. Therefore one is caught in the double bind of either being completely supportive, with little hope of modifying and perhaps even re-enforcing long-standing patterns of behavior, or attempting a treatment method to which the patient may react adversely or at the least will abandon. A possible solution to this dilemma is a treatment plan in which the therapist skillfully allows carefully measured increments of affect to emerge over a long period of time. Our experience with the most successful group indicated that this can occur but the time period is 3–4 years.

We also observed that our patients demonstrated massive dependency needs and were resentful to physicians for failing to meet these needs. These dependent demands create immediate transference-countertransference problems which must be taken into account in such apparently simple matters as to how many individual sessions should be scheduled prior to the patients starting with the group.

References

1 *Culpan, R. and Davies, B.:* Psychiatric illness at a medical and surgical outpatient clinic. Compr. Psychiat. *1:* 228–235 (1960).
2 *Hilkevitch, A.:* Psychiatric disturbance in outpatients of a general medical outpatient clinic. Int. J. Neuropsychiat. *1:* 371–375 (1965).
3 *Stein, A.:* Group psychotherapy with psychosomatically ill patients; in *Kaplan and Sadock* Comprehensive group psychotherapy (Williams & Wilkins, Baltimore 1971).
4 *Chappell, M.N.; Stefano, J.J.; Rogerson, J.S., et al.:* The value of group psychological procedures in the treatment of peptic ulcer. Am. J. dig. Dis. *3:* 813–817 (1937).
5 *Milberg, I.L.:* Group psychotherapy in the treatment of some neurodermatoses. Int. J. Grp. Psychother. *6:* 53–60 (1956).
6 *Stein, A.; Steinhardt, R.W., and Cutler, S.I.:* Group psychotherapy in patients with peptic ulcer. Bull. N.Y. Acad. Med. *31:* 583–591 (1955).
7 *Titchener, J.L.; Sheldon, M.B., and Ross, W.D.:* Changes in blood pressure of hypertensive patients with and without group psychotherapy. J. Psychosom. Res. *4:* 10–12 (1959).
8 *Fortin, J.N. and Abse, D.W.:* Group psychotherapy with peptic ulcer. Int. J. Grp. Psychother. *6:* 383–391 (1956).
9 *Sclare, A.B. and Crocket, J.A.:* Group psychotherapy in bronchial asthma. J. psychosom. Res. *2:* 157–171 (1957).
10 *Groen, J.J. and Pelser, H.E.:* Experiences with, and results of, group psychotherapy in patients with bronchial asthma. J. psychosom. Res. *4:* 191–205 (1960).
11 *Barendregt, J.T.:* A psychological investigation of the effect of group psychotherapy in patients with bronchial asthma. J. Psychosom. Res. *2:* 115–119 (1957).
12 *Mally, M.A. and Ogston, W.D.:* Treatment of the 'untreatables'. Int. J. Grp. Psychother. *14:* 369–374 (1964).

13   *Freedman, M.B. and Sweet, B.S.:* Some specific features of group psychotherapy and their implications for selection of patients. Int. J. Grp. Psychother. *4:* 355–368 (1954).

14   *Nemiah, J.C. and Sifneos, P.E.:* Affect and fantasy in patients with psychosomatic disorders; in *Hill* Modern trends in psychosomatic medicine (Butterworth, London 1970).

15   *Sifneos, P.E.:* The prevalence of 'alexithymic' characteristics in psychosomatic patients. Psychother. Psychosom. *22:* 255–262 (1973).

16   *Schwab, J.J.; Fennell, F.B., and Warheit, G.J.:* The epidemiology of psychosomatic disorders. Psychosomatics *15:* 88–93 (1974).

17   *Sifneos, P.E.:* Problems of psychotherapy of patients with alexithymic characteristics and physical disease. Psychother. Psychosom. *26:* 65–70 (1975).

Charles V. Ford, MD, Department of Psychiatry, The Neuropsychiatric Institute, 760 Westwood Plaza, *Los Angeles, CA 90024* (USA)

Proc. 11th Eur. Conf. Psychosom. Res., Heidelberg 1976
Psychother. Psychosom. *28:* 305–315 (1977)

The Problems of Group Psychotherapy for Psychosomatic Patients

J.P. Roberts

Introduction

Since the work of *Pratt* (1), 60 years ago, group methods have been used
in the treatment of psychosomatic illness. A number of workers – amongst
them *Sclare and Crocket* (2), *Groen and Pelser* (3), *Jackson* (4), *Ammon* (5),
have experimented with group psychotherapy for patients with psychosomatic disorders, and they claim varying success. Certainly, the group seems
an economic way of treating patients psychotherapeutically in a general
hospital setting. Some authors however, are pessimistic about the value of
group psychotherapy for psychosomatic patients. *Yalom* (6), in 1970, stated
that psychosomatic patients are an anathema to some group therapists and
later in the same book, says that somatizers and generally patients who use
denial as a major method of defence, are poor group referrals. Thus despite
its attractions, group psychotherapy for psychosomatic patients may offer
special problems, which we set out to explore in this pilot study.

Aims of the Work

At King's College Hospital, a London Teaching Hospital, we have
conducted two mixed groups containing psychosomatic patients in the past 4
years. Our primary aim has been to provide therapeutic facilities but,
secondarily, we hoped to observe these groups and carry out limited pilot
research studies. Initially, we hoped to include in our groups only those
patients with true psychosomatic illness, that is, those conditions in which
psychological factors are thought to contribute, through various pathways,

to the development of detectable structural abnormality. For a number of reasons we did not receive sufficient referrals of such patients and modified our aims. We thus arrived at groups composed of psychosomatic patients, together with a number of people whom, for the sake of this paper, I will call heterogeneous somatizers.

Selection of Patients

Referrals were screened and potentially suitable patients were given a 1 to 2-hour preliminary interview to ascertain suitability under the following selection criteria. (1) The patients should present with somatic complaints – with or without detectable structural abnormality. (2) The patient should show evidence of desiring help, together with overt willingness to attend weekly group therapy. (3) The patient should show no evidence of active psychotic illness at the time of referral. (4) The patient should be between 20 and 50 years old. (5) We attempted to avoid those individuals, usually with markedly schizoid characters, and often with paranoid traits, in whom there were indications of an unresolvable fear of groups.

The diagnostic make up of our two groups is set out in tables I and II.

Table I. 1st group (mixed psychosomatic) from 24. 4. 73 to 26. 3. 74

Patient	Age	Sex	Diagnosis	Attendances
M.F.	21	M	asthma	4/39
A.O.	52	M	neurasthenia	21/39
D.S.	45	F	hyperventilation/depression	14/34
V.B.	48	F	tinnitus/ 20 years chronic middle ear disease	28/35
F.F.	56	M	phantom finger (war wound)	29/32
Y.B.	39	F	obesity	18/33
L.T.	41	F	headache and backache	1/34
S.F.	23	M	asthma	2/33
J.deV.	55	M	atypical facial pain[1]	23/32
P.P.	23	F	noninfective conjunctivitis	3/25

[1] Subsequently diagnosed elsewhere: trigeminal migraine.

Table II. 2nd group (mixed psychosomatic) from 3. 6. 75 till now

Patient	Age	Sex	Diagnosis	Attendances
J.W.	35	M	compulsive sighing	26/52
B.T.	28	M	asthma	19/36
M.G.	32	M	chest pain and anxiety	27/37
Y.B.	42	F	obesity hys. dysphonia	34/52
T.G.	38	F	obesity	47/52
J.G.	28	F	uncontrolled diabetes mellitus	17/26
J.E.	26	M	Eczema	1/52
A.B.	27	F	psychogenic vomiting	27/30
E.T.	28	F	asthma	10/13
S.E.	28	M	asthma	1/8

Group Structure and Group Techniques

The groups were once weekly outpatient groups lasting for 1½ h. They were slow open groups with an optimum membership of 8, and for much of the time I was joined by a co-therapist.

Our basic technique was initially the group analytic method as developed by *Foulkes* (7). The focus of our interest was group phenomena and the majority of our interpretations were aimed at the group rather than the individual.

We did, however, interpret to an individual patient his personal conflict or experience of the repetition of early trauma, if we felt it was denied by him and was preventing his relating to the group. This we found particularly necessary with the psychosomatic patient with his apparent tendency to deny intrapsychic conflict, trauma or feelings and his tendency to disavow reality. This is however, a modification of technique which is normally used in the so-called leaderless group, which develops as a result of the group analytic technique.

I should now like to proceed to the observations we have so far made in this project. The observations fall into three categories: (1) the significant dynamics of the group; (2) some numerical observations of the attendance at the groups, and (3) two brief case studies.

The Significant Group Dynamics

The Character of the Group

A striking feature of these psychosomatic groups was their *persistent* unrealistic expectations of me, their therapist. They continued to treat me in a childlike way, as an idealized omnipotent figure, in a manner which I have never experienced in groups of patients with neuroses or personality disorders.

This required active interpretative work. Usually it was suggested that in seeking an omnipotent leader, the individual members of the group were denying the existence of the group as such and further denying its potential helpfulness. Following such interpretations. there was frequently a shift from the dependency orientated group to a group in which pairing occurred. The dependency state alternating with the state of pairing persisted for much of the group time. In an interesting way, the group seemed to take to pairing when they felt that the therapist was refusing to gratify dependency needs, by interpreting the groups dependency on him.

Usually a single pair emerged. In this pair one patient would care for another, whilst the remainder of the group looked on. We feel that this was an enactment of the primitive pairing of the ideal mother/baby unity which disavowed the existence of the rest of the group, who meanwhile regressively participated by primary identification with the mother baby pair. They thus gained vicarious satisfaction from the pairs symbiotic relating. At such times, one obese member of the group would gain additional satisfaction by sucking sweets. These phenomena bear some resemblance to, but are not identical with, *Bion*'s (8, 9) basic assumption phenomena. The sexual and aggressive components of the basic assumptions he described are, however, absent and we feel this is due to the deficits of the psychosomatic patient.

The Patient's Aims in the Group

The groups containing psychosomatic patients seem to pursue comfort as one of their main aims. This aim is often maintained at great cost. It frequently for instance, leads to a disavowal of any changes in the here and now of the groups' existence. The departure of my co-therapist went apparently unnoticed, despite his having been with the group for 9 months. To maintain the reality of this loss without having to experience psychic pain, the group decided that he was an unpleasant person and he was scarcely mentioned again. There was no sense of grief he left. In a similar way, the group totally ignored new patients for as long as 5 weeks on two separate occasions.

In conclusion, our observations suggest that these groups were seeking a need fulfilling part object to comfort them and satisfy their needs. Furthermore, in seeking to establish a comfortable environment in the group, the patients collectively and individually disavowed many events. Thus, painful feelings were avoided.

Countertransference to the Group

Our countertransference to the group was very similar to that which has been described to the individual psychosomatic patient. It was often difficult to maintain attention in the group and the feeling of meaninglessness or even frank boredom in these sessions was often overwhelming.

This experience, in my opinion, contrasts with the typical countertransference feelings aroused in groups containing schizoid patients – who may be regressed to symbiotic object relating. Here the countertransference, mirroring the close cohesiveness of the group is often intense and emotional. The sense of boredom and futility which we experienced was often trying. However, we believe this was a reflection of the strong denial of feelings and disavowal of reality by these patients. Thus, like all countertransference, it was a good guide to the group's current state.

The Individual Patient in the Group

The clinical impression of patients with psychosomatic conditions is that they are poor group attenders. Despite our small numbers, we felt it would be interesting to compare some attendance figures at group psychotherapy for four categories of patients.

Table III shows the mean attendance percentages of samples of four categories of patients attending group psychotherapy at King's College Hospital. The numbers in the samples were small – being 8, 13, 11, and 10,

Table III. Attendance percentage 4 categories of patient

PSM	true psychosomatic patient (from mixed groups)	26%
PD	psychiatric diagnosis group	66%
HS	heterogeneous somatizers (from mixed groups)	64%
AS	asthmatic group (from homogeneous asthmatic group – all women)	34.8%

respectively, each being derived from 1 year in the life of a group. The psychosomatic patients and the heterogeneous somatizers are the patients who were mixed together in the psychosomatic groups we are discussing here. Included with psychosomatic patients is the track record of an ulcerative colitic patient who attended the psychiatric diagnosis group, and incidentally, described it as the worst experience of his life! On the face of it, there appear to be considerable differences in these attendance percentages with two striking aspects – firstly, the low attendance of the truly psychosomatic patient, secondly, the relatively high attendance of the heterogeneous somatizer.

Table IV shows the results of a statistical analysis of the data which suggests that the differences in attendance percentages for these categories of patients are statistically significant.

Table V gives the figures for early drop out rates for the four categories of patient. We have taken those patients who attend 10 or less sessions to be early drop outs.

Table VI offers statistical support for the conclusion that, in our groups, psychosomatic patients tend to drop out of therapy very early.

Finally, I would like to move on and introduce two brief case studies.

Table IV. Statistical analysis – attendance percentages: analysis of variance – the differences in attendance percentages between the 4 groups significant at <0.025 level

Scheffe's Test	
PD – PSM	significant at <0.05 level
HS – PSM	significant at <0.05 level
HS + PD + AS – PSM almost	significant at <0.05 level
Other comparisons not significant	

Table V. Numbers of early drop outs (dropped out in 10 or less sessions)

Psychosomatic patients	6/8
Asthmatics	5/10
Heterogeneous somatizers	2/13
Psychiatric diagnoses	1/11

Table VI. Statistical analysis of relationship between patient type and early drop outs: χ^2 test – small samples

---

a) That psychosomatic patients tend to be early drop outs relative to psychiatric patients – significant at <0.025 level
b) That psychosomatic patients tend to be early drop outs relative to heterogeneous somatizers – significant at <0.025 level
c) The same test with asthmatic patients relative to psychiatric patients and heterogeneous somatizers – NS

Case Studies

One of our observations has been that there is a close relationship between the life situation of the psychosomatic patient and his physical status. The relationship is complex; and working in the group situation frequently made it difficult to be sure which events were related to which.

However, as he functioned in the group there seemed in the individual patient to be a close relationship between: (1) his life situation; (2) acting out; (3) his feeling state, and (4) his physical state.

We felt that we frequently identified a dynamic interaction of these aspects of the patient taking the form shown in figure 1.

I think this is self-explanatory (it is not yet a model – but an attempt to represent our observations). The occurrence of such a positive feed back situation, if our observation is correct, might be held to account in part for the chronicity of the psychosomatic conditions.

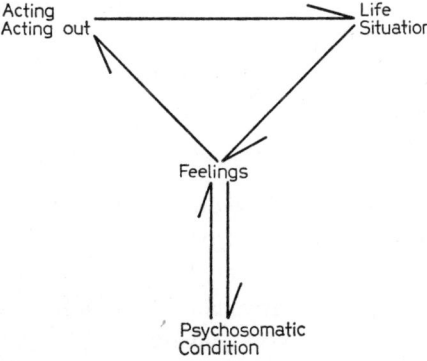

Fig. 1.

It would be impossible to demonstrate completely the interactions of these aspects of a patient in the group but perhaps two brief case studies would be helpful to illustrate the problems.

B.T.

The first case is of a 28-year-old asthmatic motor mechanic who had a lifelong history of accident proneness. He still lived with his mother whom he regarded as his best friend, although he denied any feelings of dependency on her. His father, a schoolmaster, had died 3 years after the patient's asthma started. This had developed after the patient had severely damaged his right hand in an accident at work. I saw him 6 years after the onset of his asthma when he was referred for assessment by our general physicians. They had been struck by his apparent utter indifference to nearly dying during a severe attack of status asthmaticus. At first, he seemed to do reasonably well in the group, remaining asthma free. However, the group including the conductors were struck by his apparent lack of feelings in all fields and by his overt inability to develop an attachment to the group.

After 5 months in the group he went on holiday. On his return he told a story of how, whilst away, he had dressed as an arab in a burnous and gone to a public house for a drink – as a joke. It was felt that this was an acting out, in disguise, of his unackowledged infantile dependency feelings for the group. Feelings which were remote from his consciousness and further displaced onto a public house in Cornwall. Soon after this event – at a time when he seemed to be developing the beginnings of an attachment to the group, he was prosecuted for drunken driving and lost his driving licence. This threatened his managerial post in a lorry building firm. At this time he began to show evidence of becoming depressed in the group whilst complaining that his asthma was worse between meetings. It began to appear that the group would help him contain and work through these feelings of depression – however, he suddenly left and failed to respond to all attempts to contact him.

E.T.

A second asthmatic patient, a 28-year-old woman with a markedly infantile and dependent personality, was referred from our psychiatric day hospital, She had developed asthma and eczema at the age of 18 months. Interestingly, her mother had developed ulcerative colitis within months of the birth of our patient's elder brother. There was a covertly hostile relationship between the patient and her mother, who said she found the demands of her daughter intolerable and seemed to have always done so. Consequently, the patient was sent to a boarding school from an early age and from this time had spent most of her life in schools, hospitals and hostels away from home. She denied any feelings about these separations.

Already improving in the day hospital, her asthma showed a further marked improvement soon after she joined the group. 14 weeks later she suddenly decided that she could no longer stand living in London. She decided to leave London and the group and go to live with her mother in the country. During the latter part of her time in the group, we saw that she became increasingly aware of her separation from her mother and of a longing to be with her. At the same time, she became increasingly depressed and tearful. We feel that in the group she had gained a developing insight into the problems of her longing for attachment to, and the reality of her separation from, her mother. This was accompanied by an experience of psychic pain. Unfortunately, our patient was unable to work through these feelings in the group, but took flight from them, and at the same time acted out her wish to be with mother.

Discussion

We have then had a number of problems with our groups. In brief – patients have been referred in inadequate numbers and when referred they have been reluctant to engage in therapy. In our experience, major factors leading to these problems were as follows.

Firstly, psychosomatic patients are reluctant, in a general hospital setting, to give up the role of the somatically ill person and to assume the role of the psychologically ill person.

Secondly, the patient begins to experience feelings in the group and is soon confronted with disavowed reality. This may lead in its own right to flight from the group or lead to almost compulsive acting out, for instance to delinquent acts, to rows with the boss, or extramarital sexual affairs. This frequently worsens the patient's life situation leading to an exacerbation of the experience of psychic pain. Flight from this situation, apparently caused by the group, then seems to the patient to be his only option.

Finally, the psychosomatic patient seems unable to understand the group context. The emotional ties and currents in a group seem totally beyond his comprehension, and in our groups, he will only meaningfully relate in 2-person relationships. For the patient feeling deprived of gratification by the group leader there is little in this, to him, meaningless situation which can be seen as an incentive to continuing attendance. Thus it is very difficult to hold these patients, when they begin to experience painful feelings.

Hoping to alleviate these difficulties, we have made a number of modifications in our technique.

Firstly, we have become far more active than we are in neurotic groups, usually in a supportive way.

Secondly, we have attempted to modify our interpretations to avoid interpreting the defences of denial and disavowal too early or too directly – leaving the patients defenceless. Nonetheless, within these limitations we have maintained our aims of bringing to life and containing our patient's feelings, whilst ensuring as much confrontation with reality as we felt could be tolerated.

Finally, we have made vigilant attempts to identify potential drop outs and pointed out our fears of this in the group session. We have been guided particularly by suggestions from a patient that he has acted, or is about to act, to change his life situation.

As a result of our work in these groups, we feel we have again raised questions posed previously. For instance – in what ways can group therapy help the ego – damaged psychosomatic patient who finds it hard, or even impossible, to relate to a group. Can group therapy help these patients to change from their habitual one, to one relating. Or to go a little further is a situation involving verbal relating only, the best therapy for patients feeling more at ease when they can relate non verbally or through action. Should consideration be given to using methods such as psychodrama, or encounter techniques, in which action is as important as words, and through which psychosomatic patients might slowly learn to undo the dissociation between thought and feeling.

Further, the compromise of composing homogeneous groups of patients with the same disorder might be advantageous. This can offer a setting for cross-identification, as a possible first step towards group relating proper. Our experience of a homogeneous group of asthma patients was suggestive of a more consistant attendance than at the mixed psychosomatic groups.

We were left, however, with a strong impression that it is not only modifications of technique that may be required for effective group therapy for psychosomatic patients. What we clearly need in addition, is more knowledge about such patients in terms of their capacity for object relationships.

In the 1:1 doctor/patient relationship, the psychosomatic patient frequently demonstrates the deficits of alexithymia which we have discussed at length in this conference. However, a further dimension is added to this deficit when we observe the psychosomatic patient in the group situation. Here, in our experience, he shows a marked limitation in his capacity to take part in triangular relationships, which we feel is worthy of further study in the group context.

Acknowledgements

I should like to thank Drs. *Murray Jackson* and *Margret Tonnesman*, King's College Hospital, for much help, advice and support, and Drs. *K. Hyde* and *K.R. Mayne*, my co-therapists.

References

1   *Pratt, J.H.:* The class method of treating consumption in the homes of the poor. J. Am. med. Ass. *49:* 755 (1907).
2   *Sclare, A.B. and Crocket, A.J.:* Group psychotherapy in bronchial asthma. J. Psychosom. Res. *2:* 157 (1957).
3   *Groen, J.J. and Pelser, H.E.:* Experiences with group psychotherapy in patients with bronchial asthma. J. Psychosom. *4:* 191 (1960).
4   *Forth, M. and Jackson, M.:* Group psychotherapy in bronchial asthma. 10th Eur. Conf. Psychosom. Res., Edinburgh 1974.
5   *Ammon, G.:* Analytic group therapy as an instrument for the treatment and research of psychosomatic disorders: in *Wolberg and Aronson* Group therapy 1975 an overview, p. 127 (Stratton, New York 1975).
6   *Yalom, I.:* The theory and practice of group psychotherapy, p. 157, pp. 174–175 (Basic Books, New York 1970).
7   *Foulkes, S.H.:* Group analytic psychotherapy (Interface, New York 1974).
8   *Bion, W.R.:* Experiences in groups (Tavistock, London 1961).
9   *Bion, W.R.:* Group dynamics. A review; in *Klein, Heiman and Moneykyrle* New directions in psychoanalysis, p. 440 (Tavistock, London 1955).

Dr. *J.P. Roberts,* MA, BM, BCh, DPM, MRCPsych, consultant Psychiatrist, Ingrebourne Centre, 56 Georges Hospital, *Hornchurch, Essex* (England)

Proc. 11th Eur. Conf. Psychosom. Res., Heidelberg 1976
Psychother. Psychosom. *28:* 316–322 (1977)

Behavioural Characteristics in In-Patient Group Psychotherapy with Psychosomatic Patients

A. Sellschopp-Rüppell

Psychosomatische Universitätsklinik Heidelberg

In the literature on the theory of the disease and of the personality of the psychosomatic patient there are comparatively few indications of experience in therapy. When these are given, they refer mainly to classical individual analysis and modifications of this (*Marty* 1957).

In the following address I should like to discuss observations on the behaviour of the psychosomatic patient during in-patient group therapy.

On the basis of clinical experience we have formed the opinion that in-patient therapy with analytically oriented group psychotherapy is indicated for a large proportion of those psychosomatic patients who are otherwise often given an unfavourable prognosis.

The therapeutic work with these patients in the Psychosomatic Clinic in Heidelberg comprises, besides group psychotherapy, sensual awareness therapy (konzentrative Bewegungstherapie), ergotherapy, and life in the in-patient community. The group therapy takes place for 60 min five times a week over a period of 3 months. The groups of patients are mixed with regard to age, sex and social status – as implied by their profession, and they contain both psychoneurotic and psychosomatic patients.

The ward team consist of the ward doctor, occupational therapist, sensual awareness therapist, group therapist, nurses and night nurses (*Bräutigam,* 1974; *von Rad and Rüppell,* 1975).

The empirical observations in the present paper are part of a project on group psychotherapy processes in in-patient psychotherapy which has been pursued in our clinic for the last 2 years[1]. Using the test persons involved in the project (n = 45) we formed two groups of patients. One group with psycho-

[1] We should especially like to thank Dr. *Kächele* and Dr. *Grünzig* of the University of Ulm for their advice and support.

neurotic and another group with psychosomatic patients in the narrower sense, i.e., patients suffering from organ-destructive symptoms (n = 26). The groups are comparable in terms of age, sex and social status.

The data used for comparison are:

(1) The initial prognostic data before treatment began. We compared selected interview data, Rorschach und intelligence test scores (Hamburg-Wechsler).

(2) Data from the group therapeutic process: interaction frequency and direction of interaction, and a quotient which reflects the ratio of emotional to objective content in an interaction. This quotient was won with *Bales* (1970) interaction process categories and represents the sum of the social-emotional vs. the sum of the task-oriented categories. The group data were taken by a team of observers (n = 4) by means of one-way screen and tape recordings. For the present work we assessed the first 20 min of every 7th session (n = 7). The data were compiled according to three periods (intervals) and thus the groups were compared at the beginning of the therapy, in the middle, and at the end of the in-patient treatment.

(3) Data from ward behaviour: the team – 6 raters for every patient – with no insight into the group process, filled in an interpersonal question-naire with a high correlation to Bales categories (Interpersonal Rating, Scheme A, *Bales*, 1970).

(4) A catamnestic index. This index was made by the therapists by assessment of each patient in the course of the out-patient follow-up treat-ment, in the last third of the treatment period. It represents a rather rough assessment of therapeutic success divided into five questions relating to symptoms and social behaviour. The answers were added up to give a total index of improvement for each patient (fig. 1).

We now come to the individual findings: (all the data were won with the aid of the biomedical data programme (BMDP), University of Los Angeles):

(1) The initial prognostic data:

Of the 15 Rorschach items tested only 4 showed different values for psychoneurotic and psychosomatic patients. Psychoneurotic patients give more controlled colour and shade responses (FC, FK, Fc). Psychosomatic patients give more uncontrolled colour answers and more animal movement answers (CF, AM) that is to say, they give more affect and drive-laden answers (F = 3.29, p<0.06; F = 6.30, p<0.06; F = 3.27, p<0.053).

It seemed noteworthy to us that the psychosomatic patients showed on average 8 IQ points more in the verbal theoretical part of the intelligence test than the psychoneurotic patients. (F = 3.93 p<0.025).

Catalogue of variables

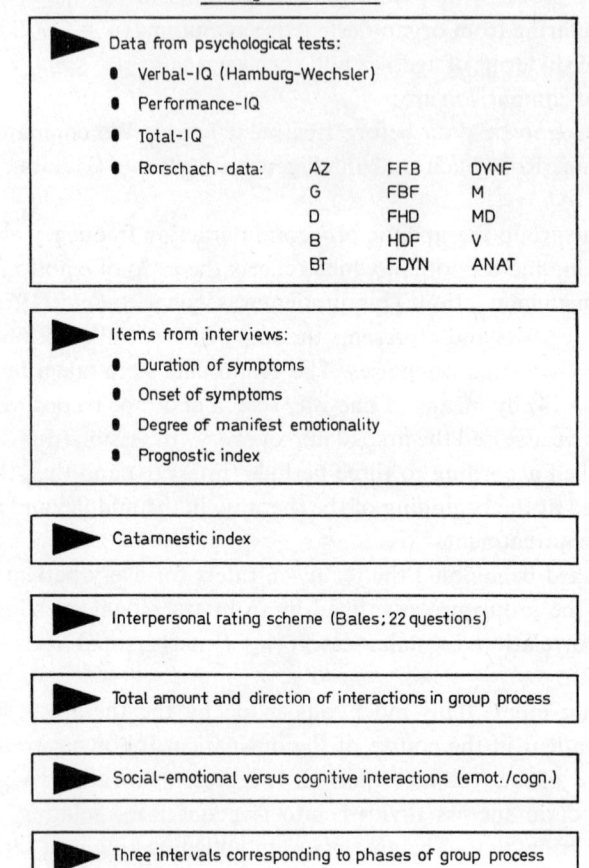

Data from psychological tests:
- Verbal-IQ (Hamburg-Wechsler)
- Performance-IQ
- Total-IQ
- Rorschach-data:

AZ	FFB	DYNF
G	FBF	M
D	FHD	MD
B	HDF	V
BT	FDYN	ANAT

Items from interviews:
- Duration of symptoms
- Onset of symptoms
- Degree of manifest emotionality
- Prognostic index

Catamnestic index

Interpersonal rating scheme (Bales; 22 questions)

Total amount and direction of interactions in group process

Social-emotional versus cognitive interactions (emot./cogn.)

Three intervals corresponding to phases of group process

1

This last finding seems to us to indicate that the average psychosomatic patient who is a candidate for one of the therapeutic groups must be more intelligent than the average psychoneurotic patient.

The only interview variable that differentiated between the groups is the prognosis given by the interviewer at the end of the initial interview in respect of the actual therapeutic chances a patient has (this is a general subjective clinical assessment). The prognoses are, namely, less favourable for psychosomatic patients than for psychoneurotic patients ($\chi^2 = 3.939$, $p < 5\%$).

(2) Results of the group sessions:

(a) The psychosomatic patient shows a greater interaction frequency than the psychoneurotic patient does (for the emotional categories F = 2.87, p<0.008, d.f. 12.12; for the task-oriented categories F = 2.38, p<0.026, d.f. 12.12). This is particularly true in the initial time interval and it declines in the course of treatment. If one looks at the who-to-whom matrix one sees the dynamics of the directions of the interactions: initially, both groups show a strong tendency to create sub-groups with their own kind. This tendency is, however, doubly strong in psychosomatic patients and it weakens less during the course of treatment than it does with psychoneurotic patients. (The absolute interaction frequencies were taken from comparison, as in the individual groups the size of the sub-groups is almost equal in respect of members. The values are calculated in a simple χ^2-test and give significances of p<0.01 for all time intervals except with the middle one with the psychoneurotic patients; fig. 2, 3).

(b) The differentiation of the contents of the interactions was expressed in a quotient – described above – which reflects the ratio of the social-emotional vs. the task oriented categories of Bales. The psychosomatic patients in these groups show more emotional contents in their interactions than the psychoneurotics do (time interval 1: F = 2.87, p<0.008; time interval 2: F = 3.07, p<0.005; time interval 3: F = 3.03, p<0,006) (fig. 4). Could this be an indication that a certain defence strategy exists in the psychosomatic patient? Or does it point to a possibility these patients have to behave in a relatively conscious way, that is controlled and appropriate to the situation, even in the psychotherapeutic setting, i.e., to show feelings as is expected of them?

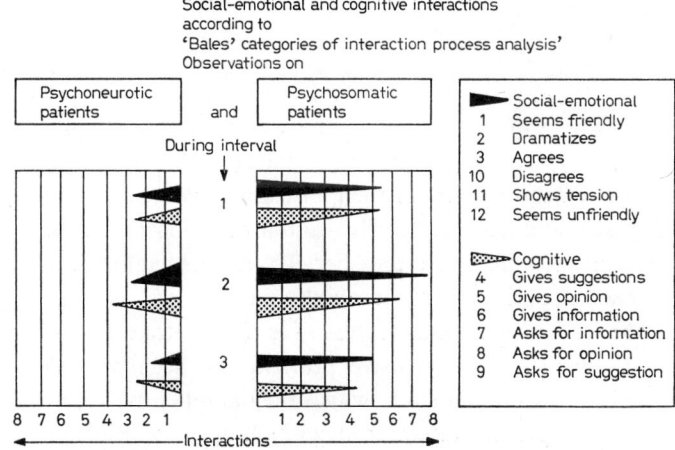

Social-emotional and cognitive interactions according to 'Bales' categories of interaction process analysis' Observations on

Psychoneurotic patients	and	Psychosomatic patients

During interval

Social-emotional
1 Seems friendly
2 Dramatizes
3 Agrees
10 Disagrees
11 Shows tension
12 Seems unfriendly

Cognitive
4 Gives suggestions
5 Gives opinion
6 Gives information
7 Asks for information
8 Asks for opinion
9 Asks for suggestion

8 7 6 5 4 3 2 1   1 2 3 4 5 6 7 8
2   ←————————Interactions————————→

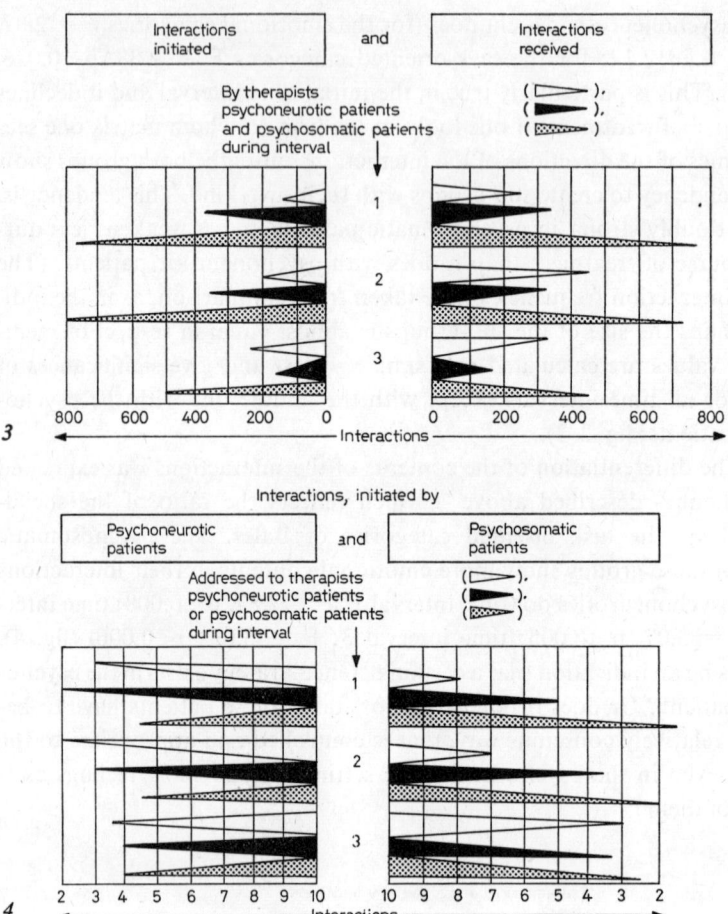

Reservations regarding the methods by which these findings were obtained should, however, also be clearly expressed: they exist in the impreciseness of the Bales categories, i.e. in their instrumental unsuitability for recording emotional contents differentially – and in the procedure described, in which the interactions were added together. To take an example: the values of the emotional categories of psychosomatic patients are very strongly influenced by the category 2 'dramatizes'. We found that psychosomatic patients very frequently give extensive positive and negative diffuse descriptions of their situation and state, which they amplify even more by the introduction of analogies and attempts at symbolisation. For instance, when a 20-year-old patient with colitis ulcerosa sees himself under attack from an older patient for neglecting his studies, he replies by telling a long and very involved story of how he once broke down the whole electric system in his parents' house by a short circuit.

The categories of Bales do not differentiate between the attitude of the speaker and the content of his verbal interaction; they do not, moreover, differentiate between different emotional aspects, e.g., emotions and feelings (*Sifneos*, 1975); i.e. no statemnets are made about the whole structural aspect.

We should, however, like to suppose that a typical characteristic of psychosomatic patients is expressed in this tendency to verbal activity in relation to verbal emotionnally-tuned contents, which points to a certain form of ego-weakness.

We found in our investigation that the most conspicuous changes in the group appear in the time between the second and the third intervals. The differences between the first and second intervals are less clear. We should like to suppose that this represents a characteristic trend of group development towards greater differentiation but also towards greater cohesion.

(3) The data of the interpersonal rating by the in-patient team:

These show that they see the psychosomatic patient as someone who adapts easily to a community when he has to, but who is often insensitive to the needs of others, demands very much time for himself and contributes less to interpersonal contentedness in group as he is very strongly interested in satisfying his own requirements, especially where status in the group is concerned. To this end he is very skilled at using strategies which arise from the actual situation. The psychoneurotic patient on the other hand is seen as a group member whose manifest group activity is less but whose inner engagement is greater and who in the course of time contributes more to the contentedness of all those in the group. (The individual items of the questionaire were provided with 'directional indicators' in accordance with a 3-dimensional calculation system drawn up by *Bales and Couch* (1970) and both groups were compared in respect of the dominant type emerging from it. The essential difference was on the upward-downward dimension.)

(4) The catamnestic index:

We found no difference in the catamnestic grading between psychosomatic and psychoneurotic patients regarding their degree of improvement as rated by the therapist during out-patient follow-up treatment.

This gives a sufficient correlation between the initial prognostic rating, given by the interviewer, and the catamnesis for the psychoneurotic but not for the psychosomatic patients. ($\chi^2 = 3.891$, p<5%). With the latter the prognoses, which were given at the end of the interview before commencement of treatment, and the catamnesis are more frequently opposed. We suppose that the treatment strategies of the therapist are oriented more to the objective findings and perhaps to a psychodynamic hypothesis sensu Malan and not so much to prognostic assessment. In this case the catamnestic index would validate the first data.

Among the group psychotherapy data we, like other authors, found no correlation between the degree of verbal activity of a patient and his treatment success.

The differentiation of the groups according to diagnosis seems in our investigation to be the most fruitful criterion. No other variable of group division which we tested yielded strictly significant results.

Finally, despite existing methodological problems which apply particularly to test defects, the time variables and the random selection in itself, we should like to draw from this first investigation the cautious conclusion that we have obtained sufficient indications justifying group psychotherapy in an in-patient setting for psychosomatic patients.

We have as yet cast little light on the actual psychotherapeutic process. Further investigations should concentrate on this in particular. In our opinion a promising starting point for this would be the psychosomatic patient's increased verbal interaction frequency.

References

Bales, R.: Personality and interpersonal behavior (Holt, Rinehart & Winston, New York 1970).

Bräutigam, W.: Pathogenetische Theorien und Wege der Behandlung in der Psychosomatik. Nervenarzt *45:* 354–363 (1974).

Marty, M.; M'Uzan, M. de et David, C.: L'investigation psychosomatique (Presses universitaires, Paris 1963).

Marty, P.: Die allergische Objektbeziehung; in *Brede* Einführung in die psychosomatische Medizin (Athenäum/Fischer, Frankfurt/M. 1974).

Rad, v.M. and Rüppell, A.: Combined inpatient and outpatient group psychotherapy. A therapeutic model for psychosomatics. Psychother. Psychosom. *26:* 237–243 (1975).

Sifneos, P.E.: Problems of psychotherapy of patients with alexithymic characteristics and physical disease. Psychother. Psychosom. *26:* 65–70 (1975).

Almuth Sellschopp-Rüppell, PhD, Psychosomatische Klinik der Universität Heidelberg, Vossstrasse 2, *D-6900 Heidelberg 1* (FRG)

Proc. 11th Eur. Conf. Psychosom. Res., Heidelberg 1976
Psychother. Psychosom. *28:* 323–329 (1977)

Group Psychotherapy of Patients with Somatic Illnesses and Alexithymia

Roberta Apfel-Savitz, Daniel Silverman, and Michael I. Bennett

Department of Psychiatry of the Beth Israel Hospital, and Harvard Medical School, Boston, Mass.

Psychotherapy for patients with somatic problems and alexithymic characteristics has been the subject of much discussion. As part of an ongoing departmental interest in the development of specific criteria of selection of patients for various modalities of therapy, Dr. *Peter Sifneos* has written about the contraindication of psychodynamic therapy in patients with psychosomatic disorders and recommended anxiety-suppressive therapeutic intervention (1). Individual psychotherapy even when supportive and intermittent can be a frustrating experience for both therapist and patient when the therapy is complicated by a chronic medical problem, passivity, regressed functioning, and difficulty in communicating affects. Group therapy offers an alternative outpatient treatment that provides a structured social environment in which new behavior can be learned. It presents the possibility of developing a social network compatible with the patient's level of functioning. This paper will discuss the authors' 2 years of experience with a group of patients which has, by means of guided talk about feelings and the use of videotape, improved interactional skills and physical functioning.

Group psychotherapy has been used increasingly for theoretical and practical reasons. Inpatient groups of psychotic, severely character disordered, and psychosomatic patients have become an established part of the milieu therapy which is so helpful with these disturbed populations (2,3). It is unusual for the alexithymic patient with a physical disorder to require psychiatric hospitalization; these patients may present at the psychiatric clinic asking for help with anxiety or coping with the medical problem and its sequelae, but more likely they are referred to psychiatry because of their multiple visits to the other clinics and emergency ward, their thick charts and the desire of the other medical staff to contain the anxiety and reduce overuse of nonpsychiatric clinic services by concentrating the transference in one place.

Alexithymia, by definition the lack of ability to express feelings, creates problems of relating to the world. Even young infants who are relatively unresponsive types have been shown to create negative responses within their environment so that coolness and rigidity are met with the same in adults who parent them (4). So, alexithymic adults tend to develop socializing patterns that defy our usual concept of a social group. Their relations are constricted and restricted to factual, minimal contact. Further attempts to relate are clumsy and often met with misunderstanding that can be inter-preted as lack of interest and further the isolation of the alexithymic indivi-dual. This communication problem may be present from infancy, a primary perhaps biological difficulty, or develop with frustrating environmental interaction later in life. The association of alexithymic characteristics with somatic illness indicates the way in which physical expressions of feelings become a modality when other means, e.g., verbal affective, are not available (5). It becomes important for people with this communication difficulty to have an experience in a social group where special techniques can be used to overcome a maladaptive pattern.

Our group of 6 patients met every other week with male and female co-therapists. All patients had somatic illnesses (thyrotoxicosis, epilepsy, ulcera-tive colitis, peptic ulcer, eye spasms, hypertension) that precluded their work-ing at regular jobs. All had been seen previously and unsuccessfully in indivi-dual psychotherapy; they were called the 'unolvables' and 'rejects'. Some had had previous psychiatric admissions and some were taking psychotropic medications (trifluoperazine, perphenazine) for paranoia and anxiety. No one was actively psychotic. Except for the woman with hypertension who related as a depressive-neurotic character, the others initially fulfilled the criteria of 'alexithymic' characteristics on our standard psychosomatic questionnaire (6). The bimonthly meetings were a major event in the lives of these patients who often reported that their days had become empty, and yet the option of meeting more regularly was perceived as a communication that their problems were serious enough to necessitate more 'help'. Members also seemed uncomfortable with the potential closeness more frequent meet-ings might bring. Cohesiveness formed around the common experience of the group itself, and the shared physical and social problems.

Interaction at first was minimal. Each member would sit in the rigid posture characteristic of these patients, making no eye contact, often not removing outdoor, barricading garments. In turn, each would offer a detailed news report. It seemed to be a kind of parallel play, directed toward no one at first. Sometimes the reports were given to the therapists, as if to tentatively relate with the parental figures. The content of each statement resembled what was said by each member the previous week and had no affectual relation to what the other members of the group were stating or experiencing. It was an anchor place for marking the passage of time, the holidays, and the months. The group served the purpose of 'a transitional object', (as *von Rad and Ruppell* (3) have reported), a consistent sheltered place within the parent hospital. There was acceptance of the patient role of each other and of the group as a unit, but few of the other values known to be important in group therapy were significantly present: self disclosure, honesty regarding feelings, nondefensiveness, and empathy (7).

Interchanges between the neurotic member, the therapists, and the 'alexithymic' members dramatically demonstrated the difficulties in communication experienced between them. The 'alexithymic' person's isolation may be furthered in attempts to relate, and the neurotic may experience the lack of understanding as a personal affront.

The neurotic woman talked with great sadness and resentfulness about her dying mother for whom she was sacrificing her life and who she was losing in spite of her efforts. The other group members sat in passive, constricted silence, apparently perplexed and withdrawing, until she yelled, 'What kind of a nut am I? Hasn't anyone here ever lost a loved one?' There was more silence and then another member volunteered that his grandmother had died just 6 weeks ago (an event he had never reported) and proceeded to give great details about her life, her role in his life, and her death. Another group member said, struggling, that he had lost his father who moved to California and then talked for a long time about the West Coast.

The neurotic woman requested an individual session in which she apologetically reported her frustration with the group, how much better she felt talking individually with an empathetic therapist, and her desire to drop out. Instead of leaving, she has had periodic individual meetings with one of the therapists, an option open to all group members but infrequently used by the others. Also, she has become the spokesperson for diffident members with problems who confide in her and allow her to speak for them in the meetings. This ability to speak for another person, to empathize to the extent of feeling or even telling another's problem is not present in the alexithymic individuals. One way of learning to cope is to become an observer of others who are not alexithymic as the group member who reported he knew he was angry only when he watched those around him and someone said 'What are you angry about?'

Rather than by verbal, empathic means, identification within the group takes place through physical symptoms.

A younger man who had peptic ulcer disease had a gastrectomy which 'cured' his ulcer pain. He began to consistently sit next to an older man in the group but never talked with him or faced him or seemed to notice and comment on the older man's legal blindness and anxiety-related blepharospasm. Within a month, the young man had a new symptom of similar eye spasms and facial grimacing which became the focus of any discomfort he felt and prevented him from working. The symptom similarity and behavior was evident and impressive to the therapists, but it was only after a year that the 2 group members shared verbally the fact that they had a common problem.

Two members who had major surgery: gastrectomy and thyroidectomy often wondered aloud when faced with a poorly-understood crisis whether more surgery, a means of active problem solution, might be necessary for them.

This young male ulcer patient, in his early twenties, has related to the group as a pet and, as members have begun to observe each other, there has been parental interest in him. He has apparently profited more than the others (all of whom are past 40 years old) from specific tutoring the therapists have done in naming feelings, discussing feeling states, and practicing these newly-developed skills. He has begun to talk about a time prior to teens when he 'felt' and refers to a re-emergence of feelings in the therapy that other group members have not so clearly recognized. This observation has raised for us the question of a secondary type of alexithymia more akin to severe repression, and different from, and perhaps more remediable in therapy than a primary biologically mediated process, similar to Dr. *Freyberger's* (5) theoretical conceptualization.

Videotape has been used to record the patients' progress and group behavior. The poignant struggle of the alexithymic patient learning to talk about feelings is demonstrated clearly on an excerpt of tape to follow. Here the questions on the schedule used to self-test for alexithymic characteristics (and reported by Dr. *Sifneos* at this meeting) is discussed:

'How would you feel if a policeman arrested you for a crime you did not commit? What thoughts do you have? Please give example.' Our young group member said he would feel *afraid* and associated to a time he had been picked up by the police for drunkenness when he was 15 years old; he launched into the pensée opératoire, typical endless details about the parole officer, his brother who is 15, etc. When pressed about the feeling by one of us *(DS)* he says he might feel *angry,* which would have in the past made his abdomen hurt and now makes his face grimace; then details about how he would lie in bed for hours concentrating all thought on the ulcer pain and forgetting the angry feeling or precipitating event. 'Pain – no one else can feel yours' he says. Other group members use appropriate words, e.g., 'indignant', 'resentful', but cannot give accompanying thoughts or fantasies. When a patient who has been silent is asked what her feelings would be, she becomes noticeably more anxious and says 'all of the above – angry, indignant, and resentful… I'm not good at expressing myself… It's hard to talk of feelings. I get sick in the stomach, trembling like butterflies…' (show video, first segment). This exercise repeatedly introduced words about feelings. Both the questionnaire and the videotaping allowed sharing of common experiences, annoyances against which the whole group united and reluctantly consented. Productive discussions first developed around something recognizable, e.g., What is a blush? Has anyone ever blushed? When? Feelings? Incidents?

While the anxiety level initially increased, the taping was done frequently enough to become an accepted part of the group process. The microphone was centered in the patient circle and the camera was outside the room on the other side of a one-way mirror. There has been great interest in reviewing the tapes, embarassment at seeing themselves on television, but also flattery and a sense of observation about individual and group behavior that is not possible to convey otherwise. The high level of anxiety is apparent to therapists who are incredulous when these patients ask 'What is anxiety?' and the videopictures convey the state in a more readily understood way than verbal descriptions can.

Meditation, as the noncultic relaxation response, has been used as a technique to reduce anxiety (8). This response usually is easily induced and similar to the hypnotic trance in its psychophysiological properties. Stokvis has previously reported on his experience using hypnosis in the treatment of psychosomatic patients (9). The striking need to deny anxiety or the lack of self-observation about it, led group members to be reluctant to try it. Comments ranged from:

'It might be dynamite for someone with a problem, but not for me', from a man with ulcerative colitis to 'I don't have anything to think of when I'm quiet' perhaps expressing the terror of the absent fantasy world.

The rigid posturing and lack of flexible interrelating body language is characteristic of the alexithymic person and becomes even more pronounced for some during the programmed attempt at relaxation. When increasing muscular tension, social grimacing, and restlessness occur, the contrast with the therapists' reaction to meditation is striking. The group experience of meditation gave a common physical experience to discuss and as such allowed people to talk about physical feelings, something more as a step in their learning about verbalizing feelings of all kinds (tape).

Group members have increasingly bound together as a social unit within and outside of the hospital setting. They share mutual suspiciousness about difficult social agencies with which they must deal for welfare income and complain about relatives and neighbors who make life difficult. Doctors and hospitals are disappointing at times but necessary and appreciated. Affective situations or potentially important events in the group such as vacation of a therapist are noted in passing as part of the monotonous dialogue. Life is hard, everyone has real problems, the stigma of psychiatric care and the 'crazy people, worse than us who don't understand psychiatry' are frequent topics. With increasing trust and contacts shared, members have revealed a few intimate thoughts especially about low esteem, e.g., never having read a book, incarceration for shoplifting or failure to finish school. Having a community of people who are all adjusting to low achievement and dependency has provided a friendlier place than the real world for most of these patients. They maintain some phone contact between sessions and have visited each other in hospitals on the few occasions that group members have required hospitalization.

A recent tragedy within the group has been the first event to focus the group affectively: a patient with thyrotoxicosis, a woman in her 40's committed suicide 3 months ago in another hospital to which she had admitted herself. The mutual shock, fear, blame, and appropriate sadness demonstrated by the group members showed the extent to which contact had been made and emotional interaction had developed. While the therapists and patients asked the inevitable questions about how we had failed and felt that the group as a therapeutic entity had disappointed this patient, there was the most genuine expression of feeling among everyone to date. The admission of despair and suicidal ideas by another patient, the recognition that doctors are not omnipotent and hospitals not totally protective seems to have been integrated cognitively as well as affectively with some resignation. There continues to be the telling paucity of fantasy when patients start talking about the dead patient in group and say that they have no thought of her between sessions, no image other than in the group itself (video excerpt).

In summary, it is our impression that a group psychotherapy experience using special techniques: guided teaching, concrete, visual feedback such as that provided by videotape, a neurotic member translator, meditation, can offer a new and important learning arena to the 'psychosomatic' patient. It was also a chance to increase our understanding of patients with 'alexithymic' characteristics and our therapeutic skills with them in an economical way. We have been impressed especially in the last episode of the suicide with the gains the individuals in the group have made. The way in which the members were able to stay together despite their fears and limitations, and to talk about the circumstances of the death and even some feelings, was well beyond their previous pattern of translating emotion to physical symptoms. The longevity of the group as a unit and continuity of therapy has provided a contrast to the usual rejection, and fragmented care experienced by these patients. Despite severe longstanding and continuing problems, the group members are starting to move out of the prison of the alexithymic character by relating to each other and the therapists over a long time.

References

1 Sifneos, P.E.: Is dynamic psychotherapy contraindicated for a large number of patients with psychosomatic diseases? Psychother. Psychosom. 21: 133–136 (1972/ 1973).

2 Jones, M.: Social psychiatry: A study of therapeutic communities (Tavistock, London 1952).

3 Rad, von M. and Ruppell, A.: Combined inpatient and outpatient group psychotherapy. A therapeutic model for psychosomatics. Psychother. Psychosom. 26: 237–243 (1975).

4 Brazelton, T.B.: Infants and mothers, afferences in development (Delta, New York 1969).

5 Freyberger, H.: Personal communication to P.E. Sifneos.

6 Sifneos, P.E.: The prevalence of 'alexithymic' characteristics in psychosomatic patients. Psychother. Psychosom. 22: 255–262 (1973).

7 Yalom, I.D.: The theory and practice of group psychotherapy (Basic Books, New York 1970).

8 Benson, H.: The relaxation response (Morrow, New York 1975).

9 Stokvis, B.: Hypnosis as a method and principle of research in psychosomatic individuals; in Jones and Freyberger Advances in psychosomatic medicine (Brunner, New York 1961).

Roberta Apfel-Savitz, MD, MPH, Harvard Medical School, Beth Israel Hospital, 330 Brookline Avenue, Boston, MA 02215 (USA)

Proc. 11th Eur. Conf. Psychosom. Res., Heidelberg 1976
Psychother. Psychosom. *28:* 330–336 (1977)

A Non-Verbal Therapeutic Approach to Psychosomatic Disorders

H. Becker

Psychosomatische Universitätsklinik Heidelberg

If one considers the current literature on psychosomatic medicine with regard to its theories on aetiology and pathogenesis on the one hand and its therapeutic efforts on the other, a considerable discrepancy becomes apparent. The therapeutic measures hardly go beyond either a modified neurosis therapy in the sense of an analytical psychotherapy or a parallel treatment by psychotherapists and somatic doctors.

I should like now to investigate these indications to a possible modification to analytical psychotherapy.

In his work 'The Infantile Personality' published in 1948, *Ruesch* writes of the necessity for a modification in the direction of child psychotherapy. He considers it important to establish a symbiotic relationship between doctor and patient in the initial phase of therapy to allow the patient to imitate the therapist and to identify with him. He compares this to the symbiotic relationship between mother and child.

In the development of a metapsychology of somatisation, *Schur* (1955) points out that it frequently becomes clear during the analysis of psychosomatic patients that a regression to a pre-verbal, pre-ego stage of development has taken place. His therapeutic procedure differs little from the classical analytical treatment. He speaks of the necessity of leading the patient out of the deep regression as quickly as possible by way of verbalisation, but mentions the difficulty psychosomatic patients have in verbalising or in keeping to the basic rule of reacting to verbal interpretation from the analyst. A clear technical instruction for the therapist, as to how he can introduce the process of desomatisation in the psychosomatic patient who is largely resistent to verbal interpretations, is not given. He does, however, mention the method described by *Kaufman* (1953) and *Margolin* (1953) of using anaclitic therapy in the severest cases of psychosomatic disorders. Apart from this he recommends a preparative therapy consisting of a combination of somatic treatment and supportive psychotherapy.

In accordance with his therapeutic concept of a common aetiology for both psychosomatic disorders and neuroses, *Mitscherlich* (1967) holds that inceptions of therapy will be the same for both. With 11–40% of psychosomatic patients, however, he finds that no therapy takes place because of lack of communication between doctor and patient. He states that with these patients the defence remained unarticulated and he speaks in this connection of so-called primitive personalities. Here he recommends medicinal treatment or suggestive procedures.

De Boor and Mitscherlich (1973) mention the possibility that our analytical treatments, which are already so long drawn-out, have not yet penetrated far enough into non- and pre-verbal level of experience. In his theoretical model of the basic fault, *Balint* (1968) included the psychosomatic disease. He speaks of the necessity of being restrained with verbal interpretations. The language of grown-ups is often misleading and useless, as the words often no longer have their conventional meaning. Interpretations are often perceived by the patients as attack, criticism, direction or stimulation. He refers to the necessity of giving the patient the time and the milieu in the first phase of the therapy to offer himself as a primary object. He also takes a largely pre-verbal communication between therapist and patient as a starting-point.

Brocher (1967) mentions *Freud's* idea that verbal communication and dialogue are of the greatest importance in the development of the earliest identifications. On the other hand, he quotes *Spitz* (1965) who has shown that motor and sensory identifications precede the verbal ones in this dialogue and that these are indispensable for the child in the parent-child relationship. *Brocher* (1967) states furthermore that the attitude to averbal expressive communication has only changed since the turning of interest from drive analysis to defence analysis. He quotes *Reich* (1948) who pointed out that the defence is manifested both in bodily movement and in the expressive gestures. While the significance of the incognito and abstinence rule for the secondary process is undisputed, *Brocher* (1967) questions whether, when keeping strictly to this rule, the averbal communication by the analyst can be perceived by the patient. He shows in case histories how significant this level of communication can be for patients in deep regression.

Extending the theory concept of the Paris psychosomatic school *Stephanos* (1973) has developed an in-patient analytical psychosomatic therapy. Here the real presence of the therapeutic team respresenting a good object, a primary object is the main thing. The regressive need of the patient for primary love is responded to and the idea is to make it possible for the patient to pass from oral-narcissistic regression to relate to the object.

If one now tries to recapitulate the methods of therapy described above for psychosomatic disorders, it becomes clear that they all, however different they may be, have two things in particular in common: (1) the assumption of a fixation on or regression to a very early stage of development, in which a pre-verbal sensorimotor level of communication is dominant; (2) communication between doctor and patient seems to be either impossible or very much reduced – at verbal level.

Some authors point out that these difficulties in communication are manifested particularly in the initial phase of a psychotherapy treatment. One can assume that despite advances in the development of theory in psychosomatic medicine, the extent to which therapeutic techniques should be modified has not been investigated enough. The attempt has been made to keep to the basic rules at secondary process level in the sense of classical analytical neurosis therapy and thus, at the verbalisation level, to interpret the speechlessness or pre-verbal expressive forms of the patient too often as resistence. The fact that the results of treatment have by no means been unsatisfactory, although often after periods of therapy lasting for several years, leads one to suppose that communication between doctor and patient took place at the pre-verbal level, but was discerned by both at best in the sense of an empathy. The phenomena which did often actually occur remained mostly blurred and unclarified.

We have now tried to do justice to the above statements in that, in an introductory phase parallel to verbal analytical group therapy, we have made available a largely pre-verbal area of communication with concentrative movement therapy.

In our clinic this therapy is part of an in-patient psychoanalytical model. The therapy range consists of analytical group therapy, analytical ergotherapy and concentrative movement therapy in the environment of the therapeutic community. There are both psychoneurotics and psychosomatic patients in the closed groups. The 3-month in-patient therapy is the initial phase which is followed by an out-patient analytical group therapy lasting about 2 years. It was in the verbal elaboration in the analytical group above all that the significance of the concentrative movement therapy became clear to us, although it was also put across to a large extent by statements by the patients. In a questionnaire the patients recorded a high opinion of the effectivity of this therapy which surprised us at first.

Now to the method of concentrative movement therapy; it goes back to *Elsa Gindler,* a kinesitherapist who died in Berlin in 1961. Her pupil *Gertrud Heller* first used the method in psychotherapy: she worked for 12 years with neurotic and psychotic patients under *Meyer/Gross* in Crichton Royal Mental Hospital in Scotland. In the last 15–20 years the circle around *Stolze* (1967) and *Goldberg* (1974) in particular have been gaining experience in out-patient psychotherapeutic practice. They tried above all to develop the method in a practical and theoretical way. *Meyer* (1972) was the first to approach it from a scientific angle.

The focal point of the therapeutic effort lies in perception and expression in the non-verbal area. The idea is to create an area which allows individual self-experience in the pre-verbal area. An absolute necessity is that the therapist has enough self-experience to be able to give sufficiently sensitive directions and interpretations. The therapist takes over a role which is markedly more active than is usual in analytical psychotherapy. In the introductory phase he has the task of preparing the ground for possible drive areas – whether intentional, oral, anal, aggressive or sexual. He offers himself as a real object and as an object for identification. The role of the therapist recalls *Ferenczi*'s (1919) active technique, in which *Ferenczi* recommends leading the patient into a tension state in order to bring the repressed instinctual drive or wish into consciousness. This conforms initially with *Freud*'s recommendation of exposing a person suffering from agoraphobia to the situation he is afraid of.

For the larger part of the sessions the patients have their eyes closed. We think that this is of special significance, as in this way that area of perception, which is usually dominant and is generally subject to a certain automatisation and habituation, is eliminated, and this gives room for new, less frequented ranges of perception. The same is true for the field of expression, in that, with the removal of speech, which is mainly consciously controlled, the unconscious bodily forms of expression come into play.

The aim of the sessions is to obtain a concentration on awareness of one's own body, and of the body in relation to the surroundings – whether lying, standing or walking, and on investigation of the surrounding area and its objects. Meetings and contact whit others occur. Here we pose the following questions: for example, how do I experience my contact with the floor, do I feel carried by it, accepted or rejected by it, do I open myself to the environment or do I close myself off, how much proximity do I want, how much distance do I need, in how far can I trust, let myself be led? The processes of attachment and separation take on a particular significance. In connection with objects it leads to qualities of emotion and remembrance, which are related to form and material, perhaps, or with giving and taking.

These descriptions, suffice to show clearly, I believe, that here a process of abstraction and symbolisation – and a process of remembrance of genetic material as well – can be introduced.

By using a few examples I should like to show how patients present that factor, which at verbal level appears more as a defence – and at non-verbal level more as the defended element – and thus make it accessible for elaboration.

A 39-year-old man with peptic ulcers which had been recurring for 10 years, who was above averagely successful in his work, came to our clinic when the stomach symptoms broke out again. The precipitating event was the separation from his wife and, no doubt connected with this, a performance drop and the loss of his job. In the verbal analytical group he quickly set himself up as co-therapist and became the recognised leader of the group. In the concentrative movement therapy he mainly lay rolled up on the floor, burst into tears on contact with co-patients and clutched them. In a situation in which he sat back to back with a co-patient the partner felt utterly overwhelmed and overtaxed by his need for support.

Another example: a 27-year-old patient with recurring cystitis and spasms described herself in the uretha and anorgasmy, who complained in the verbal group above all about constant inferiority complexes, gets in the concentrative movement therapy into a situation which I consider to be typical of the urethal drive experience. She stands with her eyes closed in a circle in which she is connected to the other members of the group by a rope. She becomes more and more tense and pulls with both hands with increasing strength on the rope until she collapses exhausted. In the verbalisation it becomes clear that she had the impression that she had to hold and support all the members of the group by herself.

I should now like to propose some hypotheses which have arisen from my experience with concentrative movement therapy up to now: in my experience one often meets the phenomenon of alexithymia described by *Sifneos* in psychosomatic patients and patients of low social status; one sees it as well, but more rarely, in neurotic patients and so-called normal population. It is possible that we have multifactorially conditioned phenomenon before us: four factors seem to me to be of importance: (1) a fixation on or a regression to a very early stage of development, where pre-verbal sensori-motor intelligence (*Piaget*, 1947) and identification processes (*Spitz*, 1965) prevail, with dependance on the real presence of objects as a result of the lack of capacity to internalise; (2) socialisation conditioned factors. *Bernstein*'s (1972) restricted code gives an indication of where the phenomena described in alexithymia are mainly reflected; (3) caused by lack of communication between doctor and patient; (4) caused by the person's 'career' as a patient with somatic symptoms.

In the combined attempt at treatment, i.e. analytical group and concentrative movement therapy, the following seems noteworthy: two verbalisation types are seen mainly with psychosomatic and low social status patients. One group tends more to verbal reservedness and the second, although it has a quantitatively inconspicuous, or possibly increased verbalisation, shows its defence mainly in denial, projection, conformity and symptom fixation. Thus communication difficulties occur to an above average extent between patient and therapist and among patients in a mixed group of neurotic and psychosomatic patients with differing social status. The non-verbal therapy attempts to overcome these initial difficulties by responding to the form of expression chosen by the patient and which it is possible for him to use. The above factor, which, in the mainly verbal therapies, was a considerable element of hindrance in the initial stages, and which can certainly be connected with the long duration of therapy, surprisingly never occurred in the non-verbal area at all. This would lead one to propose the hypothesis that the non-, or better, pre-verbal area of expression is more collective and less influenced by socialisation.

It became clear furthermore that the forms of defence which mainly occur are presented more strongly in the verbal area, whereas in the pre-verbal area the intra- or interindividual conflict constellated very early in the form of key experiences, i.e. the need side, the defended area became visible as well. One can assume that the pre-verbal area is more open to affect, closer to the unconscious and the primary processes and less subject to censure, less controlled by the consciousness. The real presence of the objects, the concrete area of expression and perception, to which the concentrative movement therapy responds, do not primarily require a process of symbolisation and abstraction. The quality of experience is, rather, intensified by the concretisation and enhances the capacity to remember genetic material. The relation to the body is integrated into this form of therapy – in recognition of the fact that it is primarily the physical symptoms which are seen in these disorders – and in this situation a connection between the patient's life history and the occurence of the symptoms becomes accessible. The process of verbalisation which succeeds it and learning of abstraction and symbolisstion take place mainly by way of help in identification by the therapist and the co-patients.

This report attempts to show that this approach to therapy which is intended as an access, connection and complement to the verbal analytical group, helps to overcome the difficulties in communication which occur in the characteristics of alexithymia.

References

Balint, M.: The basic fault (Tavistock, London 1968).
Bernstein, B.: Studien zur sprachlichen Sozialisation (Schwann, Düsseldorf 1972).
De Boor, C. und Mitscherlich, A.: Verstehende Psychosomatik, Psyche 1973).
Brocher, T.: Über averbale Kommunikation, Psyche 1967).
Ferenczi, S.: Technische Schwierigkeiten einer Hysterieanalyse. Int. Z. Psychoanal. (1919).
Freud, S.: Wege der psychoanalytischen Therapie, vol. 12 (1919).
Freud, S.: Das Ich und das Es, vol. 13 (1923).
Goldberg, M.: Über meine Therapie-Formel in der konzentrativen Bewegungstherapie. Prax. Psychother. *19* (1974).
Kaufmann, M. R.: Problems of Therapy; In *Deutsch* the Psychosomatic concept (1953).
Margolin, S. G.: Genetic and Dynamic psychophysiological determinants of patho-physiological processes; in *Deutsch* The psychosomatic concept (1953).
Marty, P.; De M'Uzan, M. et David, C.: L'investigation psychosomatique PUF, Paris (1963).
Meyer, J. E.: Konzentrative Entspannungsübungen nach Elsa Gindler und ihre Grund-lagen; in *Petrilowitsch* Die Sinnfrage in der Psychotherapie (Wiss. Buchges., Darm-stadt 1972).
Mitscherlich, A.: Krankheit als Konflikt (Suhrkamp, Frankfurt 1967).
Piaget, J.: Psychologie de l'intelligence (Colin, Paris 1947).
Reich, W.: Charakteranalyse (1948).
Ruesch, J.: The infantile personality. Psychosom. Med. *10:* 134–144 (1948).
Schur, M.: Comments on the metapsychology of somatisation; in The psychoanalytic of the child, vol. 10, pp. 119–164 (1955).
Spitz, R.: The first year of life (International Universities Press, New York 1965).
Stephanos, S.: Analytisch-psychosomatische Therapie. Jahrbuch der Psychoanalyse, vol. 1 (Huber, Bern 1973).
Stolze, H.: Selbsterfahrung und Begegnung mit den anderen durch konzentrative Be-wegungstherapie (Institut für Psychohygiene, Biel 1967).
Stolze, H.: Selbsterfahrung und Bewegung. Prax. Psychother. *17* (1972).

Dr. med. *H. Becker,* Psychosomatische Klinik der Universität, Thibautstrasse 2, D-*6900 Heidelberg 1* (FRG)

Proc. 11th Eur. Conf. Psychosom. Res., Heidelberg 1976
Psychother. Psychosom. *28:* 337–342 (1977)

Supportive Psychotherapeutic Techniques in Primary and Secondary Alexithymia

Hellmuth Freyberger

Department of Psychosomatics, Hannover Medical School, Hannover-Kleefeld

Introduction

In the majority of *alexithymic* patients, psychoanalytically orientated techniques cannot be applied because of the following three reasons:

First, *decreased inner motivation* due to reduced or failing self-reflection abilities.

This lessening of the insightful capacity includes the inability to transfer differentiated libidinous or aggressive wishes to the therapist. There frequently predominate undifferentiated feelings in the sense of the *oral-narcissistic acting-out* (with the main symptom being a labile self-esteem) on the one hand, as well as the marked mentioning of bodily sensations and hypochondriac details on the other hand. The patient's *hypochondriac self-concerns* represent a special form of substitute for the 'vacuum' in his feelings.

Second, *diminished tolerance* particularly with regard to those frustrations which are typical to the psychoanalytically orientated psychotherapeutic situation.

Third, a very marked predomination of *oral-narcissistic* needs which makes impossible the learning of new emotional behaviour.

Psychotherapeutic Situation in Primary Alexithymia

Technique

The supportive psychotherapeutic technique in *primary alexithymia* can be described by the following four steps:

First, the building-up of a stable object-relationship and the careful concern for a positive transference. This object-relationship is an *oral-*

narcissistic one which the patient tends to build up due to the doctor's offer. It results in the stabilization and lessening intensity of the *oral-narcissistic acting-out* which represents a defence formation concerning the hypersensitivity towards narcissistic trauma and the states of helplessness and hopelessness.

On the doctor's part, the careful concern for a *positive transference* concerns the offering of good advice; furthermore, the informative anticipation of eventual frustrations in the face of symbolic, threatening or real objects loss; finally, the direct clarification of the patient's wishes and displeasure to be followed by creation of possibilities for the patient to have marked cathartic-off reactions with regard to this unpleasant emotions (10). The regular carthartic-off reactions include for the patient a considerable psychic stabilization. After that, outside the sessions and in the face of object loss, most of the patients are able to imagine the superficial outlines of the doctor-patient relationship including the inherent satisfying oral-narcissistic 'climate' and the connected possibilities to have marked carthartic-off reactions. These symbolic reactions are not infrequently sufficient to give psychic relief to the patient during the waiting time before the next session. Beyond this, on the basis of the careful concern for a positive transference, there can be necessary cautions confrontations or surface interpretations. However, with regard to this limited interpretative work the doctor must be concerned to prevent a narcissistic trauma in his patient.

Second, the doctor's filling the patient's 'vacuum' in his feelings by freely and activity supplying emotional words and phantasies. This activity of the doctor aims to achieve a substitute for the patient's 'vacuum' in his feelings at least for the time being. This special technique includes the following three steps: (a) the doctor's language must be rich in phantasy and imagery; (b) the patient may be stimulated again and again to make efforts in verbalizing his feelings; (c) the doctor's ability to 'translate' the patient's anxious hypochondriac self-concerns and his utilitarian way of thinking ('operatory thinking') in somewhat more differentiated feelings. Therefore, the patient's verbalization may take on some more feeling value which will be perceived at least transitorily by the patient.

Third, the attempt in mediating conflict consciousness. The doctor should be concerned to mediate to the patient a certain amount of *conflict consciousness* by the offer of cautiously formulated and superficial interpretations.

Fourth, the constant potential availability of the psychosomaticist.

The building-up of a stable object relationship and the careful concern for a positive transference as well as the doctor's filling the patient's 'vacuum' in his feelings by freely and actively supplying emotional words and phantasies include only positive psychotherapeutic effects in so far that the patient is fully aware of the psychosomaticist's potential availability.

Effective Factors and Likely Behavior Modifications in the Patient

The supportive psychotherapy includes the following three therapeutic effects in the patient: (1) the appearance of some emotional security; (2) the limited substitution of the patient's 'vacuum' in his feelings, and (3) the eventual development of some insightful abilities.

According to our experience, in a small percentage of those patients who were treated by supportive psychotherapy we can observe the development of some abilities for self-reflection. This makes the procedure of an interpretative psychotherapy possible at a later date which is more effective than the supportive psychotherapy. In their treatment considerations, *Bräutigam and Christian* (1) in the way of psychotherapy follow up with the aim of detaching the psychosomatic patient from his oral-narcissistic fixations at least partially so that he will be a neurotic patient with the motivation to accept a psychoanalysis. In these (relatively rare) cases we can see the patient pass through three psychotherapeutic stages. The first stage concerns the application of pure supportive psychotherapy. During the next stage we can demand from the patient superficial conflict-solving psychotherapy. And in the final stage we bring the patient to accept psychoanalysis.

Psychotherapeutic Situation in Secondary Alexithymia

Definition

In the above-mentioned psychosomatic patients the alexithymia represents an important disposition factor concerning the outbreak and the further course of the somatic disorder *(primary alexithymia)*. Vice versa, the alexithymic features also frequently occur in patients with primary organic diseases; e.g. dialysis and transplant patients, patients who are suffering from cancer and patients who are transitorily suffering from a life-threatened state and are in an intensive care unit. We call it *secondary alexithymia* (9).

In these patients the secondary alexithymia is either a *transitory* state which will decrease after the disease has been cured, we call it *acute secondary alexithymia*, or the secondary alexithymia is a *permanent* state, we call it *chronic secondary alexithymia*. The latter state applies to patients whose disease tends towards a chronic development.

In these patients, the secondary alexithymic features can be explained as a *protective* factor towards the emotional significance and seriousness of the illness; namely, a defence mechanism which will be built up by the patient who is confronted with the experience of his impairing disease (9).

There are many similar details in primary and secondary alexithymia not only concerning the *phenomenal* features but also with regard to the *psychodynamic* processes. The inner pressure to accept the data of an impairing primary organic disease and to tolerate the traits of emotional exhaustion which are connected with the manifetation of the illness will be experienced by the patient as a *narcissistic trauma*. Closely united with the narcissistic traumatization are *oral-dependent* traits. As a consequence of the narcissistic traumatization the patient's *aggressive* wishes will be intensively aroused and immediately after it totally be turned against the self. The patient is obliged to *defend* his aggressive wishes for two reasons. On the one hand, this aggression defence occurs because of his emotional exhaustion due to the perception of his impairing illness. On the other hand, the aggression defence occurs because the patient is afraid of seriously endangering the interhuman relationships with the doctors and nurses insofar as he tends to exhibit aggressive wishes. Also, the patient who is suffering a primary organic disease shows *insufficient insigthful capacities*.

Technique

The supportive psychotherapeutic technique in *secondary alexithymia* corresponds with that in primary alexithymia. Additionally, to the three supportive psychotherapeutic steps there must be considered the *stabilization* of those *defence mechanisms* which are typical in primary organically ill patients, namely: (a) secondary hypochondria; (b) infantile regression; (c) denial work.

The *stabilization* of these *defence mechanisms* includes the following three supportive psychotherapeutic steps: (1) the verbalization of secondary hypochondriac self-concerns; (2) the confirmation of the infantile regressive traits; (3) the strengthening of the denial work in the direction of a realistically adapted behavior (2, 7).

A fourth important supportive psychotherapeutic step in organically ill patients is *the supplementary psychological handling of the medication and the apparatus used*. The patients develop distinctive emotional fixations to those remedies which show objectively good effects. The fixations also include certain life-saving apparatus in the outside world, e.g. the monitors and the artificial kidney and of course the transplanted kidney in the patient's inside world. On the one hand, these emotional fixations represent in the patient a marked defence formation against the anxieties due to the perception of the serious failure of his body functions. On the other hand, as the consequence of these emotional fixations in the patient the thought of an emotional security in the presence of the doctors and nurses will be strengthened for these are responsible for offering that medication and apparatus which will be experienced as effective. It is one of the psychosomaticist's tasks to strengthen again and again in a verbal way the patient's emotional fixations on the remedies and apparatus.

Patient Groups

Concerning the *primary alexithymia,* our experience in supportive psychotherapy was gained from our work in 65 *ulcerative colitis* patients (3).

Here, the period of psychotherapy lasted from 1 to 7 years; 50% of the patients underwent therapy for more than 3 years.

With regard to *secondary alexithymia* our experience in supportive psychotherapy was gained in the following three patient groups:

(1) 60 *myocardial infarction* patients who were in an intensive care unit for the duration of 3–8 days (6).

(2) A hemodialysis group which was made up of 58 center dialysis patients and 15 home dialysis patients (4).

In our center dialysis patients, the period of psychotherapeutic supervision lasted from 1 to 6 years. In our home dialysis patients the period of psychotherapeutic supervision took from 6 months to 3 years, in 50% more than 2 years.

(3) Various patient groups in critical illness situations who simultaneously showed certain symptoms and failure adaptations which were highly endangering and required *emergency psychotherapeutic relief* (5). The *emergency psychotherapy* reprensents a particular variant of the supportive psychotherapy.

In 36 patients we observed the main symptoms to be *serious anxieties* and *serious hopelessness* which occurred in the following units: (1) general surgical and medical wards, 10 patients; (2) intensive care departments, 10 patients; (3) dialysis center, 12 patients; (4) cancer ward, 4 patients.

The four main reasons which made the emergency psychotherapy necessary were the following: (1) dialysis patients object loss in relatives; (2) severe anxieties caused by the somatic state; (3) insufficient cooperation during the intensive therapy; (4) functional anorexia.

Auxiliary Therapists' Pools

In connection with the mentioning of supportive psychotherapeutic techniques in alexithymic patients there arises the question in which way can the great discrepancy be solved between the high number of patients who use supportive psychotherapy on the one hand, and the number of available therapists on the other hand. This discrepancy comes to light particularly in the medical inpatient clinics. Here, the majority of patients shows the typical *alexithymic* characteristics. In our opinion, at present the best way to reduce this discrepancy is the foundation of students' pools who act as auxiliary therapists and will be supervised by fully trained therapists within Balint groups. So far, is there a sufficient number of supervising therapists at our disposal, then the alexithymic patients of greater medical institutions can be systematically supplied by supportive psychotherapy. I will be obliged to postpone my statement concerning the auxiliary-therapist pool to the later Round Table.

References

1 *Bräutigam, W. und Christian, P.:* Psychosomatische Medizin (Thieme, Stuttgart 1975).
2 *Cassem, N. H. and Hackett, T. P.:* Psychiatric consultation in a coronary care unit. Ann. intern. Med. *75:* 9 (1971).
3 *Freyberger, H.:* The doctor-patient relationship in ulceratice colitis; in *Pierloot* Recent research in psychosomatics (Karger, Basel 1970).
4 *Freyberger, H.:* Six years' experience as a psychosomaticist in a hemodialysis unit; in *Freyberger* Topics of psychosomatic research (Karger, Basel 1973).
5 *Freyberger, H.:* Psychosomatic aspects of an intensive care unit; in *Howells* Modern perspectives in the psychiatric aspect of surgery (Brunner/Mazel, New York, 1976).
6 *Haan, D. und Freyberger, H.:* Ergebnisse der Intensivbehandlung des Herzinfarktes unter gleichzeitiger Berücksichtigung psychosomatischer Gesichtspunkte. Verh. dt. Ges. inn. Med. *74;* 990 (1968).
7 *Hackett, C. P. and Cassem, N. H.:* The coronary care unit in an appraisal of its psychological hazards. New Engl. J. Med. *279;* 1365 (1968).
8 *Kimball, C. P.:* Medical psychotherapy. J. Psychother. Psychosom. *25;* 103 (1975).
9 *Nemiah, J. H.; Freyberger, H., and Sifneos, P. E.:* Alexithymia: a view of the psychosomatic process; in *Hill* Recent advances psychosomatic medicine (Butterworths, London 1976).
10 *Sifneos, P. E.:* The prevalence of 'Alexithymia', characteristics in psychosomatic patients; in *Freyberger* Top. psychosom. res. (Karger, Basel 1973).

Prof. Dr. med. *H. Freyberger*, Medizinische Hochschule Hannover, Abteilung für Psychosomatik, Postfach 610180, *D–3000 Hannover 61* (FRG)

Discussion

Dr. Meyer: Although I have no personal experience with psychosomatic patients I suppose that concentrative movement therapy is very valuable, particularly when combined with analytic group therapy. The different results compared to meditation may be due to the fact that vigilance in concentrative movement therapy is not impaired and in certain respects even increased. Two questions: what do you say to the psychosomatic patient about the aim of this treatment? Do you think that psychosomatic patients have initially more difficulties than others in following the verbal suggestions of this therapy?

Dr. Becker: We have up to the present time been working in concentrative movement therapy combined with analytic group therapy in mixed groups of neurotics and psychosomatic patients. The initial stipulations and my therapeutic instructions are the same for everybody. In the course of therapy, one gets the impression that both groups (psychoneurotics and psychosomatic patients) profit from one another; at first this is most conspicuous amongst the psychosomatic patients as against the neurotics which can also be observed in the verbal analytic groups. The nucleus here is that with psychosomatic patients for the first time basic conflicts can be definitely observed and witnessed, whereas in the case of neurotics, who tend to intellectualize, an emotional experience through body contact and objective treatment is made possible. A considerable ambivalence is often noticed with psychosomatic patients in a 'near – far' need and amazingly early an until now dormant emotionalness and, most important of all, aggression, becomes visible.

Dr. Wolff: I would like to comment on these very interesting papers which seem to me to point towards new developments in groups psychotherapy. We have previously heard from Dr. *Sifneos,* Dr. *Nemiah* and the Boston group how important it is to help alexithymic patients in groups to get in touch with their feelings. I entirely agree with this. Now some of these patients have, as Dr. *Tonnesmann* and others have said, regressed to or have remained stuck at a preverbal which essentially means a physical level of functioning and communication. Most group therapists on the other hand have been conditioned by their training to function only in terms of words through interpretations. Clearly this would correspond to a situation in which a mother whose child needs her to hold or feed and play with him decides instead only to talk to him before he is ready to use language as a means of communication. It is, similarly, not surprising that in group psychotherapy we remain relatively ineffective if we restrict ourselves to verbal communication only. In London there used to be the Bion school of group therapy where the therapist only made group interpretations and never even dealt with the problems of individual patients. This is now gradually being given up. In group-analytic psychotherapy, more attention is now being given to individual group members and their interaction as well as to group phenomena as a whole. I was delighted this morning to hear that more attention is generally being paid to individual patients, and that in Boston other methods like videotape replay are being introduced into group therapy. Dr. *Becker*'s paper from Heidelberg makes the crucial point that if a patient has regressed to a preverbal level of functioning and, therefore cannot communicate in words what he feels, the therapist needs to use bodily communication and work at a body-feeling level with the patients in the group. To do this kind of work the therapist must have had similar experience in a training group in order to be fully aware himself of the links between psychic and somatic experience.

Dr. Apfel-Savitz: We have had different experiences in teaching meditation to the psychosomatic and neurotic patients; the principal difference was the suspiciousness with which meditation was looked upon by the psychosomatic patient. The level of denial of the anxiety and need for relaxation of body muscles was much greater in the somatic patient and we found it necessary to use more verbal reassurance and time to prepare the psychosomatic patients for this experience than we did with neurotic patients. In the preparation we spoke to the fact that this was normal, that all people, including ourselves, had body tension and found relaxation useful. This enabled the psychosomatic patients to go along with the meditation whereas they were quite reluctant to do so initially.

Dr. Groen: To begin with: I think that the main conclusion which emerged from all the papers of this session is that group therapy can be practiced with benefit with patients with so-called psychosomatic disorders. It took a long time before group therapy was introduced into this field and it is interesting that the internists who learned this technique from the psychiatrists were the first to go ahead and apply group therapy to their patients with internal diseases. These were in our own first studies mainly asthmatics. Lately, we have also been working extensively with diabetics. It took the psychiatrists a much longer time before they dared to treat psychosomatic patients with group therapy. We have some suggestion why that is so. In the first place I always felt at home among people who had asthma or diabetes. I was not afraid of their questions because I knew more or less, through my own profession in internal medicine what was medically wrong with them. But several of our psychiatric colleagues did not feel at home with these patients. The second reason may have been the disappointment of the psychiatrist when he found that these psychosomatic patients take such a long time before they are willing (or able) to talk about their anxiety, insecurity, infantile fixations and regressions. And yet this is just what I had been taught from my psychiatric teachers (Dr. *Bastiaans* has been the main one), namely: 'Do not be impatient with patients. Just as you should never be impatient with a child when it does not develop quickly enough along the way you want it to develop, but trust it, give it confidence, don't frustrate it by your impatience, don't push it, and then the child will develop naturally and show normal behavior.' The same rule applies to the behavior of our groups. Many a time, let me tell you, after the session was over, *Bastiaans* interpreted to me what was wrong with me, so that I did not have to interpret the behavior of the patients but could continue to accept them as they were. This confidence that the group, if you only leave it to itself, will develop along its own way into emotional maturity, is still the main principle which guides Dr. *Pelser* and me.

Moreover, as you know we regard alexithymia as a way of 'detached intellectualized' communication which our modern western society induces in its members and which some people only exaggerate more than others. We all communicate in a matter of fact way with each other – we ourselves show alexithymia: we do not tell each other about our fantasies, our feelings when we go to scientific meetings. Instead we give each other facts, figures, so-called important factual data and statistical probabilities. And yet we and all the people who behave similarly, before we start giving our papers, we sweat in our hand-palms, we have high pulse rates and you can see by the way we behave how emtional we are. So we cannot blame our asthmatic patients when they spend sometimes weeks of group sessions in discussing allergy or drugs instead of their emotions because that is just what the doctors who have been treating them have taught them by their example. Only very gradually the patients discover and learn in their own way, the importance of feelings in general and for the development and case of their diseases as well.

Another major point in our behavior as discussion leaders is that we feel very much that although we are the discussion leader, we are also ourselves a member of the group. We learn from the patients in the group and if necessary, we let them modify our behavior. If, for instance, these patients – asthmatics or diabetics – ask in the first stages mainly instructions to understand their disease and, if this appears to be a common wish of the group (which you notice because they all want to know, and look at you, and because there is a silence in the group when they put certain questions straight to us), well, we then answer them. In other words, not all intellectual discussions in the group are interpreted by us to the group as defense mechanisms. That this attitude has advantages has been proved by the number of drop-outs. In the first paper which *Pelser* and I published in 1956 on the asthma group therapy, we did not mention that we had two control groups in those days (1952–1956) which were run by psychiatrists. Both these psychiatrists, when the patients asked purely somatic questions like 'why do I spit up so much sputum', or 'what does it mean when this sputum is yellow or white?' or 'why do I wheeze so much when there is snow in the air?' answered in a psychiatric interpretetive language or most often asked 'why do you ask that question?' It did not take a long time, however, before in these groups the patients began to tell these psychiatrists 'But when we ask you a question, why do you always answer by saying "why do you ask that question?"!' Both these groups, considered from the increasing number of drop-outs, were failures. We have now three groups of diabetic patients, two are run by internists like *Pelser* and me, one is run by a psychologist. Dr. *Pelser* lost 2 out of 15, I lost 0 out of 16. The psychologist, who refused to give purely intellectual instruction when the patients asked him about diabetes, and kept on insisting that these questions were defence mechanisms, got out some very interesting emotional material, but he lost five out of eleven patients and we regard the drop-out, the loss of any patient, as a failure.

Another of our guidelines is that we are inspired very much by *Kurt Levin*'s experiments of the democratic class. We let the patients, as much as possible, run the group themselves. Their influence on us has been so great that when I begun to report in the medical staff meetings of our department about what happened in the asthmatic group, my colleagues became so interested that they said 'Why don't you let us talk out, why don't you let us behave as we want?' Gradually there was also an indirect influence of the patient group, on the behavior of the staff in our department. Now, if you can achieve as a group leader the feeling that you learn at least as much from the patients in the group as they from you and by feeling yourself an actual group member, you have also shown to the patients that we are really meaning to be one of them and that we accept them as they accept us. Actually, learning to accept yourself, and each other as you really are, is part of emotional maturation and this is one of the ways along which our group therapy seems to work.

We have no experience with so-called psychoneurotic patients. I am sorry I have to apologise for this, so that I cannot give any comments on the comparisons which some of you have been contributing to the discussion.

Dr. Crisp: Ladies and gentlemen, coming from England, which is a small country, I have always been impressed by the scale of things on the Continent and particularly your great river, the Rhine and it seems sad to me that a trout, which starts at Rotterdam, and eventually gets into the Neckar, should subsequently be fished out of the water and served up for lunch. But I propose to overcome my grief because Dr. *Bräutigam* tells me that it is trout for lunch at the Mensa at 1 o'clock.

Varia

Proc. 11th Eur. Conf. Psychosom. Res., Heidelberg 1976
Psychother. Psychosom. *28:* 346–356 (1977)

Beyond the Psychosomatic Phenomenon

Reflexions on the Life of Blaise Pascal

S. Stephanos and U. Auhagen

The term 'psychosomatic phenomenon' could, in our view, be defined as the characteristic 'inner emptiness' or 'lack' of the psychosomatic patient, that is, his meagre fantasy, poor interpersonal relationships and his inability to experience and elaborate in the psychic sphere (*Stephanos*, 1973, 1974, 1975, 1976/77b). This phenomenon is rooted in disturbances in the area of primal identity (*Lichtenstein*, 1964) and primary identifications, which have resulted in the subject remaining bound to his primary significant object in an inescapable relation of dependence throughout his life.

The lack of adequate 'primary maternal preoccupation' (*Winnicott*, 1956) in very early infancy is a major factor contributing to the establishment of this primary deficiency in the patient and to the corresponding psychosomatic fixation mechanisms: he responds to tensions directly with somatic disturbances, which can lead to organ lesions and even death. This is what we call the pathological disorganisation. Disorganisation and reorganisation processes work together to determine the specific economy of the individual, influencing the development of his illness and with it his fate.

The hypothetical scale in figure 1 shows how a person can be characterized according to the degree to which he is dominated by the primary deficiency or filled with psychic life, as the case may be. The primary structural 'lack' is localized at the lower end of the scale. Here we find the patients who, with no neurotic defence processes at their disposal, are always more or less at the mercy of destructive forces. At the upper end of the scale are the character-neurotic patients whose primary deficiency is embedded in a psychic organisation, remaining largely compensated. Between these two extremes are the patients with 'allergic fixation mechanisms' and the 'mechanistic character neurotics'.

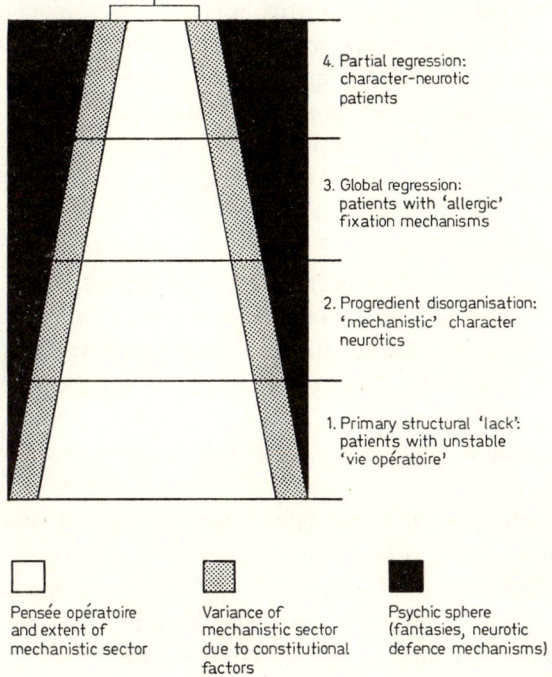

4. Partial regression:
   character-neurotic
   patients

3. Global regression:
   patients with 'allergic'
   fixation mechanisms

2. Progredient disorganisation:
   'mechanistic' character
   neurotics

1. Primary structural 'lack':
   patients with unstable
   'vie opératoire'

Pensée opératoire and extent of mechanistic sector	Variance of mechanistic sector due to constitutional factors	Psychic sphere (fantasies, neurotic defence mechanisms)

Fig. 1.

The concept of the psychosomatic phenomenon has recently brought about a number of misunderstandings. It has often been mistakenly assumed that the entire personality, and not just a sector of it, is claimed to be affected by the primary deficiency. For this reason it seems to us to be especially important to stress how very complex the psychosomatic phenomenon can be, and in particular to show how the extent to which a person's life is influenced by it depends upon how far his individual capacity for elaboration has been able to develop. If he is able to suffer from his inner emptiness and, through experiencing it, to work it over on a psychic level, his primary deficiency and psychosomatic affliction can help him towards a differentiated form of reorganisation and so even to creativity.

The life of Blaise Pascal, the 17th century religious philosopher and genius in physics, offers us a good illustration of this thesis.

Blaise Pascal was born on 19th June 1623 in Clermont-Ferrand as the third child and only son among four children. His eldest sister died as a small child. His second eldest sister, Gilberte, was 3½ years older than Blaise, while Jacqueline was 2½ years younger. His father was a high-ranking civil servant with a passion for mathematics, whose house was a meeting place for the highest intellectual circles. His mother, Antoinette, well known for her piety and self-sacrificing love for the poor, died when Blaise was 3½ years old. Towards the end of his first year Blaise was taken ill with a disease which decisively moulded his psycho-biological evolution. He suffered from 'cramps' which lasted 12 months and then spontaneously disappeared. In his biographies (by Gilberte Pascal-Périer, his sister, and Marguerite Périer) we find the reference: 'il tombe en chartre' (*Anzieu*, 1975). These biographies provide detailed descriptions of his symptoms: 'He screamed, kicked violently and fell into a state of agitation.'[1,2] Conditions were also described which showed signs of death: 'He had neither pulse nor voice nor feeling, and became increasingly colder; after a while he returned to his senses.'

Two situations precipitated these conditions: when he came in contact with water, or when his parents approached each other in his presence.

In our view, this indicates in all probability a typical example of infantile affective spasms, in this case of the serious pallid form which, according to *Lombroso and Lerman* (1967) comprises 19% of the affective spasms known to occur in childhood. The more frequent cyanitoc form (81%), which particularly affects the respiratory system, is seldom accompanied by generalized muscle cramps.

The pallid spasm is usually caused by pain or excitement and is accompanied by a standstill of the heart for 8–10 sec and a cerebral anoxia. The child turns pale and loses consciousness, with tonic-clonic fits often to the point of episthotonus. This functional disorder, typically occurring in the second year of life, is described by *Kreisler et al.* (1974) as a deep-rooted pathological disorganisation which is comparable to the experience of the 'petite mort' (the temporary 'little death'). The involvement of the entire social environment is another important element of the syndrome.

Blaise's illness leads us to suppose that his relationship to his mother during his first year of life was full of tension and that there were conflicts

---

[1] Translater's note: In the absence of original English translations at the time of publication, all quotations are translated from the German sources cited in footnotes [2] and [3].

[2] Gilberte Pascal-Périer: Das Leben des Blaise Pascal (*Rüttenauer*, 1938).

[3] Guardini, R.: Einführung zu 'Blaise Pascal-Gedanken' (*Rüttenauer*, 1937).

between his parents. His mother showed two typical sorts of behaviour – one overly careful and hectically oppressive, the other hysterical and phobic – which exerted a pathological influence on his development. On the one hand, as an overprotective object she smothered him with exaggerated care and attention ('pare excitation') which aroused unendurable unpleasure in him. At the same time, however, she clung anxiously to her son, whom she strongly eroticized, in order to avoid sexual contact with her husband. Various incidents that have been recorded are evidence of the discord between Blaise' parents. For example, his father once publicly accused one of his wife's protégées of having bewitched his son.

The mother had conveyed an idea of the primal scene to her son too soon, at a time in which he was still unable to assimilate the oedipal tensions. The result was a defective establishment of the primal repression, whereby his body underwent a pathological autoerotic cathexis.

In accordance with our conception of psychosomatics the affective spasm can be seen as a form of disorganisation which established itself on the basis of the primary deficiency. On the one hand it represents the violent experience of somatic deterioration, on the other a mechanistic, orgiastic discharge in the relationship to the erotisizing mother. In other words, through the attacks the intolerable sexual stimuli are released directly on a somatic level, without any psychic involvement. Thus, in the course of his second year Blaise Pascal had to acquire character-neurotic defence mechanisms to enable him to keep his objects at a tolerable distance and to manipulate his environment according to his needs.

The death of his mother one year after the birth of his sister Jacqueline meant for Blaise the loss of his primary significant object. After experiencing the 'petite mort' in his own body in the affective spasms he suddenly found himself confronted with death in the outside world. His feeling of inner emptiness could now no longer be compensated. At the same time his mother's death aroused in him the guilt-ridden fantasy that he had destroyed his sexual object. This is the basis for the repression of his dependency wishes and his feminine identification. For the rest of his life he never fully cathected another sexual object and strongly resisted offering himself as such to others. On a piece of paper which he always kept on his person in later life he had written: 'It would be unjust if others were to become attached to me, however joyfully and freely they may do it. I would be misleading those in whom I aroused such a desire, for I am no object for another person and have nothing with which to satisfy them. Am I not destined for death? Thus, the object of thier attachment would die. For if I am guilty when I cause another to believe an untruth, however winningly I may speak and however much pleasure it may give me (to be believed), so too am I guilty if I stir up love in another or if I attract other people to my person, for they should use their lives and endeavours to please God or to seek Him.'[2]

After his mother's death, Blaise was taken care of by his fond father and a governess who went by the name of 'ma fidèle'. Soon afterwards his father gave up his post in the Royal Treasury for a number of years in order to devote himself entirely to the education of his son. Thus Blaise never attended a school. The fact that he was caught up in a 'facilitating environment' (*Winnicott*, 1965) saved his unstable energic equilibrium. In addition, he now began to develop a close relationship to Jacqueline, the 'worthy sister'[2] whom he looked upon as his own daughter, later even as a substitute for his mother. Gilberte describes their relationship as follows: 'He could love nobody more than he loved my sister ... for their feelings were so alike that they agreed in all things; and their hearts were surely one heart.'

His childhood passed until puberty without further disturbances. At 11 years of age his self-taught studies in mathematics had progressed to such an extend that, without any help, he discovered Euclid's 32nd theorem. Thereupon his father offered to let him join in with the activities of his learned circle of mathematicians, a group which he had kept closed to him until then. In so doing he demonstrated anew his readiness to open up his intimate world – the highly cathected mathematics – to his son and so enabled Blaise' awakened spirit to find its first reality in the world of theoretical science (*Loch*, 1976). In this way Blaise found security and stimulation, even if this rational truth was not yet embedded in a sensory dimension.

The following description of the illness which began in his adolescence shows the nature of Pascal's specific psycho-biological economy.

From earliest childhood he was sickly, weak and feverish and in Gilberte's account we find that along with many neuro-vegetative symptoms he also suffered from a feeling of emptiness in his body. At 18 a series of functional disorders and hypochondrial anxieties appeared. The records mention anorectic symptoms, loss of appetite, epigastric pains, heat in the bowels, unbearable headaches and many other ailments; at times he could only take liquids administered in drops. According to his own accounts he did not live another day without pain from that time on, although this did not prevent him from continuing his work in science and mathematics. With his illness he subtly achieved a new control over his environment, for he was now dependent on special care and attention. The onset of this new bout of symptoms coincided with the marriage of his sister Gilberte and his father's arrangements for Jacqueline's marriage. That there was an inner connexion between these events and Blaise' somatic labilization seems highly probable.

In the remarkable libidinal relation to his illness that he had developed over the years, Blaise Pascal had found a psychic mechanism which protected him from the progredient disorganisation. In her biography, Gilberte writes: 'It was evident that he loved this condition, which few others could have done, for such a love demands a humble and peaceful submission.' He was inspired by the thought: '. . . to desire suffering, for this is the condition in which a Christian should always live.' He repeatedly prayed to God not to take his illness away from him.

In January 1646, when Pascal was almost 23, his father suffered a dislocation of the hip through a fall. We also know that about a year later Blaise was similarly using crutches on account of a hip complaint. The feelings of guilt that his father's accident aroused in Blaise threw him into a crisis which threatened to upset his inner equilibrium. He had to fear losing both his significant objects: his father through death and his favourite sister Jacqueline, by now a great social success, to another man. Through two uncles of his who came to take care of his sick father Pascal was introduced to the Jansenists, a religious sect which adhered to a strict, ascetic Christianity. Their views convinced him and he gave himself over to an intense faith. This was the time of his first conversion. He also succeeded in winning Jacqueline over to the teachings of Jansenius, thereby getting her away from her societal ambitions, and later converted the rest of the family.

Religious faith and the stabilization of his object relations in the family gave him a new inner security which allowed him to turn his attention to experimentation in physical science. In two theoretical essays which resulted from this work he refuted Aristotle's postulate of the 'horror vacui' and proved that vacuum exists as an entity in nature, although it is kept within limits and is maintained in economic equilibrium with opposing forces, such as gravity. The recognition that vacuum is no longer merely absence, or the unthinkable or unnameable, but is a definite and circumscribable reality represented a further step towards overcoming his feeling of inner emptiness, his psychosomatic phenomenon. With his thesis Pascal formulated a universal law of nature which stood in opposition to the prevailing view of the time, whose most brilliant advocate was Descartes. To this emptiness he attributed an economic function counteracting matter.

Blaise Pascal's father died unexpectedly in 1651. A few months later Jacqueline, against the will of her brother Blaise, became a nun at Port Royal de Champs, a cloister near Versailles which was well known as the stronghold of Jansenism. Pascal was very much affected by these events. Shortly before his father's death a new chapter in his life had already begun, which his biographers referred to as the 'worldly period' ('la période mondaine'); this lasted for about another two years but then a growing restlessness and sense of helplessness drove him to seek refuge with his sister at Port Royal. It was in a cell there, in a nocturnal enlightenment, that he experienced his 'second conversion'. He recorded the experience of this enlightenment, a decisive moment which he apprehended as an encounter with God, on a piece of paper and sewed it into the lining of his suit. This 'memorial' was found by his servant only after his death and became an important document on the life of Pascal the 'homo religiosus'. He became a member of Port Royal and remained so until shortly before his death, despite frequent polemical confrontations with some of the leading Jansenists there. However, he spent considerable periods of time outside the cloister as well and it is interesting to note that he always chose to use a pseudonym in the inns where he stayed during his times in Paris. Together with his sister he was very active in bitter struggles in defence of Jansenism. At this time he wrote the famous 'Provinciales', a series of letters in which 'he publicly exposed his adversaries with the utmost vehemence and tied them in knots with the most insoluble dialectical reasoning' (*Beguin*, 1959). Now began his last great creative period (1656–1658) during which he produced his most important philosophical reflexions, the 'Pensées'. These are 'really fragments of a complete work, at least of a larger undertaking' (Guardini)[3], which he had conceived as a whole and wanted to make into an apology. Due to his illness and early death, however, he was unable to combine these fragments. In the Pensées, Pascal reflects on the Christian faith and the existence and mind of man in his relation to God, especially to the 'suffering Christ'. In Guardini's view, the Pensées arise from the intuition of a genius, are of high aesthetic quality and are guided by ethical and religious aspirations together with a will to truth.

In some of the Pensées, Pascal applied his physical postulates on the nature of external reality to the inner psychic world of man: in man, too, he discovered the inner emptiness, the fundamental dependency, which on the one hand through the act of thinking, on the other by striving towards the Godly – the infinite object – can be filled and overcome. The acquisition of understanding and sensual union with God, the eternal truth, set limits to the inner emptiness and thereby annul it. So he writes, for example: 'Man is only a swaying reed, the most fragile in all nature, but he is a reed that thinks', or: 'Through space the universe seizes me and devours me . . . ; through thinking I seize it.'

These insights of Pascal's correspond to our economic conception of psychosomatics: inner emptiness, illness and an unstable energic equilibrium can lead to resignation, progredient disorganisation and even death. However, if the individual succeeds in finding basic support with his objects and in mobilizing his psychic adjustment mechanisms, he can restore his inner equilibrium. If he is further able to become aware of his inner emptiness and face up to experiencing it, this elaboration process can lead to the discovery of the 'libidinal object' (*Stephanos*, 1976/77a, b). Thus he internalizes a libidinal object constancy, a stable 'inner possession' and so finds the way to his own creative potential. Our analytic approach to psychosomatics aims to bring about just such a psychic maturation process (*Stephanos*, 1973, 1974, 1975, 1976/77a, c).

In the last 4 years of his life, Blaise Pascal's physical condition declined to such an extent that he was forced to give up his scientific work. According to his sister Gilberte these years were 'one long, uninterrupted process of wasting away'. There was no new illness involved but merely a grave intensification of the many ailments which had plagued him since his youth. For Pascal himself this was a time of vacillation between meditation and helplessness; however, little by little, he was consciously preparing himself for the death in which he saw the possibility of consummating his sacrifice to God.

On the 4th October 1661 his sister Jacqueline died and Pascal showed as few signs of mourning at this loss as he had at the death of his father. Two months later he renounced his membership of Port Royal following a quarrel with some of its leading members and abandoned his struggle for Jansenism. The beginning of 1662 saw him totally emaciated and prey to intensely painful colic attacks and on the 19th August 1662, at the age of 39, he died – 10 months after his sister. The autopsy revealed a 'gangrene' of the colon.

A review of this life history shows us an interesting series of connexions. Pascal's genius could unfold because he had overcome his primary deficiency. We are aware that it is impossible for psychoanalysis alone to comprehend the complexity of a highly gifted constitution and our aim in this study is to concentrate only on Pascal's 'vital economy' (*Marty*, 1976). His biography shows us his progression from absolute dependence, through abstract science (mathematics and physics) to self-knowledge and thus to his sensual truth (*Loch*, 1976). In the course of this development he was continually oscillating between his psychosomatic phenomenon, character neurotic defence and creativity.

Blaise Pascal remained throughout his life close to a maternal object, first his father's wife and later his father's daughter. The interest in mathematics he developed during puberty can be seen as a part of his search for the father's feminine partner, the 'femme amante' (*Braunschweig and Fain*, 1971; *Stephanos*, 1976/77a, c). His unconscious archaic bond to his mother led to a number of reaction formations, such as his refusal ever to utter the word 'I'. Pascal's intellectual eminence stood in contrast to his infantile personality traits. Shortly before his death a friend of his, a priest, described him as naive: 'He is a child; he is humble and submissive like a child.'[2] His behaviour towards his adversaries was quarrelsome, arrogant and obstinate in the extreme, which can be seen as an expression of his defence against the bad introject. A few days before he died he begged his sister Gilberte to arrange for him '. . . to be brought to the "hôpital des incurables", for he had a great longing to die in the company of the poor.'[2] Now that his strength had left him he wanted to seek refuge among his mother's 'friends', the social 'outcasts'.

Pascal had an idea of his need for support but also of his fragile basal homeostasis. He managed his relations with his external objects strategically, in order to protect himself from excessive stimulation, possessive claims and eroticism, and resisted every form of attachment. To quote Gilberte, 'He distinguished between two sorts of compassion, one rooted in sentiment and the other in reason, and while admitting that the former may be of some use in the world, yet he maintained that merit has no part in it and that virtuous people should value only reasonable compassion which, he said, consists in sharing all that befalls our friends in every way that reason dictates – at the price of our property, our convenience, our freedom, even our life, if the object of our compassion is deserving of such sacrifice; and that he is always deserving of it if it is made for God, who must be the only aim of the compassion of Christians.'

Filled with an inexorable severity towards himself he further renounced every form of bodily gratification, in order to sublimate his drives in thinking and to deepen his inner life. Gilberte tells of the spiked belt he wore against his bare skin and of how he would strike against it whenever he felt himself threatened by vanity or pride.

The repression of his dependency, on the one hand, and the elaboration of his death fears – the 'fear of breakdown' (*Winnicott*, 1974) – and with it his psychic emptiness, on the other, helped him to develop his ego functions and to attain to creative thought. In this way he was able to prevent the psychosomatic phenomenon from gaining total control over his life, even if the constant struggle against his primary lack – the 'nothing' in him ('le néant dans l'homme') – exhausted his bodily strength early in life and the loss of his object Jacqueline, along with the parting from Port Royal, meant the final breakdown of his biological equilibrium. But did he not find refuge in the death he had so much longed for? For in the finality of death he could at last achieve an eternal union with his 'objet infini'.

References

Anzieu, D.: Naissance du concept de vide chez Pascal. Nouv. Revue Psychol. *11:* 195–203 (1975).

Beguin, A.: Blaise Pascal in Selbstzeugnissen und Bilddokumenten. Rowohlts Monographien (Rowohlt, Hamburg 1959).

Boutroux, E.: Blaise Pascal (1900).

Braunschweig, D. et Fain, M.: Eros et Antéros (Payot, Paris 1971).

Cresson, A.: Pascal, sa vie, son œuvre (1938); 4e éd. (Paris 1956).

Faugère, P.: Lettres, opuscules et mémoires de Madame Périer et de Jacqueline, sœur de Pascal et de Marguerite Périer, sa nièce (Faugère, Paris 1845).

Giraud, V.: Pascal, l'homme, l'œuvre, l'influence (Paris 1898).

Kreisler, L.; Fain, M. et Soulé, M.: L'enfant et son corps (PUF, Paris 1974).

Lichtenstein, H.: The role of Narcissism in the emergence and maintenance of a primary identity. Int. J. Psych. Ass. *45:* 49–56 (1964).

Loch, W.: Psychoanalyse und Wahrheit. Psyche *30:* 865–898 (1976).

Lombroso, C.T. and Lermann, P.: Breath-holding spells (cyanotic and pallid infantile syncope). Pediatrics *39:* 563–581 (1967).

Marty, P.: Les mouvements individuels de vie et de mort (Payot, Paris 1976).

Rüttenauer, W.: Blaise Pascal – Gedanken, Vol. 7 (Dieterichsche Verlags-Buchhandlung, Leipzig 1937; Neuausgabe, 1955).

Rüttenauer, W.: Blaise Pascal – Vermächtnis eines grossen Herzens – Die kleineren Schriften, Vol 16 (Dieterichsche Verlags-Buchhandlung, Leipzig 1938; Neuausgabe, 1947).

Stephanos, S.: Analytisch-Psychosomatische Therapie. Beiheft zum Jahrbuch Psychoa., No. 1 (Huber, Bern 1973).

Stephanos, S.: Die Krankenschwester als therapeutische Bezugsperson und das Nachbehandlungsarrangement im Stationsmodell der Psychosomatischen Klinik Giessen. Psychother. med. Psychol. *24:* 117–131 (1974).

Stephanos, S.: A concept of analytical treatment for patients with psychosomatic disorders. Psychother. Psychosom. *26:* 178–187 (1975).

Stephanos, S.: Überlegungen zur analytisch-psychosomatischen Therapie. Medsche Welt *9:* 441 (1976).

Stephanos, S.: Sexualobjekt, libidinöses Objekt und Übertragungsprozess. Jahrbuch Psychoa. (Huber, Bern, in press 1976/77a).

Stephanos, S.: Die Problematik des 'psychosomatischen Phänomens' im Zusammenhang mit dem Konzept der 'pensée opératoire'; in *Uexküll:* Lehrbuch d. Psychosomatischen Medizin (Urban & Schwarzenberg, Munich, in press 1976/77b).

Stephanos, S.: Theorie und Praxis der analytisch-psychosomatischen Therapie; in *Uexküll:*

Lehrbuch d. Psychosomatischen Medizin (Urban & Schwarzenberg, Munich, in press 1976/77c).

Winnicott, D. W.: Primary maternal preoccupation; in Collected papers – through paediatrics to psycho-analysis (Tavistock, London/Basic Books, New York 1956).

Winnicott, D. W.: The maturational processes and the facilitating environment (Hogarth, London 1965).

Winnicott, D. W.: Fear of breakdown. Int. Rev. Psychoa. *1*: 103 (1974).

Prof. Dr. med. *Samir Stephanos,* Zentrum für Innere Medizin, Arbeitsgruppe Psychosomatik, Gaffkystrasse 14, *D-6300 Giessen* (FRG)

Proc. 11th Eur. Conf. Psychosom. Res., Heidelberg 1976
Psychother. Psychosom. *28:* 357–360 (1977)

Pinocchio – a Psychosomatic Syndrome

A. Sellschopp-Rüppell and M. von Rad

Psychosomatische Universitätsklinik Heidelberg

In this address we should like to tell the story of Pinocchio, as it appears
to us to have a number of elements in common with the case history of the
psychosomatic patient. Thus – despite the risk that we shall have Pinocchio's
donkey's head put on ourselves – we shall be referring to our earlier term,
the 'Pinocchio syndrome', which we should like to explain and clarify here.

Pinocchio is a fairy-tale figure, who first appeared almost 100 years ago
(1881) in a series by the Italian writer and journalist *Carlo Lorenzini* in the
'Giornale dei Bambini'. The story quickly spread all over the world (1).

Lorenzini, the son of a cook and a seamstress, lost his father while he was
very young, and, as the oldest of nine children, he had to look early for a job.
All his life he remained a fighter whose ideals were the improvement of
education and the political struggle for independence. But at the time when
Pinocchio was published he was already so debilitated by asthma that he
could no longer do regular work. He was also looked on as an idler and vaga-
bond and thus as a constant source of annoyance. Apparently it was difficult
for him to make close emotional attachments. He did not have a familiy of
his own – in honour of his mother he later named himself after her birthplace,
Collodi (2).

It thus appears that the creation of Pinocchio in Collodi's old age is an
expression of his desire to master his conflicts. The story of Pinocchio is full
of wise humour and contrariety, in fact it is so unfeigned and true to life
that it occasionally has something disconcerting about it and, in it, the same
theme recurs again and again as if in counterpoint: in each wayward attempt
to become a real person Pinocchio misjudges himself and his counterpart –
each apparent step forward turns out to be a blunder; and it seems a real
question as to whether the unhappy beginning of the story – freeing oneself

with a kick and not looking back – is not, in fact, a better solution that the seemingly happy ending with its superficially successful adaptation.

In the following we should like to tell you the story of Pinocchio in short extracts. Then we shall pinpoint some essential characteristics of the psycho-somatic patient as they are shown up in the story. Furthermore, we should like to indicate some particularities of the parent-child relationship in psycho-somatic patients. Finally, we shall deal with some thoughts on these patients in the therapeutic situation.

The Story

Pinocchio's birth begins with a quarrel, followed by a verdict – he alone is guilty. Immediately afterwards he gets a 'warning' which is given him as a 'great truth' (p. 16) – 'Woe to those boys who turn against their parents and run away (p. 16) from home for no reason whatever; they will never come to any good in this world, and sooner or later they will repent bitterly.' The first time he tries to eat he fails absurdly: the saucepan is not real, it is only painted on the wall; instead of yolk and white the egg contains a chick, which mocks him.

Now he is to go to school. On the way he meets the marionettes who would like to play with him as their brother. He forgets school, but gets everything mixed up, himself into mortal danger, and calls in utter despair for his father for: 'I never knew my mother'. In real love for his father he intends to return home. But his incapacity to experience emotions and feel-ings and to differentiate between real and false friends – and to hold on to this differentiation and use it for his actions – is his downfall again. The fox and the fawning cat chum up to him, take advantage of him and finally hang him. Dying he murmurs 'Oh, papa! papa! if only you were here.' The story seems to have come to an end. But this is not to be, and a motherly fairy appears to save him, who – how could it be otherwise? – calls the most famous doctors of the region to her aid. They state that 'the wisest thing a prudent doctor can do, when he does not know what he is talking about, is to be silent' and that 'when a dead person weeps it is a sign that he is on the way to getting well' (p. 76). But Pinocchio does not turn out to be a good subject for their therapy. He refuses to take the medicine: 'We children are all like that! We are more afraid of the medicine than of the illness' (p. 80). He takes up the search for his father once again and ends up in prison. The paradoxes con-tinue: in the same way as it is not the parents who may not leave him, but he who may not leave his parents, he gets into prison as the person who has been robbed and not as the thief. Thus everything he does gets confused and disharmony prevails: he runs away when he is excpected to learn; he steals when it would be good to earn money. But there is also repentance and despairing efforts to make reparations for his own salvation and to please his parents: it is high time for him to become a real person like everyone else (p. 125). But despite the additional warning that his manner of living will put him in prison or in hospital he cannot keep to his resolutions.

At last he seems to have seen reason and gone to school. A large tea-party has already been arranged to celebrate his becoming a human being. But on the night before he makes a last attempt to escape into toyland, which ends cruelly. He is laughed at and mocked there, they try to drown him and sell his skin. He finally ends up inside the whale, where he meets his father who was shipwrecked looking for his son. The end is quickly told. During a fit of coughing of the asthmatic (!) whale he is thrown back into the sea with his father, whom he carries on his shoulders to the shore. At last he goes to school, works and earns money, with which he supports his parents. A happy ending?

If we look at the Pinocchio story in the light of some typical reactions which we find in psychosomatic patients, we notice the following: (1) He is made of wood; apart from his uncoordinated motor ability, it is obvious that he is totally unfamiliar with emotions. The only ones which occasionally break through are aggressive destructivity or abrupt despair. (2) An incapacity to relate inner experiences meaningfully to action is also conspicuous. The formation of experience takes place, rather, by performance training. (3) He exhausts himself in constant efforts to bring his desires into harmony with stubborn reality (toyland). (4) He has an overconcrete association with reality (painted saucepan) and the mechanical character of this makes his inner retreat obvious. (5) Losses give rise to panic and are life-threatening. (6) Lack of introjects leads to the repeated attempt to establish contact with transitional objects, which must fail.

We now turn to the structure of the parent-child relationship, which seems to us to be similar to that of many psychosomatic patuents. (1) An exaggerated demand for loyalty binds the patients to his family, and this leads to an insoluble conflict with other love objects. The parents cannot live without the child (one aspect of parentification); the patient is, however, left alone when he himself needs help. (2) We often find a pseudostrong father and an instable, unreliable mother. (3) An overstated and unyielding ideology of what is right and good, and a belief in their own selflessness, hardly allow any feelings of guilt to arise in the parents.

Finally, we should like to point out that the therapeutic work with these patients must take the opposite direction; away from their compulsion to adapt to the norm – this implies an offer of a concrete, reliable, emotional attachment with strict observance of the countertransference as well as making available possibilities for representing conflicts scenically (group therapy, semiverbal methods) (3). We shall go into this in further detail elsewhere.

References

1 *Collodi, C.:* Pinocchio – the tale of a puppet; translated by *M. A. Murray,* revised by *G. Tassinari* (London 1975).
2 *Eichhorn, B.: Carlo Collodi* – der Mensch, sein Leben und sein Werk. Z. Jugendliteratur, Heft 5 (1968).
3 *Rad, M. v. and Rüppell, A.:* Combined inpatient and outpatient psychotherapy: a therapeutic model for psychosomatics. Psychother. Psychosom. *26:* 237–243 (1975).

Almuth Sellschopp-Rüppell, PhD, Psychosomatische Klinik der Universität Heidelberg, Vossstrasse 2, *D–6900 Heidelberg* (FRG)

Panel- and Plenum-Discussion:
Psychotherapeutic Problems with Psychosomatic Patients

Dr. Bräutigam: Quite apart from the concept of alexithymia, the question of special treatment techniques for psychosomatic patients is prompted by the general experience that psychosomatic patients have difficulties in the classic psychotherapeutic interview situation. The difficulties lie in the fact that the patient, with help from his therapist, be confronted with himself. He should not take his experience as given and his behavior for granted, but see it as open, as being susceptible to new alternatives. The situation, and course of his life as well as his own reactions should become matters of critical, clarifying reflections. Thus, it is hoped that the psychosomatic patient's verbalization will lead to his desomatization. The neurotic patient is characterized by highly ambivalent attitudes, fluctuating self-esteem and fixations as revealed in current memory bits, fantasies and other infantile material. Thus, he presents ideal conditions for a dialogue – particularly if he can reenact his infantile situation in his relationship with a doctor he experiences as a parent figure. The psychoanalyst needs only facilitate such dialogue by listening and responding sympathetically to the patient – perhaps by helping him along with interpretations when he falters in working through his past.

The psychosomatic patient does not usually share the neurotic patient's initial advantages: his symptoms and complaints are very much more bound up with current stresses and losses, etc., i.e. with external events. At the same time, his physical symptoms, whether based on destructive organic processes or not, are viewed as real physical conditions rather than as expressions of intrapsychic forces. Another impediment, if the concept of alexithymia is correct, consists in his 'concrete' thinking, lack of fantasy and incapacity to recognize alternatives.

Therefore, special therapeutic techniques must aim at helping the psychosomatic patient overcome his difficulties to enter into a dialogue with himself. He must learn to view from the outside the life which he now takes for granted; by disengaging a part of himself and an observer role vis-à-vis himself, he must become able to encounter himself and outgrow his limited and concretitic understanding of himself and of his world. For the neurotic patient, who can utilize fantasies, thoughts and spoken words, this appears a manageable task; for the psychosomatic patient this is extremely difficult, if not impossible.

How can one help the psychosomatic patient to enter into a dialogue with himself and to view himself from the outside? How can one widen his narrow and overconcrete perspective of himself and his world?

In their papers, members of my clinic staff have indicated the lines along which we are working. Group therapy seems to offer good start. Here one can enlist other patients in the group, who suffer from similar problems but are further on the road to progress to help the given patient in discovering something about himself. For example, these other patients may provide parallels from their own lives and thus help in the verbalization of one's experiences.

The external dialogue with equal partners in the group can lead to a dialogue with oneself. Initially, the group therapist and other members can represent the yet fragile new self in such a dialogue; they serve not only a reflective function, but they can also compensate in various other ways for the patient's own weakness in emotional awareness and in verbal fluency.

Another approach we found useful is 'sensual awareness therapy' (konzentrative Bewegungstherapie). Generally, touching the patient is taboo in psychoanalysis and body awareness is usually not much fostered. Here, however, we foster such awareness deliberately and encourage the patient to perceive and express bodily feelings in a differentiated manner. We may either address him directly or utilize the resources of the group.

A third approach toward an inner dialogue is analytical ergotherapy (Gestaltungstherapie). Here we encourage patients to deal with emotionally charged material by way of creative expression, i.e. by drawing pictures or modelling clay of other materials. Thus, anxieties, desires, memories but also the significant persons from the patient's life become accessible in an elementary fashion. These creations expose a part of the patient's own self. This part can then become to interpretation and clarification during the sessions with the analytical ergotherapist and other members of the group. Thus, a dialogue with a part of the self is facilitated. We have had our least experience with the modifications of standard psychotherapeutic techniques for psychosomatic patients. We refer to techniques by which the psychotherapist may alert his patient to new perspectives and alternative attitudes during critical and conflictual situations. By 'borrowing ego functions' from the analyst, the patient may then experiment with a new self-image and new behavior. Thus, he is released from the restrictive stranglehold of his concrete and own-dimensioned perceptions of reality. Here we should include what *Fürstenau* has called the 'vicarious exercise of ego functions by the analyst' a preparatory step toward a more classical analysis and dialogue with himself. We still know too little about the variable of the psychotherapeutic process as a whole to be able to say more exactly under which conditions of therapy the physical symptom itself enters into the healing process, i.e. the cathartic and comforting effects.

All these techniques are intended to counteract the psychosomatic patient's limited capacity for self-exposure and self-reflection – either by interpreting a part of his past life, or by developing for his current life, a new experimental matrix.

Dr. Shands: My first analyst, Hanns Sachs, had an aphorism that the analysis ends when the analysand realizes it will never end. This means to me that the analysand takes over the analyzing function in a self-reflective or *reflective* manner. The patient who cannot describe feelings cannot 'take a point of view' outside himself, one must first become an object to oneself by taking the point of view of the other. This is an ability the psychosomatic patient does not demonstrate; he does not develop the same kind of describable 'transference' reaction. In *Piaget*'s language, this reflexive maneuver is an 'operation upon operations' or a second-order descriptive system. One most interesting aspect of this problem is that of accessibility to the 'private world' of emotional states. *Cannon*'s classic work was based upon 'invading' the privacy of the body with electrocardiographs, electroencephalographs, blood samples and the like. In a concrete metaphor, it is possible to suggest that a 'linguistic probe' is another form of instrument for invading the privacy of the inner world so as to render the otherwise invisible events there into an 'objective' or described form through verbalization.

Jakobson describes two polar ways of describing; that using metonymy with a basic relation of contiguity, and the other uses metaphor, with a basic relation of similarity. These two are as well the two modes of association in association psychology. Exploratory forms of psychotherapy use both modes, asking 'What was that like?' and 'Under what circumstances have you felt these feelings before?' using metaphor and metonymy alternatively. *Lacan*'s famous analysis of *Freud*'s 'Signorelli' dream analysis explores the dialectical relation of the two in great detail.

In my experience, the psychosomatic patient is unable to use the therapist as a symbol for other persons in his life in a conscious sense, that is, 'in the transference'. To the psychosomatic patient, 'doctor' is an idea he cannot play with, and the doctor who is there is a 'real' rather than an 'imaginary' relative. It sometimes happens that patients may learn or develop feelings after a long period of work; recently a patient I have seen sporadically for 17 years suddenly developed describable feelings for the first time in his mid-30s! To me, the implication is that there is a great deal of quite unconscious learning implicit in a relation with a preceptor that may continue long after the period we usually think of as that of learning.

Dr. Nemiah: I should like to make a couple of brief comments that perhaps go beyond the subject of psychotherapy, but which are, I think, needed to correct some misconceptions about alexithymia that appear to have arisen during this conference. I am concerned particularly at the view that has been expressed that the concept of alexithymia implies that those who manifest the characteristics are unresponsive, and that consequently nothing can be done to help them.

Nothing could be further from the facts. The essence of the psychosomatic concept is that patients with psychosomatic disorders are responding to environmental stresses and strains with a disturbance in psychophysiological processes. The questions to be answered are: *How* are they responding? What is the nature of the internal biological and psychological processes which are set in motion by environmental stimuli to result in a bodily illness? Do these processes differ from those found in neurotic patients and, if so, in what way? This is, after all, the basic theme of this conference, and it is to these questions that the concept of alexithymia is addressed.

It should also be pointed out that alexithymic patients with psychosomatic disorders are responsive to their environment in ways that are therapeutic. All of us know from experience that many such patients improve by merely being hospitalized – a procedure that removes them from a pathogenic stressful situation and provides them with a supportive and helpful human environment. This provides us with an important clue as to the kind of psychotherapeutic approach indicated for such patients – that is that a supportive relationship with their physician and other caretakers is central to their clinical management.

This leads me to a final comment. We have been tending to talk about psychotherapy today as if it were a single unified procedure involving the exploration of feelings and fantasies as a means through insight of resolving internal psychodynamic conflicts. Such insight psychotherapy, based on and derived from psychoanalysis, is, of course, a major form of psychotherapy highly effective for many patients. But it is not applicable to all of the clinical problems with which we have to deal, and the skilled psychotherapist employs, or should employ, a variety of procedures, his choice of technique being based on the needs and psychological characteristics of his patient. It is our contention, based on our experience thus far, that patients with alexithymic characteristics do not generally respond well to insight psychotherapy, and that other kinds of psychotherapeutic measures must be devised to help them. It is a value of the concept of alexithymia that it focuses attention on the psychological characteristics and needs of the individual who manifests them and challenges us to look for more effective psychotherapeutic techniques that will take these characteristics and needs into account.

Dr. Köhle: I am working at a department of psychosomatic medicine which is part of an internal medicine center. With this setting in mind, I would like to focus on the problem of establishing a working alliance with hospitalized psychosomatic patients. Apart from the problem of developing adequate modifications of the psychotherapeutic approachs suitable for this group of patients, we have to solve the task of winning the patients for psychosomatic treatment. Whatever psychotherapeutic or behavioral approach we wish to apply, the prerequisite for bulding up a working alliance with these patients is the establishment of an environment that facilitates the recognition of psychic processes. In our country the psychosomatic patient is generally first confronted with a general practitioner or a medical doctor in a hospital who has not had any training in psychosomatic medicine. The approach towards his illness is therefore likely to be an illness-centered one. This implies a learning procedure for the patient who is successively taught to think and speak in illness-centered terms. At this point the theory of alexithymia comes in on which, in my opinion, there is not yet enough research material available in order to discuss the point of 'alexithymia' of the members in an institution or the alexithymogenic potency of institutions any further right now.

The psychosomatic consultant's task of building up a working-alliance with the psychosomatic patient is often so difficult because the individual patient's resistances are reinforced by the resistances inherent in the medical institution. Keeping this unpleasant fact in mind, it seems to be a necessary and meaningful policy to experiment with modifications of the setting in medical institutions. We have, therefore, concentrated our efforts in Ulm in this direction on a 15-bed ward of the University Department of Internal Medicine. It was our major aim to structure medical and nursing routine in such a way so as to allow a continuous development as well as a reflection of the relationship with the patient.

We reorganized the doctor's interview and developed an interview for nurses; we discuss these interviews every morning in a ward-conference and try to modify the daily ward rounds in a patient-centered way. In addition to this development in the organization of the regular ward events, we have established a 1-year training course in 'patient-centered nursing'. In our concept, medical and nursing care form the basis for the establishment of a relationship in which a patient, who experiences himself as primarily bodily ill, can feel secure enough to open up to a psychosomatic approach to his illness.

It is our experience that more patients can be reached in such a setting. The setting allows a continuous connection of bodily complaints and the patient's interactional experiences and emotional situation.

Dr. Wolff: I only want to make a few comments to illustrate my basic approach which I described on the first morning. When we are treating a patient in psychotherapy who has a psychosomatic symptom, be it functionally or structually determined, the first thing we have to remember is that we are not treating a disease but rather that we are working with a person who is ill. How do we treat the *person?* Here I want to remind you of the notion which I quoted from *Winnicott* that for psychotherapy to be effective, both patient and therapist have got to learn to play together and find the right way of doing so. By this I mean that the patient and I have to play with fantasies, thoughts, feelings and experience. I entirely agree with *Sifneos and Nemiah* that in some psychosomatic patients the characteristics described as alexithymic are often a considerable obstacle to this kind of work as the patient may be out of touch with his fantasies and feelings. The question which I as a therapist then have to ask myself is not 'has he got no feelings', but rather 'where has he put his feelings?'

I will give you an example to illustrate this. A few months ago I was asked to see an asthmatic boy of 19 who had had asthma for many years, but who had recently also started to cut himself. The referring doctor had sent him to me with the comment that he doubted whether psychotherapy could help him as he seemed to be completely out of touch with his feelings. That seemed to be a correct description when he came to see me. The patient gave me a brief account of his asthma and of the fact that he cut himself, but when I asked him 'Why do you cut yourself?' he replied 'I don't know, I just do'. 'What do you feel when you cut yourself?' 'I don't know'. Some enquiry into his family and personal life also only elicited some factual information but without any relevant feelings. So I knew his feelings had got lost and I asked him simply 'Which arm of yours cuts which arm?' 'I always use my right arm and cut my left'. 'Right, I want you please to imagine yourself to *be* your right arm and later on to tell me what that feels like'.

Until then he had looked collapsed and bored and I had felt bored too, but when asked to describe what it felt like to *be* his right arm he got excited and said 'I could cut anything in the world, I'm feeling incredibly angry when I'm that – I don't like it, it's frightening ,I prefer to be my left arm'. I said 'Alright, please be your left arm' and he said 'I feel very passive and completely at the mercy of anybody who would attack me. I don't like this at all'. Then he suddenly said 'I feel awful' and put his hand on his stomach. I said 'What is going on in your stomach?' 'I don't know'. Then I said 'Alright, shut your eyes and be your stomach and tell me what that feels like'. Then he said in a frightened voice 'very vulnerable, as if I'm going to go to pieces completely', at which moment both his legs began to shake and tremble. I commented 'Something else is happening to your legs, isn't it?' And he said 'Yes, yes, that's right'. He looked at his legs and said 'It feels as if they couldn't support me'. 'So you want to collapse' I said, 'is there any part of your body where something is going on at the moment?' He replied, 'Well, I'm getting a headache'. I said 'Right, what's happening up there in your head?' to which his reply was 'I feel terribly confused'.

The lesson I learned from all this, and which I want to get across to you, is that when I work with an alexithymic patient, I use every means at my disposal to try and locate where his feelings have been projected into. To this young man, who by now seemed to have come alive, I was now able to say: 'We seem to have learned a lot about you. Your anger is in your right arm, your passivity and receptiveness in your left arm. Vulnerable and frightening feelings are in your stomach, the wish to give up completely is in your legs and, as a result of all that, you feel confused; but you don't feel that either but your confused feelings are put into your head. We will have to do a lot of work, in order to try and put all these bits and pieces together to make you into one whole human being.' He is now in psychotherapy where that process is slowly beginning.

I have given you this example to illustrate how playful and inventive one sometimes has to be when working with patients of this kind. Once one has helped them get in touch with their feelings and fantasies, one can in my experience continue working with them in analytically oriented therapy, often for a long period, provided one is prepared again to use similar methods if progress gets blocked by loss of contact with feelings and fantasies.

One last comment: during ongoing therapy it is essential to make continuous use of one's own countertransference because the patient instead of projecting his feelings into his body may project them into the therapist. Dr. *Taylor* has already described this to us; when the therapist feels bored or sad or angry he may be experiencing the patient's feelings and fantasies. This gives the therapist frequent opportunities of suggesting to the patient what he may be feeling or what fantasies he may be avoiding so that further work can be done in therapy.

Dr. Pierloot: After all the different contributions we have heard during this conference and this afternoon, it is hard to imagine that something new can still be said on the subject of psychotherapy and psychosomatic patients. So I would like to limit myself to a few remarks which I consider as a result of the opinions I have heard at this conference confronted with my own experience.

The first remark will be very complimentary to what Dr. *Wolff* has said. It concerns the term 'psychosomatic patient'. I wonder if, from the point of view of therapy, it is opportune to stress this term too much. Psychotherapy is after all always directed to the person and not to the complaint or disease. Moreover, every psychotherapy is a unique form of interaction between a given therapist and a given patient. What is important is the total personality of patient and therapist. And I am somewhat afraid that the labelling of a patient on the basis of one aspect of his functioning, the formation of psychosomatic symptoms, may create a negative bias towards this patient. The choice of a given form of psychotherapy should be based on the whole personality of the patient on the one side and the attitude of the therapist towards his patient on the other side. And I would like to complete this statement with the remark that sometimes it can be better to ignore or not to take into account the specific symptomatology. An example is the group psychotherapy for anorexia nervosa patients. In our experience, groups composed uniquely by anorexia patients are very hard to run. Since we simply ignore the anorexia label and treat these patients in groups consisting of different sorts of neurotic patients, the results are much better. A second remark regards the meaning of the presentation of the somatic symptom in psychotherapy. Whatever the value of the symptom may be in the total economy of the psychological function of the patient, the presentation of the symptom to the psychotherapist has a meaning in itself. It may, for instance, be a form of seduction, but very often it appears as a barrier. It disturbs the communication between the patient and the therapist. The patient speaks another language than that the therapist would like him to speak, but it also disturbs the communication between the psychological experience and the somatic functioning in the patient. *Heinz Wolff* has spoken of a splitting of psyche and soma. In the same sense alexithymia can be considered as a splitting between emotional experience and verbalized feeling. The concept of splitting has been advanced by *Melanie Klein and Fairbairn* and has been elaborated by *Otto Kernberg* as the essential feature of the so-called borderline personality. It seems attractive to suppose a connection between different forms of splitting but I think we must be very careful not to make the term splitting to a new magical term that sounds good and explains almost nothing. Still it can be interesting to note that splitting, as described by the mentioned authors, is a mechanism that cannot be overcome by interpretation which is a classical tool in dynamic psychotherapy.

What is needed are procedures with rather integrative effects and in many contributions at this conference it has been proclaimed that the phenomena of alexithymia should be overcome by specific therapeutic procedures. I would only like to refer to our experience with the autogenic training of *Schulz*. Although I cannot confirm it in exact numbers, we have the impression that some alexithymic patients after completing the lower cycle of relaxation can proceed to the higher cycle described by *Schulz* and based on inside and interpretation.

And that leads me to my last remark, more specifically with regard to the phenomena of alexithymia. From the point of view of therapy, the primary question seems to me in how far the phenomenon is irreversible. In the paper I presented yesterday I mentioned the puzzling finding that alexithymia correlates with drop-out in short-term dynamic psychotherapy, but not with less success in the completed therapies. That leaves open the supposition that in these completed therapies alexithymia had been overcome. What is lacking is a comparison of the rating of patients for alexithymia before and after certain therapeutic procedures. Therefore, we have to refine our measurement tools to plan new research designs and to provide data. I think that this conference has stimulated us in that direction and I am grateful to all the contributors who provided perhaps different but always interesting ideas.

Dr. Heiberg: I would like to share with you the experience that made me, so to speak, believe in the concept of alexithymia and in how to deal with it therapeutically:

Three years ago when I was giving a lecture in the Norwegian Psychiatric Association with our young residents, I had just come to learn about this new concept of alexithymia and I was very enthusiastic about it, ending up by saying triumphantically: 'Isn't it nice that this defect that others call lack of communication is no longer our fault, it's a deficiency in our patients! Would there be any questions or comments?' There were none.

Then we had a break of a quarter of an hour; one of my colleagues came up to me and very quietly said 'I didn't make any comments to what you presented to us because I recognize myself in that you spoke about. I think I am alexithymic the way you described it'. I went red and felt very embarassed, keeping in mind what I had just said about deficiencies, but she took it very well and went on just telling me about it. She said that she used to be bothered by an ulcer that had really been incapacitating her for several years. She graduated from medical school and she was always somewhat interested in psychiatry because she was curious about feelings and emotions. So she started to train to talk about feelings, to learn what feelings really are and she said that by this process, by sharing with her patients, she had herself gained new ideas, new awareness of what they were really talking about and she very nicely said 'You know, my ulcer has not been bothering me since I entered psychiatry'. She ended by saying 'but my family never talk about emotions and feelings at all and they all have hypertension or ulcerative colitis or ulcer or whatever you'd like to mention'.

To me that was a kind of turning point because for one thing it made me really believe in the concept and for another, she gave such a beautiful example of a spontaneous way of learning how to deal with it. I think that this learning concept is probably a very important part of the whole procedure of therapy with alexithymic patients.

Dr. Freyberger: My contribution concerns auxiliary therapist pools which consist of medical students who are able to deal with supportive psychotherapy in selected psychosomatic patients. In connection with the mentioning of supportive psychotherapeutic techniques in alexithymic patients, the question arises in which way the great discrepancy can be solved between the high number of patients who use supportive psychotherapy on the one hand, and the restricted number of available therapists on the other hand. In my opinion the best way at present to reduce this discrepancy is the foundation of students pools acting as auxiliary therapists and supervised by trained therapists within Balint groups. The application of supportive psychotherapy by an auxiliary therapist presupposes in the patient the following four psychodynamic processes which are the typical marks of the pregenital arrest and can be almost always found in alexithymic patients. The first psychodynamic process derives from a narcissistic conflict with the following oral-narcissistic acting out and the inability to transfer differentiated libidinous and aggressive wishes to the therapist; secondly, we observe marked oral-regressive fixations; thirdly, there arises – on the basis of an aggression conflict – an aggression defence and the resulting depressive traits, and fourthly, markedly insufficient insightful capacities. As a consequence of these four psychodynamic processes, which make a psychoanalytically oriented psychotherapy impossible, the following four supportive psychotherapeutic steps result which I described in this morning's session in my paper 'Supportive-psychotherapeutic techniques in primary and secondary alexithymia'. Up to now, we cooperated on the campus with a group of eight students for the duration of four semesters (Department of Psychosomatics, Eppendorf Hospital, University of Hamburg, Hamburg) and with a second group of eight students for the duration of two semesters (Department of Psychosomatics, Hannover Medical School, Hannover). For the purpose of supervision, the group met twice weekly for a period of 2 h each time. On the basis of this procedure we survey in 14 patients the supportive psychotherapeutic treatments, performed by students, which lasted from 6 months up to 2 years. If the patient was in the inpatient clinic, two sessions weekly took place. In the outpatient clinic, the frequency of the patients' sessions depended on the intensity of the patient's oral-narcissistic needs. When the patient was not able to come in weekly or at 2 weekly intervals, then, in the meantime phone contacts were established. The supervisors and the students were all very impressed with the high supportive-psychotherapeutic effectiveness of these phone contacts. As to the outpatient clinic patients during the semester holidays, the sessions did not regularly take place. This was not a disadvantage when the patients were sure that the therapy would be continued later on, and a substitute therapist would be at their disposal if suddenly an object-loss experience occurred. Originally we founded the auxiliary therapist's pools as a consequence of the urgent demand of the colleagues in the medical departments. These colleagues have had psychological difficulties with their patients during the somatotherapy. These difficulties particularly occurred in patients who were suffering from ulcerative colitis and morbus Crohn; furthermore, in dialysis and transplant patients as well as in patients who were suffering from cancer, and finally in those patients with functional somatic disorders who showed alexithymic features. Because of the work overloading of the doctors of our psychosomatic department, we saw no other supportive psychotherapeutic possibility than the organization of the students' group.

Dr. Sifneos: I would like to comment very briefly on three aspects which are mostly clarifications of some of the things which I have said here last Tuesday. The first one is on the alexithymic phenomenon, the second one is on psychotherapy, and the third one is on my own particular position as far as some of the criticisms which have been directed at me from various people are concerned. The first point is about the alexithymic phenomenon. The word was simply used to describe certain clinical observations that were made over very many years. I tried appropriately to use a Greek word or a pseudo-Greek word for descriptive purposes. Alexithymia is a nasty phenomenon. It is a nasty concept, but so is cancer. The fact is that they exist and that all the wishing in the world will not make them go away and it is up to us to fight against them. Now alexithymia presents such a challenge to our psychotherapeutic abilities, or to our own narcissism, that we want to deny it, or we want to rationalize it, or we want to relegate it to the lower classes, or we want to forget it. As Dr. *Shands* said the other day, for 30 or 40 years we have managed to forget it. We have succeeded unfortunately. It's up to us, up to you, ladies and gentlemen, to recognize it. The fact is, as I said on Tuesday, that alexithymia is here to stay whether we like it or not and it is going to be with us for the rest of our lives. It is up to us to be honest, to be scientific, to observe it, to study it and to do something about it.

The second responsibility I have is to the notion of therapy in general and particularly to psychotherapy. Dr. *Wolff* mentioned, on the day about psychodynamic psychotherapy, that my countertransference was involved. The only defence I can have to this criticism is that I like psychodynamic psychotherapy, I am a psychoanalyst and the major contribution of my professional life, small as it may be, has been on short-term psychodynamic psychotherapy. So I believe in psychotherapy very much but I also believe that it is a major mistake to offer certain kinds of psychotherapy when they are contraindicated, in the same way as it is to operate on the thyroid gland if the appendix has to be removed.

As pious as we may be about how much we like the patients, we do them a disservice when we make global generalizations about the patient. The fact is that we know that there are certain individuals who have low IQs and certain individuals who have IQs that are very high. This is a fact. Similarly, there are certain factors, certain genetic and developmental constellations which influence the psychodynamic makeup of our patients and which is our responsibility to evaluate. There are good psychotherapy candidates and bad psychotherapeutic risks.

Appropriate therapeutic techniques to fit specifically with the idiosyncratic needs of these particular individuals must be developed. A global offer of 'psychotherapy for all' is not the answer, popular as it may be judging on the applause. Finally, I want to clarify one misconception about my personal attitude which has been criticized. I have listed, and fortunately it has been recorded on this tape recorder, four different etiological factors for the explanation of the alexithymic phenomenon. Furthermore, I mentioned that Dr. *Freyberger* has contributed other factors as well. The alexithymic phenomenon in my opinion is challenging. In addition, there might be several kinds of alexithymia. The fact is, as I have mentioned, that it could be due to a variety of etiological factors: (1) a neuroanatomical deficit; (2) a neurophysiological deficit; (3) a developmental or sociocultural deficit, and (4) a psychodynamic paucity of defence mechanisms. I do not want to be put into a cubbyhole and I do not want my opinion to be distorted, namely, I favor only one, i.e. that alexithymia is a neurological deficit and that nothing can be done about it. This is only one of the four possibilities. I would very much like at present to have the audience participate in our discussion particularly since some of you have expressed the desire to have members of the panel discuss their ideas with each other as well as with the audience.

Dr. Pelser: Referring to the introduction of Prof. *Bräutigam,* I would like to point out that we have long ago given up expecting psychosomatic symptoms to disappear by causing the patient to verbalize his emotions. But only because these symptoms are produced by repression of an emotional conflict rather than by an inability of the patient to express emotions, but also because the psychosomatic patient expects from his doctor in the first place that he will treat his somatic condition. The asthmatic patient may well have emotional problems, but he has also a deficient and faulty breathing, from which he wants to be cured. Only after he discovers that medication and breathing exercises are not sufficient to stop his asthmatic attacks, he will become motivated to discuss *why* this treatment is not sufficient to cure his asthma and then he will appear to be no longer alexithymic and discuss his emotional problems with his doctor. The same goes for the ulcer patient who, in spite of all medications and dietary prescriptions, is still suffering from his stomach and only *then* becomes inclined to discuss the emotional tensions of his work and family situation. In conclusion, I think that what we should aim at in therapy is not a verbalization of emotional conflicts, but rather to help the patient in changing his attitude in these conflicts. Unless we have achieved such a change in behavior, we have done nothing for our patient essentially.

Dr. von Rad: One often gets the impression here that there are such things as people who are alexithymic and that there are others who are not. I have not had this experience. The people I have seen have, if you want to give it such a name, always been more or less 'alexithymic'. I feel this makes a great difference as it is of such importance for the theoretical considerations and, for example, the etiological problem. There are individuals who are alexithymic in certain situations and not in others. Others are alexithymic in a certain part of their personality ('psychosomatic sector'), again others perhaps only in respect to a certain conflict area. This is one of the reasons why I want once more to urge Prof. *Sifneos* to standardize his questionnaire because we are obviously so often talking about completely different patients under the same heading 'alexithymic'. With the varied selection of patients we have, our experiences are consequently so varied and for this reason we do not know what we can call an alexithymic patient.

Dr. Kimball: My comments will follow those of the previous speaker. I think that there is no question that alexithymia exists as a phenomenon, as described. It is described, therefore it is. I think the question is whether it is a fixed behavior type related to a specific disease, or group of disease, or whether it is a defensive stance that occurs at a particular time in a particular situation with a significant other. I think this has great implication for research in these patients manifesting psychosomatic illnesses. Do they act differently in different positions with authoritary, than they do in their families or with those that they are very close. Thus, we would need to see them in different situations. It would also apply that we would need to, in our researches, see these patients at different points of time. Now I think that this is particularly so when we try to relate this concept to the 'holy seven' psychosomatic diseases of *Alexander,* can we really say that these individuals have defensive patterns all of a kind? I would merely ask you to see an asthmatic patient in juxtaposition with a patient with an essential hypertension, and I would defy you to identify many similar characteristics in terms of defenses. *Engel* in his careful observations of patients with ulcerative colitis described different defensive patterns when the patient was in a state of remission or in a state of exacerbation. So I would ask those of us who would look at the concept or the phenomena of alexithymia that we look at what is common, if there is a common element, if there is a trait, or a behavior or a pattern than can be identified both during the stage of remission and the stage of exacerbation. I cannot pull this out of my clinical experience at this time. In my current thinking about alexithymia, I see it as a phenomenon that is seen quite frequently in psychosomatic patients in different stages in the development of the disease and at different times depending upon the course of that disease and as probably having something to do with stress correlationships with significant others at a particular point of time.

Dr. von Kries: I want only to make a few remarks about the psychoanalytic treatment of the so-called psychosomatic patients. One of the main traits of alexithymia is the inability to express emotions. If there is an inability to develop and express emotional reactions, this must have to do with a very early disturbance of the mother-child relationship. This has been mentioned several times during this congress as well. We know that these early disturbances later in life bring about a definite lack in object relationships. The object cannot be perceived as a human being different from oneself. Indeed these persons are disturbed in a narcissistic way; in contrast to the era of *Freud,* we now assume that it is possible to help those patients and to bring about a change in their approach to others and of course towards themselves as well. I wonder whether the reduplication symptom of the French authors is not the same phenomenon we encounter in the treatment of narcissistic patients. The other person is merely used to fulfill one's own needs and, over a long period, we have to accept this. This narcissistic defect can be altered only if a person becomes capable of developing psychic pain and grief and anxiety. Qualities which in the mother-child relationship obviously could not be developed or had to be repressed immediately. But, and that is the crucial point, we have to have tremendous patience in those treatments. *Balint* speaks of the basic fault, a term which describes the above-mentioned symptoms, and he wrote that it is not important to make the patient speak, that it is much more important to create an atmosphere of tolerance and acceptance. I had patients who could not verbalize at all and I just said 'We both have to accept that and we must try to understand later why it is so'. And by starting to speak first, just making casual remarks about something, eventually the patient started to join in with what I was saying. Procedures like these of course take a tremendous time. I would like to quote *MacDougall,* who in her marvellous paper in 1974 described the psychic state of an alexithymic patient in the following way: she used lines of a modern folk song – it goes like this.

'I touch no-one and no-one touches me. I'm a rock. I'm an island and a rock feels no pain and an island never cries.' She concludes by saying '. . . the analytic process can produce overwhelming change even though to do this it may lead the rock to feel great pain and the island to cry for many years to come'.

Dr. Philippopoulos: '...I would like to have Dr. *Sifneos*' opinion on the role that cultural factors play in the development or in the genesis of some neurotic and/or psychosomatic manifestations including alexithymic phenomena. Personally, I feel that they do play a role *not* only among people of the same national structure but also among minorities of ethnic groups existing far away from their national trunk (immigrants etc.).

In a personal communication some years ago, Professor Paul Kielholz of Basel, Switzerland, to lay stress of the importance of socio-cultural milieu as a causative factor in the genesis of emotional, neurotic and psychosomatic disorders, told me the following story:

"Two Swissmen were having their evening beer in a Weinstube in Basel. They were sitting there for about an hour quite, silent and stiff. Then a third man comes in, approaches them, says 'good evening' and joins them to have his beer too. He remains speechless for an hour or so, pays for his beer, says 'good night' and goes away.

Then, one of the two men left behind said: 'Well, this man talks too much!' "

It is, I think, apparent that the point I wanted to make is being supported by Prof. *Kielholz*'s story!'

Dr. Sifneos: In terms of the question regarding the cultural factor I think that it should be looked into just as much as any of the other factors. Under my 'develop-mental hypothesis' on the etiology of alexithymia, social, anthropological and cultural factors would be of course included.

Dr. Gaddini: A remark on the concept of somatization and desomatization as it has been used by Dr. *Bräutigam* in connection with learning and education. The point I am raising is that learning and education imply ego functions and ego functions imply a substrate on which to build themselves. This substrate is, for me, the *self* in the sense of *Winnicott*. The *self* is the result of the total experience of that which has gone on between mother and child in the early months. The concept of the *self* brings me back to the 'safety concept' that Dr. *Bastiaans* presented this morning. The elements which enter in the realization of safety as he describes it are the very elements which we find developmentally as basic to the process the infant in his first months undergoes in building his own *self* and subsequently in relating to his mother and to the outside world. Also, Dr. *Bastiaans*' idea that the 'psychosomatic' way of reacting to fear and stresses is a 'deficient coping strategy' which originally has established itself in the early interactions with mother is develop-mentally convincing. The moment this 'deficient strategy of interactions' between mother and child has established itself, it is, however, hard to go back. I agree with Dr. *Nemiah* that the exploration of feelings in adult psychosomatic patients is extremely difficult and not often useful; I do not know whether it may be harmful too. This is the problem of soma-tization as I see it: it comes to exist as a distorted form of communication early in life. This ivew implies that the only sort of intervention we may expect to be successful in the field of psychosomatic medicine is of a preventive order.

Another point which has interested me in the 'Panel Discussion' is that raised by Dr. *Shands* on the object and the subject. I am sorry he is no longer here. He said that in his view language is *objective* in respect to the subject's *private* world: for him, 'free association go between metanomy and metaphore'. In my view, if I look at the process of development, I can see the object which is there since birth but is not recognizable as such by the subject. From the point of view of psychology, the object starts to exist when the mental structure enables the subject to experience it as such. *Winnicott's* concept of subjective object, which I find clinically enlightening, refers to the intermediary stage when the subject moves to-wards the object and withdraws from it.

Dr. Heiberg: I have been impressed with how many people in this congress have actual experience in the field of alexithymia. As you have been the first outstanding child therapist to speak here, I would like very much to know whether you know about any studies in these traits in children.

Dr. Gaddini: If you meant to ask me whether I worked with a special group of children called 'alexithymic', my answer is 'no'. I have not studied them as a group. I am not sure the characteristics we find in patients – adults and children – suffering from psychosomatic illnesses may enter one group. My own experience indicates that fantasy life is particularly poor in autistic children and, in a different way (mostly limited to its *expressive* capacities) with a few children suffering from psychosomatic disorders but not selected on the basis of this diagnosis. You may recall the project which I mentioned at a different part of this conference. It is on the basis of this long itudinal study that I have noticed a correlation between evocative capacities at 8, 10 and 12 months as expressed by the presence of a transitional object or phenomena and the capacity of playing at the age of four. This correlation points out to me an existing continuum of self-creativity (the transitional object is the creation of the subjective object) and the capacity of playing (and of sharing) later in life.

Inspired by these observations of mine, my allergological colleagues – with whom I work closely – have retrospectively noticed that in severe cases of asthma and/or atopic dermatitis transitional objects or phenomena are not usually found. In my study which was prospective, I have followed from birth to 8 years, children belonging to three different social groups (rural, urban and foreigners living in Rome) focusing on their going-to-sleep pattern at the end of the 1st year and on their capacity to play at the age of four. Nearly 40% in the urban group and over 70% of the foreign group had a transitional object (blanket, nylon, teddy, etc.) or phenomenon (a rhyme, a prayer, being rocked), while in the rural group where the child sleeps close to the mother the incidence of transitional objects is only 4%. The working hypothesis of this longitudinal study was that the transitional object is the first expression of evocative imaginatively (as contrasted to nonimaginative play, such as acting out and running around) comes next, as a derivation from it. The play of the severe cases of asthma observed by our allergologists, in whose past histories no transitional object had been found, had also been found to have more the character of motor discharge and/or testing out than that of a creative dramatization. Of course when we talk about asthmatic or atopic dermatitis children, we ought to clearly define the type and the severity of the illness. But this will be done more thoroughly on a different occasion.

Dr. König: The question is still under discussion as to whether you can get psycho-somatic alexithymic patients into psychoanalytically oriented treatment. There were several speakers today who said they could do it. I may mention the names of *Sellschopp, Wittich* and *Stephanos;* perhaps you can also remember *Cremerius'* presentation yesterday and I might join these people because I have had similar experiences. What these authors all have in common is that they all work, as I do, in a psychoanalytically oriented hospital. Further, they all practice analytically oriented group methods either doing group psychotherapy or running the ward and the team as a group or by group methods. And they all more or less employ auxiliary methods as mentioned by Dr. *Bräutigam.* What is it, however, that makes it work with some patients – not with all – but with some? Is it group psychotherapy alone? We have listened to Dr. *Ford*'s and Dr. *Roberts'* presentations which told us about very low attendance figures and a very boring and unproductive therapeutic process. As I said previously, the authors I mentioned getting psychosomatic, alexithymic into treatment all have in common that they work in a hospital and I think that in addition to the possi-bility of combining analytic group methods with auxiliary methods it may be the provision of a different set of social norms, counteracting previous social influences that makes hospital treatment effective. The fact that it is indeed effective has come to the notice of quite a few psychoanalytic practitioners who send us patients to initiate treatment which they later continue in their private practice. Therefore, if initiating treatment in a hospital setting is a feasible way of making these patients treatable, why don't you try it – and if you don't have the hospitals, put them up.

Dr. Freyberger: Dr. *König's* remarks were indeed very important. There are obvi-ously psychosomatic patients who only show 'partial' traits of alexithymia. These patients should be suitable for psychoanalytically orientated group psychotherapy. According to my experience, however, there is also occurring a larger group of 'total' alexithymic patients who cannot be treated by pschoanalytically orientated group psychotherapy. Possibly a smaller group of these patients may be finally suitable for group psychotherapy after they have been processed by 1 or 2 years of individual supportive psychotherapy. I regard these therapeutic considerations as very relevant. Therefore, during every long-term supportive psychotherapy it will be advantageous to discuss closely the question of whether the patient can be expected to cope with merely a group psychotherapy or if other forms of interpretative psychotherapy are needed.

Dr. Taylor: I'll be brief. I would like to respond to the remarks made by Dr. *Wolff* and Dr. *Sifneos* because I agree that there do seem to be some misconceptions at this conference. First, I think that the phenomenon of alexithymia is not in dispute at all and I agree with Dr. *Kimball* on that point. Second, it is refreshing that Dr. *Nemiah* and Dr. *Sifneos* have emphasized the third and fourth possible explanations for alexithymia. I think that one of my own misconceptions came from reading their earlier papers in which a much greater emphasis was placed on the neurophysiological and neuroanatomical explanations but this conference has clarified that. Third, I think that what we mean by the term 'counter-transference' must be clearly defined because it is not employed in a perjurative way nor intended to offend. In fact 'counterresponse' may be a more acceptable term. The plea here is to consider the countertransference as an instrument of research which would help clarify the third and fourth possible explanations for alexithymia. The focus is on becoming more aware of the feelings, fantasies and dreams evoked in us by our patients and asking ourselves what further information these may provide about the inner worlds of the patients and how this information may be used in the treatment. Finally, in response to Dr. *Frankel*'s comments, I would agree that many psychosomatic patients do become physically sicker when treated with analytical psychotherapy. However, many such patients also become sicker when they do not receive analytical psychotherapy.

Dr. Bräutigam: I would like to make some comments on Dr. *Pelser's* remarks. The first point Dr. *Pelser* made was that he stresses the importance of accepting the patient's physical complaint. I think it is most important with the psychosomatic patient to accept this kind of communication and to meet him on the level on which he understands his illness. Unfortunately, a psychoanalyst or psychotherapist treating psychosomatic patients as outpatients hardly has a chance of having physical contact with them. Therefore, I think it is better for some of these patients to start their treatment by coming to the wards where they can have physical examinations, can experience a medical setting and can get into physical contact with their therapists. For the time being, at least, we have to accept the preverbal levels of that communication and understanding. A great number of patients have learnt to speak only about physical complaints and it takes a long time to shift their attention from physical complaints to feelings.

The second point that Dr. *Pelser* mentioned concerns their learning experience. It is an important item for the psychoanalysts to know about. As a young analyst I was very puzzled when I saw a patient used the same words as I did, made the same kinds of movements – that he imitated me. I always thought that I was not a good analyst for having such patients that I had to be more distant and treat them in another way. I learned later that we have to accept such needs of patients to get in touch with us as real persons and, accordingly, to have an opportunity to imitate us. However, what may be necessary in the beginning of treatment may later become resistance on the road to autonomy and needs to be worked through.

I would not follow Dr. *Pelser* in giving up hope on the psychosomatic patient's ability to learn cognitively through the exploration of their conflicts and personal history. He may experience that new cognitive learning is also an emotional process and may lead to behavioral change. Therefore, I may say that I am as optimistic as Dr. *Pelser* seems to be about the possibility of treating psychosomatic patients with psychotherapy on a verbal level. Evidently in this regard Dr. *Sifneos* and Dr. *Nemiah* are much more sceptical than we are. As to the treatment and research that Dr. *von Rad* mentioned, we possibly deal with a very selected sample of patients. It seems to me that you are dealing in Boston with patients whose physical complaints, education and abilities of verbalization differ from those of our patients. In order to overcome this problem Dr. *Sifneos* and Dr. *Nemiah* should come back to Heidelberg and study our patients with us – and we should go to Boston to observe their patients with them.

Dr. Nemiah: Let me just make a brief response to Dr. *Wolff,* whose remarks have been very stimulating for all of us. Dr. *Wolff* suggests that in treating psychosomatic patients it is essential to get at their feelings. I would agree with this as a general psychotherapeutic principle, but in dealing with the group of patients under discussion here, there appears to be a basic problem. As we have tried to stress throughout the conference, such patients have a fundamental difficulty in experiencing affect and, in our therapeutic attempts at least, it has often been impossible to get at their affects by the usual therapeutic procedures. I should like to stress, however, that much more clinical experience is necessary before one can confidently state this as a valid generalization. Clinical investigation should be aimed in the future at systematically exploring the effectiveness of analysis and analytically oriented psychotherapy in a large number of patients with psychosomatic disorders. Only then will it be possible to determine whether one can uncover in them a capacity for experiencing both affects and fantasies.

Proc. 11th Eur. Conf. Psychosom. Res., Heidelberg 1976
Psychother. Psychosom. *28:* 376–388 (1977)

The Concept of Alexithymia and the Future of Psychosomatic Research

H.H. Wolff

It certainly is a challenging and anxious-making task to summarize this stimulating and exciting conference. I hope you will, therefore, follow Dr. *Murray Jackson*'s advice and act as a container for my anxiety; otherwise I might go down with some psychosomatic illness before the evening is up which I hope to avoid.

To begin with I would like to say how honoured I feel to have been asked to summarize the conference. I would particularly like to thank Prof. *Bräutigam* and Dr. *von Rad* and their organising committee for having given us the opportunity in these 3 days to discuss and share our views on many important and controversial aspects in the field of psychosomatic medicine and research.

I would especially like to thank Dr. *Sifneos* and Dr. *Nemiah* for having provided us through their research and publications with a theme around which we were able to concentrate our thoughts and deliberations. The theme of alexithymia has certainly stimulated a great deal, and at times heated exchange and controversy and I hope in this summary to resolve some of the more controversial issues. During the workshop this afternoon Dr. *Sifneos,* himself, has made this task easier for me by making it clear that his view on alexithymia is by no means a closed one. Some of us, me included, had perhaps to some extent misunderstood him from his earlier writings, and thought that he regarded the phenomenon of alexithymia as an entity due to an irreversible neuro-anatomical deficit in which case there would have been very little one could do about it therapeutically. Dr. *Sifneos* has made it clear that whilst he is interested in the possibility of a neuroanatomical and neurophysiological explanation for some of these phenomena he is equally concerned with exploring their developmental and psychodynamic aspects.

Dr. *Nemiah* assumed a similar standpoint in his paper on theories and models of alexithymia. Having cleared up this misunderstanding we can try to integrate the different views expressed more easily. Let me start, therefore, by summarizing what has been going on during these last 3 days.

The first problem which I think is important and kept recurring during the discussion, is the problem of definition. Some contributors have used the term 'psychosomatic disorders' in the restricted sense of a small group of specific disorders with structural organic lesions; we all know which they are so that I need not enumerate them here. Others included under the same term various functional physiological disturbances related to stress. Others still used the term psychosomatic in an even wider sense and included behavior disturbances and conversion hysteria. If *George Engel* had been here he might have contributed something to this problem of definition at the beginning. When I last heard him talk about it he was, I think, coming round to the view which I also hold, namely, that the concept of a small number of specific psychosomatic disorders is too narrow and that it might be better to think of every patient we see, whether he is physically or psychiatrically ill, with a psychosomatic approach; this means that in each case we ask ourselves the important question: how do physical, psychological and social factors contribute to bringing about this particular condition, symptom or behavioral abnormality in this particular person at this time in his life and how do they affect the course of the disorder. Linked with this psychosomatic approach is the problem of how the illness affects the patient and his family; and finally, how these various interrelated factors can be taken into consideration in the patient's treatment.

Whatever definition anyone of us may prefer, it is clearly essential in research and theoretical discussion to define exactly what conditions have been studied and in what sense the term psychosomatic is being used. I hope, therefore, that in future we shall not talk about psychosomatic disorders without stating what particular disorders we have in mind. We have, of course, heard several excellent papers in the conference in which this has been done. There are first of all some studies on patients with peptic ulcers. *Overbeck* from Frankfurt, in his studies on alexithymic phenomena demonstrated that only 15% of a group of ulcer patients had alexithymic characteristics. So, we know something about the frequency of the incidence of alexithymia in patients with peptic ulcers. It is a small but no doubt a significant proportion of them.

Other contributors have studied patients with ulcerative colitis, especially *Murray Jackson* from London and *Hellmuth Freyberger* from Hanover.

Again, we knew exactly what condition they were talking about. We learned from *Murray Jackson* that some patients with ulcerative colitis at the initial interview may show no evidence of psychopathology; this apparent normality may, however, turn out later to be a pseudonormality. The psychopathology may, as it were, have been expressed entirely in the patient's physical illness; his psychopathology, especially in terms of his object relationships, may only reveal itself gradually when the patient is in psychotherapy, for example, in a group. Many of the ulcerative colitis patients had some alexithymic characteristics but these were often reversible during psychotherapy.

Another condition discussed was anorexia nervosa. Prof. *Weiner* from New York stressed its heterogenous etiology, various psychological and neural factors all playing their part; I was surprised to hear that so many of the patients with anorexia nervosa he saw had Turner's syndrome, a finding different from that of most of us. Prof. *Groen* in discussion commented on his observation that the symptomatology of anorexia nervosa has been changing since the introduction of the contraceptive pill, an interesting finding worth further study. None of us would doubt that in anorexia nervosa alexithymic characteristics are common; these patients are almost totally preoccupied with their bodily appearance, their fear of getting fat and their dietary habits, and yet they have very remarkable fantasies about their bodies and body image so that they are not, in fact, devoid of fantasies and are able to express them. Some are depressed and use words to express their sadness; others find it much more difficult. The degree of alexithymia seems to vary from patient to patient, and often changes in the course of treatment.

I will mention a few other specific disorders that were discussed. The personalities of patients with psoriasis were investigated by Dr. *van der Schaar,* using psychometric tests. Dr. *Musaph* and Dr. *de Korte* gave us a report on a follow-up study of group therapy for patients with psoriasis; they stressed the importance of regression in some of the patients, and the need for team work in treatment, combining psychological and physical treatment methods. Dr. *Heiny,* using a personality inventory, demonstrated that patients with an irritable colon, the irritable bowel syndrome, are more nervous, depressed and emotionally unstable than a healthy control group. Dr. *Carmona* from Brussels described how behavioral therapy may aid the return of repressed memories in patients with colonic irritability. The phenomenon of alexithymia was not specifically studied in the papers just referred to. Time prevents me from mentioning other papers on specific disorders discussed, e.g., obesity, hypertension and coronary disease. The advantage of all these papers was that we knew exactly what condition the authors were referring to. I hope in future conferences each author will clearly define which patients or disorders, he has studied and in what sense he is using the term 'psychosomatic'.

I would next like to say a few words about the definition of 'alexithymia' itself and about its meaning. Dr. *Peter Sifneos* has done us a very good turn by coining a term to describe some people's inability to express in words what they feel; similarly *Marty and de M'Uzan* have usefully coined the term 'pensée opératoire' to describe a state of mind characterized by pragmatic, operational thinking and absence of fantasy life.

The value of such words as alexithymia and 'pensée opératoire' is that they help us more easily to communicate with each other, to convey with a single word instead of lengthy descriptions what phenomena we are talking about. Like all words in language they stand for and are abstractions or symbols of a number of related phenomena and thus make it easier to communicate to others what we mean. There is, however, a real danger that a concept like alexithymia might become reified, be thought of as a thing or concrete object to be located, as it were, in space or in this case in the brain. Coining the term alexithymia does not mean that a new object or structure has been discovered but rather that we have recognized certain functional psychological disturbances which are worth studying in detail from the point of view of their nature, their origin and their significance in individual patients, and in so-called normal people including ourselves. Similarly, it is essential not to regard alexithymia as an all-or-none phenomenon, as was pointed out by Dr. *Heiberg* in the course of her genetic studies, but rather to recognize that there are degrees and varieties of alexithymic characteristics in different individuals and that they may be evident to different degrees at various times in the same person's life.

Several papers were concerned with detailed analysis of alexithymic characteristics. Dr. *von Rad* and his colleagues, studying the verbal behavior in interviews confirmed that psychosomatic patients used fewer affect-laden words than psychoneurotic patients; Dr. *Gottschalk* described the use of content analysis of speech in psychophysiology, neuropharmacology and psychotherapy. Dr. *Overbeck* using linguistic tests also showed that in psychotherapy psychosomatic patients were silent for longer periods whilst the therapists tended to be more active. Dr. *Singer* from California studied the transactions in the families of psychosomatic patients and showed that alexithymic patients showed various clusters of personality traits; she drew attention to the influence of selection of patients and to the need for more accurate tests for the study of alexithymic personality traits. There was general agreement that tests for alexithymia, for example the questionnaire devised by *Sifneos,* needed to be properly validated and applied to a normal population.

Another aspect of alexithymia I would like to comment on is the impoverishment of fantasy life in some of these patients. Dr. *Shands* in his paper spoke of the lack of interest of these patients in their inner private world which is of importance in considering their suitability for psychotherapy. As an analytical psychotherapist I would like to know more about this aspect of alexithymia; what fantasies are they in touch with and what is their content; and how can we during psychotherapy help them get in touch with other aspects of their fantasy life? Then there is the importance of finding out more about the frequency or lack of frequency of dreaming in these patients and the content and meaning of their dreams. Many so-called normal people have difficulty in remembering their dreams and show little interest in this aspect of their inner world. Those of us who have been in analysis or psychotherapy have learnt to value our dreams and what they signify. I will take the risk of telling you a dream I had last night. It would be out of place if I analyzed it in detail here but some aspects of it seem relevant to my present task of summarising the conference. I dreamt that there was somebody standing near me who held a hacksaw in a menacing manner close to a baby and a white pussy cat; I felt very angry with him for endangering the baby and the pussy cat. No doubt it was my own aggression I was disturbed by, and when on waking I considered the meaning of my dream, I took it as a warning not to be aggressive in my talk today, not to saw various aspects of the conference to pieces and to tear them apart. In fact, I do not feel at all aggressive now; if anything I want to be reparative and bring about some consensus among all of us. I am giving you this example to point out how essential it is to be interested in our own inner world, our dreams and fantasies if we are to help our patients to do the same. How many of us wake up in the morning and ask ourselves 'what did I dream last night?' and perhaps share the dream with someone close to us? If in this way we remain in touch with our own inner world it becomes easier to get our patients interested in theirs and make their fantasy life less impoverished. What I am stressing is that if we are to help alexithymic patients to become less alexithymic, we must become less alexithymic ourselves and take a real interest in our own fantasies and dreams.

I want next to say a word about another important and controversial issue that arose in the conference. This concerns the relationship between the different aspects of psychosomatic medicine, the psychological, social and the neurophysiological and neuroanatomical aspects. It seems easier nowadays than it used to be to integrate the different psychological approaches, especially the psychodynamic and behavioral approaches and to correlate these with the interpersonal and social approaches; some analysts, however, still find it difficult to integrate some aspects of classical theory with more modern, including Kleinian concepts and to correlate these with a social approach in their work with patients. The main problem, however, concerns the relationship between the physical, mainly the neurophysiological aspects of our discipline and the psychosocial or experiential aspects. *MacLean* gave us a fascinating and detailed account of the neuroanatomical basis of human experience and emotional functioning; and *Hoppe* described the development of alexithymic characteristics, especially impoverishment of dreams, fantasies and symbolization in 12 patients who had a commissurotomy done for epilepsy. The degree of alexithymia was greater than in patients with psychosomatic disorders; *Hoppe,* therefore, postulated that alexithymia in psychosomatic patients could be looked upon as a 'functional commissurotomy'.

The problem that concerns me is the relationship between the neuroanatomical findings and our clinical findings when dealing with alexithymic patients and their limited experience of fantasy and feeling. In essence we are faced with the problem of the relation between human experience and brain function. Every human experience can be studied at a psychological *and* at a neurophysiological level of abstraction, and as Harre in his book *The Principles of Scientific Thinking* has put it 'to every mind-state there is a corresponding brain-state'. Discovering that certain brain lesions, as after a commissurotomy, can lead to the development of alexithymic characteristics does not mean that we have discovered the *cause* of alexithymia; it only tells us something about underlying cerebral *mechanisms*. It tells us nothing about the personal meaning of the experience of being to a greater or lesser extent alexithymic, or about the multiple psychological determinants which may lead to the development of alexithymic characteristics in a particular person whose brain is structurally normal but is functioning in a particular way as a result of his personal life experience and present life situation.

I will illustrate this with a personal example. If I tell you that last night when I was preparing this summary, I felt very anxious, this, I am sure, means a lot to you; but I am sure that if Dr. *MacLean* were to describe to you in detail the neurophysiological changes in my cortex or limbic system, this would not tell you anything about how I felt last night. In other words, whilst the study of brain structure and function is of profound interest and importance it can never be a substitute for the description of human experience nor can it serve as an explanation of such experience. This problem of the relation between neurology and psychology was one *Freud* already struggled with when he wrote *The Project for a Scientific Psychology*. It is also essential to remind ourselves of the distinction between mechanisms and meaning in this central area of psychosomatic research; and of the difference between causal and meaningful connections to which attention was first drawn by *Jaspers* here in Heidelberg. This is important because knowledge of the mechanism of a condition does not necessarily mean that we have understood its cause, not does it provide us with an understanding of its psychological meaning.

As I am considering some theoretical or philosophical issues just now there is one further point I want to make. *Wittgenstein* pointed out that no right answer can be given to a wrong question. If the question 'what is *the* cause of alexithymia' were to be the wrong question then we cannot give a meaningful answer to it. I have pointed out already that alexithymia is a concept which comprises several facets; it is not a single entity and may, therefore, have a number of different, though interrelated causes. This may well be the reason why we cannot give a single answer to the question 'what is *the* cause of alexithymia'. Instead we have to look for multiple reasons why a particular person cannot find a word for a particular feeling or is out of touch with certain, though not with all, aspects of his fantasy life. In some patients or normal individuals their previous life experience, in others their present social situation or their relation to the interviewer, and in others still neurological factors may singly or jointly play a part in producing certain alexithymic characteristics. In the whole field of psychosomatic medicine we must be careful to ask clearly defined, specific instead of global questions; otherwise we shall get lost in useless discussion or research.

In this context I wish to comment on some of the papers which dealt with the influence of the social environment and of the interview situation on the behavior of patients with psychosomatic symptoms and disorders. The reason why I turn to these papers now is that they demonstrated that alexithymia is often not a mode of behavior determined by the patient in isolation but rather that alexithymic behavior may be determined by the social and interview situation in which he finds himself. Thus, Dr. *Brede* from Frankfurt pointed out that patients who express their emotional conflicts in psychosomatic symptoms and by adopting the sick role through the development of a physical illness may do so because in this way they can comply with the expectations of society; a physical illness being more acceptable than complaining of emotional problems or conflicts. In other words, the conformity aspect in the social and sociological sense is an important factor in determining alexithymic behavior. Dr. *Schneider* from Lausanne similarly stressed that when studying the phenomenon known as 'pensée opératoire' it is essential to know in what setting the patient is being seen. Prof. *Cremerius* showed us that patients referred to a physician or psychiatrist in a hospital setting and seen together with students behaved in a more alexithymic manner than patients who came on their own initiative and were seen on their own in a relaxed atmosphere by a psychotherapist or a person-oriented physician. Prof. *Stierlin* also pointed out that the alexithymic phenomenon needs to be studied from the point of view of family dynamics, including the process of individuation and different modes of family transaction, rather than in terms of the individual patient in isolation, a point also made by Dr. *Wirsching, Dr. Knauss,* and by Dr. *Waring.* Dr. *Kimball* drew attention to the influence of cultural differences and pointed out that words to express feelings may not be equally available in different languages.

In my own paper I drew attention to the fact that when a patient is being interviewed the attitude of the interviewer and the way he handles his countertransference will have a profound effect on whether or not the patient's alexithymic behavior is reinforced or at least partly abandoned; Dr. *Taylor* described in detail how proper use of the therapist's countertransference, in terms of object relations and fantasy can help one understand and modify the patients' alexithymic characteristics.

In other words in the study of these phenomena more attention needs to be paid to the selection of patients, their social class, their cultural background, their family structure, the setting in which they are being seen and the nature of the interview situation. As *Cremerius* put it 'the psychosomatic structure may not be disease-specific' but may be dependent on social factors and the setting in which the patient is being interviewed. Equally important are considerations of the patient's childhood development in the family in which he grew up, a point to which Dr. *Gaddini* and Dr. *Mitscherlich* drew our attention; they dealt particularly with the significance of the early infant-mother relationship and the way children handle transitional objects in *Winnicott's* sense. More longitudinal studies are needed to investigate the influence of early childhood development on the future appearance or absence of psychosomatic symptoms, and on fantasy life and emotional functioning.

Next I would like to make some comments on some of the papers which dealt specifically with the treatment of the psychosomatically ill patient. I take it for granted that in many of these patients physical, psychological and social treatment methods need to be combined, an approach which is the basis of psychosomatic medicine. Prof. *Aitken* gave us an account of the team approach including physicians, psychiatrists, nurses, physiotherapists and social workers, in a medical rehabilitation service in Edinburgh; and Dr. *Wittich* discussed the clinical aspects of working in an integrated psychosomatic hospital. The group of workers from Giessen dealt more specifically with the psychoanalytic team approach in their University Clinic for Psychosomatics where detailed attention is paid to the patients' object relations and how these are manifested, and modified through their relationship to different staff members.

Most of the papers concerned with psychotherapy indicated that alexithymic behavior can be modified by appropriate psychotherapeutic means. *Sifneos* pointed out that brief analytically oriented psychotherapy is often not effective, a view with which I am in full agreement but this does not mean that longer, more intensive and flexible methods are necessarily ineffective in alexithymic patients. Thus, *Savitz* and co-workers from Boston described how long-term group psychotherapy, sometimes combined with videotape, relaxation and meditation techniques may help alexithymic patients, especially when they are treated together with psychoneurotic and less alexithymic patients in the same group. *Becker* from Heidelberg showed how attention to preverbal phenomena and bodily behavior in action groups can be used in combination with or in preparation for analytical psychotherapy, and I drew attention to similar methods, including bodily movement which can be used in association with individual and group psychotherapy. The classical, purely interpretative psychoanalytical approach may often not be appropriate by itself for alexithymic patients but a more flexible analytical approach with proper use by the therapist of his countertransferential response is often more effective. As alexithymia may be based on very early disturbance in the patients' development, later reinforced by his social environment, it must be acknowledged that in treatment attention needs to be paid to preverbal phenomena and that long-term therapy may be needed to help some of these patients.

To give an example, I once treated a patient in a group who had various psychosomatic symptoms, an isolated man with a schizoid personality disorder and many alexithymic characteristics. During the first year he always sat outside the circle, hiding behind a newspaper. After 6 months he occasionally responded by lowering his paper and making some brief comments. Later he began to participate more, brought his chair into the circle of patients and after about 2 years he would smile, or look sad and even get angry. He stayed in the group which was an open one with several changes of patients, for 10 years gradually becoming more and more alive both in the group and outside. When he ultimately left the group having lost his somatic symptoms and being able to relate to people with real feelings, he said with tears in his eyes 'I know I am ready to go but I feel very sad because this is the only family I have ever had'.

I learnt from him and other patients since that given plenty of time and a safe therapeutic environment, alexithymic characteristics can be modified or even cured; of course, I am aware that this raises serious problems in terms of the availability and cost of long-term psychotherapy but groups are relatively inexpensive; desirable though it would be if we could help these patients with briefer forms of psychotherapy the fact is that some of them need longer treatment on account of the depth of their psychopathology and its origin at very early developmental stages.

From the point of view of research this means that such a question as to whether or not alexithymic patients are amenable to psychotherapy is too global a question to ask. We need to know exactly what kind of patients with what particular alexithymic characteristics are being treated with what form of psychotherapy, for how long and by what kind of therapist before we can hope to get meaningful answers in research on psychotherapy. The therapist's personal qualities may, I believe, turn out to be of special importance in determining the outcome. His theoretical understanding of how the mind works, his interest in every detail of his patients' biographical data and personal development, his self-awareness and his skill to establish a trusting therapeutic relationship and to use this in a reliable and flexible manner throughout may turn out to be among the most important factors. In my own paper I drew your attention to *Winnicott's* view that the therapist needs to learn to play creatively with his patient just as a mother plays with her infant or child. This may be especially important when we treat psychosomatic and alexithymic patients. These same factors may also determine the outcome of diagnostic interviews. Our medical training hardly ever emphasizes the importance of taking a detailed biographical history, and even less does it emphasize the significance of our subjective reactions to our patients and what we can learn from them. When I take notes during a diagnostic interview I not only write down what the patients tells me but also what I feel at certain moments, e.g., when I feel sad or sympathetic; or bored frustrated and angry which is, of course, the usual response to an alexithymic patient.

Even the training of psychiatrists does not lay enough stress on the need to be aware of and to understand the meaning of one's subjective experience in interviews. Training in psychoanalysis and psychotherapy does, of course, emphasize these aspects.

I would, however, like to suggest that there are additional ways of getting in touch with the significance of personal development and experience, and of human conflict, feelings and fantasy life. I am thinking here of what we can learn from some of the greater works in literature. Readers familiar with the British author *Mervyn Peakes'* trilogy, *Titus Groan, Gormenghast* and *Titus Alone* will readily remember the sensitive account, full of feeling and fantasy, of Titus' struggle for freedom and individuality from his birth into early adulthood. Speaking here in Germany I would remind you of *Hermann Hesse's* novels; I am thinking especially of '*Narziss and Goldmund*'. Narziss is a good example of the man who leads a monastic, ascetic and intellectual life devoid of intimate feelings and alienated from his body while Goldmund represents the opposite, the sensuous man, living a life full of emotional experience in the outer world. At the very end Narziss is able to express his love for Goldmund and his deep sadness at his death; symbolically the two characters could be said to represent the mind and the body aspects of each human being; their increasing closeness represents the gradual achievement of what we in our less expressive language would call 'psycho-somatic integration'. And then most of us will be familiar with *Thomas Mann*'s '*Death in Venice*'. Here we have an account of Aschenbach, the lonely man in his 50s who shares his longings, his love and his sadness with no one. Ultimately, even though he knows that there is a cholera epidemic he goes into the side streets of Venice, buys and eats strawberries and dies. We might speak of his having reached the stage of the giving up-given up complex which leads him to self-destructive behavior but such a description in psychological terms is infinitely less meaningful than *Thomas Mann*'s vivid story, or the beautiful film version which many of you will have seen.

As doctors and scientists we should not forget how much we can learn from creative artists when it comes to that aspect of our discipline which demands a deep understanding of the individual patient we are trying to help, and of our own psychological reactions and makeup which is so important when we are involved in work with psychosomatic and other patients. We owe it to *Freud* that we have learnt to concern ourselves with each patient's biographical history and with our own subjective, if you wish, countertrans-ferential responses; to integrate these aspects of our professional task with the equally important scientific aspects is a challenge which confronts everyone who uses a psychosomatic approach. Clearly defined psychophysiological and psychopharmacological investigations and well-designed follow-up studies are, of course, an essential part of our discipline but so are individual case studies and their careful documentation. There has been a tendency to limit the process of scientific investigation to methods which use measurement, statistical analysis and experimentation but I would remind you that these methods of scientific investigation must be preceded by observation and by the formulation of a testable hypothesis. As the British scientist Sir *Peter Medawar* once put it 'the mental events which lead up to it (the formulation of a hypothesis) happen below the surface of the mind'. We might say they are derived from the unconscious. Work in the psychosomatic field demands equal attention to objective, measurable phenomena and to subjective, including unconscious mental processes. We who are working in this field must, therefore, respect both and not limit investigations only to the former. This conference which had alexithymia as its central theme has, I hope, reminded us all of the importance of fantasies and feelings which are part of everyone's inner private world, that of ourselves as well as of our patients.

These thoughts bring me to my concluding comments on the future of psychosomatic medicine and research. *Lipowski* has pointed out that psychosomatic medicine not only has a scientific but also a 'missionary' function. It started in part as a reaction against the development of a purely technological approach to patients; we have all benefited and will continue to benefit from these scientific advances in medical knowledge but the emphasis on the psychosomatic approach arose out of the need not to forget the person who is ill, including his social environment and his psychological experience. I see some danger in the possibility that we in our own discipline might again lose sight of the experiential aspects of our patients by only emphasizing the measurable physiological and anatomical data. Although we have a great deal to learn from brain research, as *MacLean*'s paper showed us, it would be a mistake, to put it in extreme terms, to look for the cure of psychosomatic and alexithymic phenomena in purely pharmacological or even neurosurgical procedures. If this were to happen, psychosomatics would also become a purely technological discipline, and yet another field of enquiry would have to be created to remind us of the fact that patients are people and not only machines. The challenge we are faced with, therefore, consists of the need to integrate enquiry into physiological and anatomical with the study of social and psychological, including inner world phenomena. This conference has shown us that this is, indeed, possible.

I look forward to our next conference in Norway where we shall learn about further developments. I hope we will have the opportunity there to concern ourselves, perhaps in small group discussions, also with aspects of our own personal experience, even our fantasies and dreams. Otherwise we might forget that in treating our patients an important tool of treatment is ourselves and what we personally experience in relation to them.

H.H. Wolff, MD, Department of Psychological Medicine, University College Hospital, Gower Street, *London, WC 1* (England)

List of Contributors